Myeloproliferative Disorders

Myeloproliferative Disorders

Biology and Management

Edited by

Richard T. Silver
Weill Medical College of Cornell University
New York City, New York, USA

Ayalew Tefferi
Mayo Clinic Cancer Center
Rochester, Minnesota, USA

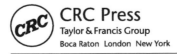

CRC Press
Taylor & Francis Group
Boca Raton London New York

CRC Press is an imprint of the
Taylor & Francis Group, an **informa** business

First published 2008 by Informa Healthcare, Inc.

Published 2019 by CRC Press
Taylor & Francis Group
6000 Broken Sound Parkway NW, Suite 300
Boca Raton, FL 33487-2742

First issued in paperback 2019

No claim to original U.S. Government works

ISBN 13: 978-0-367-45291-9 (pbk)
ISBN 13: 978-1-4200-6162-8 (hbk)

Visit the Taylor & Francis Web site at
http://www.taylorandfrancis.com

and the CRC Press Web site at
http://www.crcpress.com

Library of Congress Cataloging-in-Publication Data

Myeloproliferative disorders : biology and management / edited by Ayalew Tefferi, Richard T. Silver.
   p.; cm.
Includes bibliographical references.
ISBN-13: 978-1-4200-6162-8 (hb : alk. paper)
ISBN-10: 1-4200-6162-3 (hb : alk. paper)
1. Myeloproliferative disorders. I. Tefferi, Ayalew. II. Silver, Richard T., 1929–
[DNLM: 1. Myeloproliferative Disorders. WH 380 M99857 2007]

RC645.75.M94 2007
616.1'53 – dc22
                                           2007023432

Preface

What an exciting age for those of us interested in the myeloproliferative diseases!

Myeloproliferative diseases—a term first used 55 years ago by the famous hematologist William Dameshek—include chronic myeloid leukemia, polycythemia vera (PV), essential thrombocythemia (ET), and primary myelofibrosis (PMF). These are clonal hematopoietic stem cell disorders characterized by the expansion of one or more cell lines accompanied by varying degrees of marrow fibrosis.

Slumbering in the diagnostic and therapeutic advances of other areas of hematology, explosive interest in them began with the exploitation of the molecular understanding of chronic myeloid leukemia and by the development of the small molecule, imatinib. This drug not only revolutionized the treatment of chronic myeloid leukemia, but also stimulated interest in the Philadelphia-chromosome–negative (Ph$^-$) myeloproliferative diseases because of their clinical and hematologic similarities. The Ph-negative diseases nevertheless remained in relative hematologic limbo until the discovery of a molecular abnormality now found in all patients with polycythemia vera and in about half the patients with essential thrombocythemia and primary myelofibrosis. This abnormality, found in the regulatory domain of JAK2, is denoted as $JAK2^{V617F}$.

In addition to the intellectual appreciation of the biologic relevance of the Ph-negative diseases, are these diseases appropriate to study with intensity, owing to their relative infrequency? The answer is an unequivocal "yes." The model of *BCR-ABL*/imatinib has provided enthusiastic impetus for understanding the mechanisms of action of $JAK2^{V617F}$ and for developing drugs effective against this abnormality. This has applicability not only for the more common Ph-negative MPDs, PV, ET, and PMF, but also for the less common ones, mast cell disease and the hypereosinophilic syndromes. This textbook has been prepared both for the more casual student of the MPDs as well as for those of us who are particularly interested in these disorders. We have also selected topics of interest to the clinician treating these patients and to laboratory scientists studying the molecular and cytogenetic abnormalities of these illnesses. As our understanding unfolds, specific inhibitors of the JAK2 pathway may be discovered, which are uniquely useful in the clinic. Until that time, more traditional treatments, which are reviewed, such as phlebotomy, anagrelide, hydroxyurea, interferon, and marrow transplantation, will continue to be employed in a rational manner, acknowledging the limitations of our current therapeutics.

We are very grateful to our contributors for their scholarly and timely contributions that have made this volume possible. This is particularly important because of the rapid advances that are currently being made. Hopefully, this book will serve as a repository and summary of recent information relevant to the field.

Richard T. Silver, M.D.
Weill Cornell Medical College, New York, New York

Ayalew Tefferi, M.D.
Mayo Clinic, Rochester, Minnesota

Contents

v

Contributors

Cem Akin   Division of Allergy and Clinical Immunology, University of Michigan, Ann Arbor, Michigan, U.S.A.

Tiziano Barbui   Department of Hematology, Ospedali Riuniti, Bergamo, Italy

Giovanni Barosi   Unit of Clinical Epidemiology and Center for the Study of Myelofibrosis, IRCCS Policlinico San Matteo, Pavia, Italy

John M. Bennett   Professor of Laboratory Medicine and Pathology, James P. Wilmot Cancer Center, University of Rochester Medical Center, Rochester, New York, U.S.A.

Francisco Cervantes   Hematology Department, Hospital Clinic, IDIBAPS, University of Barcelona, Spain

Guido Finazzi   Departments of Transfusion Medicine and Hematology, Ospedali Riuniti, Bergamo, Italy

Curtis A. Hanson   Professor of Laboratory Medicine and Pathology, Mayo Clinic College of Medicine, Rochester, Minnesota, U.S.A.

Hans-Peter Horny   Institute of Pathology, Klinikum Ansbach, Ansbach, Germany

Hans Michael Kvasnicka   Institute for Pathology, University of Cologne, Cologne, Germany

Ruben A. Mesa   Division of Hematology, Mayo Clinic, College of Medicine, Rochester, Minnesota, U.S.A.

Dean D. Metcalfe   Laboratory of Allergic Diseases, NIAID/NIH, Bethesda, Maryland, U.S.A.

Vesna Najfeld   Departments of Pathology and Medicine, The Mount Sinai School of Medicine, New York, New York, U.S.A.

Attilio Orazi   Department of Pathology, Indiana University, School of Medicine, Indianapolis, Indiana, U.S.A.

Animesh Pardanani   Division of Hematology, Mayo Clinic College of Medicine, Rochester, Minnesota, U.S.A.

Josef T. Prchal   University of Utah, Hematology Division, Salt Lake City, Utah, U.S.A.

Richard T. Silver   Leukemia and Myeloproliferative Disease Center, Division of Hematology-Oncology, Weill Medical College of Cornell University, New York, New York, U.S.A.

Shireen Sirhan   Department of Hematology, McGill University, Montreal, Quebec, Canada

Radek C. Skoda   University Hospital Basel, Department of Research, Experimental Hematology, Basel, Switzerland

Ayalew Tefferi   Division of Hematology, Mayo Clinic College of Medicine, Rochester, Minnesota, U.S.A.

Juergen Thiele   Institute for Pathology, University of Cologne, Cologne, Germany

Peter Valent   Division of Hematology & Hemostaseology, Medical University of Vienna, Vienna, Austria

Srdan Verstovsek   Department of Leukemia, MD Anderson Cancer Center, Houston, Texas, U.S.A.

1

Modern Classification, Diagnostic Criteria, and Practical Algorithms in Myeloproliferative Disorders

Ayalew Tefferi

Division of Hematology, Mayo Clinic College of Medicine, Rochester, Minnesota, U.S.A.

INTRODUCTION

William Dameshek (1900–1969) is credited for introducing the term myeloproliferative disorders (MPDs) as well as the first classification scheme in MPDs; he nominated chronic myelogenous leukemia (CML), polycythemia vera (PV), essential thrombocythemia (ET), and primary myelofibrosis (PMF) as the original members of the group (1). These four classic MPDs are now part of a broader category of "chronic myeloid neoplasms," which also includes the myelodysplastic syndrome (MDS) and the operationally named "nonclassic" MPDs (Table 1) (2,3). The latter include chronic myelomonocytic leukemia (CMML), juvenile myelomonocytic leukemia (JMML), chronic neutrophilic leukemia (CNL), chronic eosinophilic leukemia (CEL), hypereosinophilic syndrome (HES), systemic mastocytosis (SM), the 8p11 myeloproliferative syndrome (EMS, a.k.a. stem cell leukemia and lymphoma syndrome), chronic basophilic leukemia, atypical CML (aCML), and "MPD not otherwise classified" (MPD-NOC) (Table 1). The World Health Organization (WHO) classification system for chronic myeloid neoplasms is different from that depicted in Table 1; the WHO system includes four subgroups of chronic myeloid neoplasms: MDS, MPD, MDS/MPD, and SM (4). The WHO MPD category includes the four classic MPDs as well as CNL, CEL, HES, and "MPD, unclassifiable." The WHO MDS/MPD category includes

Table 1 Modern Classification of Chronic Myeloid Neoplasms

Main categories	Subcategories	Molecular signatures
Myelodysplastic syndrome	*According to WHO classification system*	
Classic myeloproliferative disorders	1. Chronic myeloid leukemia	100% BCR-ABL[+]
	2. Polycythemia vera	~95% JAK2V617F[+]
		~4% JAK2 exon 12 mutations[+]
	3. Essential thrombocythemia	~50% JAK2V617F[+]
		~1% MPLW515L/K[+]
	4. Primary myelofibrosis	~50% JAK2V617F[+]
		~5% MPLW515L/K[+]
Nonclassic myeloproliferative disorders	1. Chronic myelomonocytic leukemia	~3% JAK2V617F[+]
	2. Juvenile myelomonocytic leukemia	~30% PTPN11 mutation[+]
		~15% NF1 mutation[+]
		~15% RAS mutation[+]
	3. Chronic neutrophilic leukemia	~20% JAK2V617F[+]
	4. Chronic eosinophilic leukemia	~100% FIP1L1-PDGFRA[+]
	i. *PDGFRA*-rearranged	100% various PDGFRB
	ii. *PDGFRB*-rearranged	translocations
	iii. Molecularly undefined	
	5. Hypereosinophilic syndrome	
	6. Systemic mastocytosis	~90% KITD816V[+]
	i. *KIT*-mutated	
	ii. Molecularly undefined	
	7. 8p11 Myeloproliferative syndrome	100% various FGFR1 translocations
	8. Chronic basophilic leukemia	
	9. Atypical chronic myeloid leukemia	~20% JAK2V617F[+]
	MPD not otherwise classified (MPD-NOC); includes the WHO categories of "MPD, unclassifiable," "MDS/MPD, unclassifiable," and "RARS-T"	~20–50% JAK2V617F[+]

Abbreviations: SCLL, stem cell leukemia and lymphoma syndrome; MPD, myeloproliferative syndrome; MPD-NOC, MPD not otherwise classified; MDS, myelodysplastic syndrome; RARS-T, refractory anemia with ringed sideroblasts associated with marked thrombocytosis; WHO, World Health Organization.

CMML, JMML, aCML, and "MDS/MPD, unclassifiable." In the classification scheme outlined in Table 1, both MPD, unclassifiable, and MDS/MPD, unclassifiable, are listed under "MPD-NOC."

The diagnosis of CML requires a demonstration of *BCR-ABL*. The diagnostic criteria for the other *BCR-ABL*–negative classic MPDs (i.e., PV, ET, and PMF) are discussed later in this chapter. The CNL represents *BCR-ABL*–negative mature granulocytosis with < 10% immature granulocytes, < 1% myeloblasts, and < 1 × 10^9/L monocytes in the peripheral blood. In addition, the diagnosis of CNL requires the absence of diagnostic criteria for another myeloid neoplasm. The WHO definition of HES requires the presence of a sustained (> 6-month duration) absolute eosinophil count of > 1.5 × 10^9/L and evidence for target organ damage as well as the absence of aberrant phenotype or clonal T cell population. An HES-like phenotype associated with either a molecular/cytogenetic clonal marker or excess myeloblasts in blood (> 2%) or bone marrow (> 5%) is designated as CEL, which may (i.e., *PDGFRA/B*-rearranged) or may not be molecularly defined (Table 1).

The diagnoses of CMML and JMML require the presence of peripheral blood monocytosis (1 × 10^9/L) as well as the absence of *BCR-ABL*. In addition, at least two of the following are needed for JMML diagnosis: increased hemoglobin F, left-shifted granulocytosis, abnormal cytogenetics, and in vitro GM-CSF hypersensitivity. I prefer the term "*PDGFRB*-rearranged CEL" instead of "CMML associated with a *PDGFRB* mutation" because prominent eosinophilia and not monocytosis is the laboratory marker that is invariably associated with this imatinib mesylate–sensitive clinicopathologic entity (5). I use a similar argument in my designation of the term "*PDGFRA*-rearranged CEL," fully recognizing the fact that the majority of such cases are characterized by clonal bone marrow mastocytosis (6,7). The diagnosis of SM is based on bone marrow histology and requires the presence of dense aggregates of morphologically and phenotypically aberrant mast cells. However, I would make a working diagnosis of SM even in the absence of dense mast cell aggregates as long as a typical clinical scenario is accompanied by some molecular (*KIT*D816V) or immunophenotypic (CD25-expressing mast cells) evidence for abnormal mast cells in the bone marrow (8).

According to the WHO, MPD, unclassifiable, is used to refer to a clinically and histologically MPD-like phenotype that does not fulfill the standard diagnostic criteria for CML, PV, ET, PMF, CNL, HES, or CEL. Some of these cases represent early stages of *BCR-ABL*–negative classic MPDs. Similarly, the WHO defines MDS/MPD, unclassifiable, as a clinical phenotype that displays histological characteristics of both MDS and MPD and yet does not fulfill the diagnostic criteria for CMML, JMML, or a CML. Some place the WHO provisional entity of "refractory anemia with ringed sideroblasts associated with marked thrombocytosis (RARS-T)" in this category of MDS/MPD, unclassifiable. It is important that one does not confuse RARS-T with either ET/PMF with ringed sideroblasts or RARS with thrombocytosis but without the MPD-like megakaryocyte features. I consider MPD, unclassifiable, MDS/MPD, unclassifiable, and RARS-T all under one category—MPD-NOC (Table 1).

TOWARD A MOLECULAR CLASSIFICATION OF MPDs

The prospect of molecular classification in MPD started with the discovery of *BCR-ABL*—the disease causing mutation in CML (9,10). It is to be recalled that CML is the first leukemia to be described (11) and also the first to be associated with a consistent cytogenetic abnormality, the Philadelphia chromosome (Ph[1]) (12). Ph[1] is a shortened chromosome 22 that is the consequence of a reciprocal translocation between chromosomes 9 and 22, t(9;22)(q34;q11) (13). In the mid-1980s, the Philadelphia translocation was molecularly characterized and the CML disease-causing *BCR-ABL* identified. Accordingly, the four "classic" MPDs are now further subclassified as being either *BCR-ABL*[(+)] (i.e., CML) or *BCR-ABL*[(−)] (i.e., PV, ET, and PMF) (3). Such classification is now molecularly validated. An activating *JAK2* mutation (*JAK2*V617F) is found in the majority of patients with *BCR-ABL*[(−)] classic MPDs (14–17), whereas it is either absent or occurs infrequently in other myeloid disorders. Other relevant mutations in MPDs include *JAK2* exon 12 mutations in PV (18), *MPL*W515L/K in ET or PMF (19,20), *FIP1L1-PDGFRA* and other *PDGFRA* mutations in *PDGFRA*-rearranged CEL (21), *ETV6-PDGFRB* and other *PDGFRB* translocations in *PDGFRB*-rearranged CEL (22), *ZNF198-FGFR1* and other *FGFR1* rearrangements in EMS (23), *KIT*D816V and other KIT mutations in SM (24), and RAS pathway mutations, including *RAS*, *PTPN11*, or *NF1*, in JMML (25–27). Such discoveries in the molecular pathogenesis of MPDs will ultimately lead to a predominantly genetic classification system that is also treatment-relevant (Fig. 1).

DIAGNOSTIC CRITERIA FOR PV, ET, AND PMF

The first formal attempt in establishing diagnostic criteria for MPDs focused on PV and was undertaken by the Polycythemia Vera Study Group (PVSG) in 1967 (Table 2) (28). The PVSG subsequently published similar diagnostic criteria for ET (Table 3). The PVSG "diagnostic" criteria for PV and ET were formulated, primarily, to exclude other causes of erythrocytosis and thrombocytosis, respectively, and to establish uniformly applied practical criteria for entering patients into clinical studies. The WHO Committee for the Classification of Myeloid Neoplasms incorporated bone marrow histology and made additional refinements to these criteria and published in 2000 the first WHO diagnostic criteria for these diseases (Tables 4–7). In March 2007, proposals for the revision of the WHO criteria were submitted by an international panel of experts and presented to and endorsed by the majority of the members of the Clinical Advisory Committee for the Revision of WHO Criteria for the Classification of Myeloid Neoplasms, at a meeting in Chicago, IL, U.S.A. (Tables 8–10).

The new proposals for the revision of the WHO diagnostic criteria for PV, ET, and PMF were instigated by the discovery of *JAK2* mutations (*JAK2*V617F and *JAK2* exon 12 mutations) in virtually all patients with PV (14–18). *JAK2*V617F is also found in approximately 50% of patients with either ET or PMF and at

Table 2 Polycythemia Vera Study Group Diagnostic Criteria for Polycythemia Vera[a]

Category A
A1. Increased red cell mass: males $\geq$ 36 mL/kg, females $\geq$ 32 mL/kg
A2. Normal arterial oxygen saturation: $\geq$ 92%
A3. Splenomegaly

Category B
B1. Thrombocytosis: platelets $\geq$ 400 $\times$ 10^9/L
B2. Leukocytosis: white cell count $\geq$ 12 $\times$ 10^9/L; in the absence of fever or infection
B3. Elevated leukocyte alkaline phosphatase score: $>$ 100 in the absence of fever or infection
B4. Elevated serum B$_{12}$ or unbound B$_{12}$-binding capacity: B$_{12}$ $>$ 900 pg/mL; UB$_{12}$ BC $>$ 2200 pg/mL

[a]Diagnosis requires all of the three A criteria or the first two A criteria and two of the four B criteria.

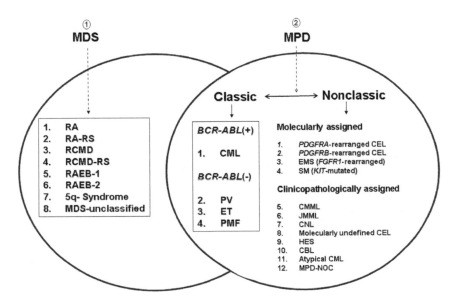

Figure 1 Semimolecular classification of chronic myeloid neoplasms. MDS, myelodysplastic syndrome; MPD, myeloproliferative disorders; RA, refractory anemia; RA-RS, RA with ringed sideroblasts; RCMD, refractory cytopenia with multilineage dysplasia; RCMD-RS, RCMD with ringed sideroblasts; RAEB, refractory anemia with excess blasts; CML, chronic myeloid leukemia; PV, polycythemia vera; ET, essential thrombocythemia; PMF, primary myelofibrosis; SM, systemic mastocytosis; EMS, the 8p11 myeloproliferative syndrome; JMML, juvenile myelomonocytic leukemia; CMML, chronic myelomonocytic leukemia; CNL, chronic neutrophilic leukemia; HES, hypereosinophilic syndrome; CEL, chronic eosinophilic leukemia; CBL, chronic basophilic leukemia; MPD-NOC, MPD otherwise not classified.

Table 3 Polycythemia Vera Study Group Diagnostic Criteria for Essential Thrombocythemia[a]

1. Platelet count $\geq 600 \times 10^9$/L and megakaryocytic hyperplasia
2. No evidence of reactive thrombocytosis
3. A normal red cell mass or hemoglobin < 13 g/dL
4. Stainable bone marrow iron present or < 1 g/dL increase in hemoglobin following 1 month of oral iron therapy
5. No Philadelphia chromosome
6. Bone marrow collagen fibrosis absent or $\leq$ one-third of the cross-sectional area of the marrow biopsy. A lesser degree of fibrosis should not be accompanied by both splenomegaly and leukoerythroblastosis

[a]Diagnosis requires meeting all listed criteria.

a lesser frequency in other myeloid neoplasms (29–32). These mutations are, however, absent in patients with reactive myeloproliferation, including secondary polycythemia and reactive thrombocytosis (33–41). Therefore, a *JAK2* mutation constitutes a sensitive diagnostic marker for PV, and *JAK2*V617F complements histology in the diagnosis of early cases of ET with lower than the WHO-threshold

Table 4 Current World Health Organization Criteria for Polycythemia Vera[a]

A criteria
1. Elevated red cell mass $> 25\%$ above mean normal predicted value, or hemoglobin > 18.5 g/dL in men, 16.5 g/dL in women, or > 99th percentile of method-specific reference range for age, sex, and altitude of residence.
2. No cause of secondary erythrocytosis, including
   a. absence of familial erythrocytosis
   b. no elevation of erythropoietin due to
      i. hypoxia (arterial $pO_2 \leq 92\%$)
      ii. high-oxygen-affinity hemoglobin
      iii. truncated erythropoietin receptor
      iv. inappropriate erythropoietin production by tumor
3. Splenomegaly
4. Clonal genetic abnormality other than Philadelphia chromosome or *BCR-ABL* fusion gene in marrow cells
5. Endogenous erythroid colony formation in vitro

B criteria
1. Thrombocytosis $> 400 \times 10^9$/L
2. Leukocytosis $> 12 \times 10^9$/L
3. Bone marrow biopsy showing panmyelosis with prominent erythroid and megakaryocytic proliferation
4. Low serum erythropoietin levels

[a]Diagnosis requires the presence of the first two A criteria together with either any one other A criterion or two B criteria.

Table 5   Current World Health Organization Criteria for Essential Thrombocythemia

Positive criteria
1. Sustained platelet count $\geq 600 \times 10^9/L$
2. Bone marrow biopsy specimen showing proliferation mainly of the megakaryocytic lineage with increased numbers of enlarged, mature megakaryocytes

Criteria of exclusion
1. No evidence of polycythemia vera
   a. Normal red cell mass or hemoglobin < 18.5 g/dL in men and 16.5 g/dL in women
   b. Stainable iron in marrow; normal serum ferritin or normal MCV
   c. If the former condition is not met, failure of iron trial to increase red cell mass or hemoglobin levels to the PV range
2. No evidence of chronic myeloid leukemia
   d. No Philadelphia chromosome and no *BCR-ABL* fusion gene
3. No evidence of chronic idiopathic myelofibrosis
   e. Collagen fibrosis absent
   f. Reticulin fibrosis minimal or absent
4. No evidence of myelodysplastic syndrome
   g. No del(5q), t(3;3)(q21;q26), or inv(3)(q21q26)
   h. No significant granulocytic dysplasia, few, if any, micromegakaryocytes
5. No evidence that thrombocytosis is reactive due to
   i. Underlying inflammation or infection
   j. Underlying neoplasm
   k. Prior splenectomy

Table 6   World Health Organization Criteria for Prefibrotic Stage Primary Myelofibrosis

Clinical findings		Morphological findings	
Spleen and liver	No or mild plenomegaly or hepatomegaly	Blood	No or mild leukoerythroblastosis No or mild RBC poikilocytosis Few, if any, dacryocytes
Hematology	Variable but often; Mild anemia Mild to moderate leukocytosis Mild to marked thrombocytosis	Bone marrow	Hypercellularity Neutrophilic proliferation Megakaryocytic proliferation Megakaryocytic atypia[a] Minimal or absent reticulin fibrosis

[a]Clustering of megakaryocytes, abnormally lobulated megakaryocytic nuclei, and naked megakaryocytic nuclei.

Table 7   World Health Organization Criteria for Fibrotic Stage Primary Myelofibrosis

Clinical findings		Morphological findings	
Spleen and liver	Moderate to marked splenomegaly or hepatomegaly	Blood	Leukoerythroblastosis Prominent RBC poikilocytosis Prominent dacryocytosis
Hematology	Moderate to marked anemia	Bone marrow	Reticulin and/or collagen fibrosis
	WBC decreased to elevated		Decreased cellularity Dilated marrow sinuses
	Platelet count decreased to elevated		Intraluminal hematopoiesis Neutrophilic proliferation Prominent megakaryocytic proliferation Megakaryocytic atypia New bone formation (osteosclerosis)

platelet count (42). Accordingly, the aforementioned international expert panel recommended that the presence of a *JAK2* mutation be listed as a major criterion for PV diagnosis (Table 8) and the platelet count threshold for ET diagnosis be lowered from the 600 to 450 × 10^9/L (Table 9). Bone marrow histology and other biological markers remain integral components of the newly revised WHO criteria, which also allow identification of early cases of PV with a documented increase in their baseline hemoglobin level in excess of 2 g/dL, without reaching the diagnostic threshold (Table 8). On the other hand, the concern about underdiagnosing inapparent PV, because a red cell mass (RCM) measurement is not routinely recommended, has been mitigated by the questionable value of aggressive phlebotomy in aspirin-treated PV, within hematocrit ranges of 40–55% (43).

The utility of mutation screening for *JAK2*V617F for the diagnosis of ET or PMF is limited by suboptimal negative predictive value and lack of diagnostic specificity within the context of myeloid neoplasms (32,44). However, the presence of the mutation effectively excludes reactive thrombocytosis or bone marrow fibrosis and thus confirms the presence of an underlying myeloid neoplasm. Regardless of this, a bone marrow biopsy is still required to differentiate ET from other chronic myeloid neoplasms, including cellular phase/prefibrotic PMF and MDS (45).

Table 8   Proposed Revised World Health Organization Criteria for Polycythemia Vera[a]

Major criteria
1. Hemoglobin > 18.5 g/dL in men and 16.5 g/dL in women, *or* other evidence of increased red cell volume[b]
2. Presence of *JAK2*V617F or other functionally similar mutation, such as *JAK2* exon 12 mutation

Minor criteria
1. Bone marrow biopsy showing hypercellularity with trilineage hyperplasia (panmyelosis) with prominent erythroid, granulocytic, and megakaryocytic proliferation
2. Low serum erythropoietin level
3. Endogenous erythroid colony formation in vitro

[a]Diagnosis requires the presence of both major criteria and one minor criterion *or* the presence of the first major criterion together with two minor criteria.
[b]Hemoglobin or hematocrit > 99th percentile of method-specific reference range for age, sex, and altitude of residence. *Or*, hemoglobin > 17 g/dL in men and 15 g/dL in women if associated with a documented and sustained increase of at least 2 g/dL from an individual's baseline value that cannot be attributed to correction of iron deficiency. *Or*, elevated red cell mass > 25% above the mean normal predicted value.

Table 9   Proposed Revised World Health Organization Criteria for Essential Thrombocythemia[a]

1. Sustained[b] platelet count $\geq$ 450 × 10^9/L.
2. Bone marrow biopsy specimen showing proliferation mainly of the megakaryocytic lineage with increased numbers of enlarged, mature megakaryocytes. No significant increase or left-shift of neutrophil granulopoiesis or erythropoiesis.
3. Not meeting WHO criteria for polycythemia vera,[c] primary myelofibrosis,[d] chronic myelogenous leukemia,[e] myelodysplastic syndrome,[f] or other myeloid neoplasm.
4. Demonstration of *JAK2*V617F or other clonal marker, *or* in the absence of a clonal marker, no evidence for reactive thrombocytosis.[g]

[a]Diagnosis requires meeting all four criteria.
[b]Sustained during the work-up process.
[c]Requires the failure of iron replacement therapy to increase the hemoglobin level to the polycythemia vera range in the presence of decreased serum ferritin. Exclusion of polycythemia vera is based on hemoglobin and hematocrit levels, and a red cell mass measurement is not required.
[d]Requires the absence of relevant reticulin fibrosis, collagen fibrosis, peripheral blood leukoerythroblastosis, or markedly hypercellular marrow accompanied by megakaryocyte morphology that is typical for primary myelofibrosis—small to large with an aberrant nuclear/cytoplasmic ratio and hyperchromatic, bulbous, or irregularly folded nuclei and dense clustering.
[e]Requires the absence of BCR-ABL.
[f]Requires the absence of dyserythropoiesis and dysgranulopoiesis.
[g]Causes of reactive thrombocytosis include iron deficiency, splenectomy, surgery, infection, inflammation, connective tissue disease, metastatic cancer, and lymphoproliferative disorders. However, the presence of a condition associated with reactive thrombocytosis does not exclude the possibility of ET if other criteria are met.

Table 10 Proposed Revised World Health Organization Criteria for Primary Myelofibrosis[a]

Major criteria
1. Presence of megakaryocyte proliferation and atypia,[b] usually accompanied by either reticulin and/or collagen fibrosis

Or, in the absence of significant reticulin fibrosis, the megakaryocyte changes must be accompanied by an increased bone marrow cellularity characterized by granulocytic proliferation and often decreased erythropoiesis (i.e., prefibrotic cellular-phase disease).

2. Not meeting WHO criteria for polycythemia vera,[c] chronic myelogenous leukemia,[d] myelodysplastic syndrome,[e] or other myeloid neoplasm
3. Demonstration of *JAK2*V617F or other clonal marker (e.g., *MPL*W515L/K)

Or, in the absence of a clonal marker, no evidence of reactive bone marrow fibrosis[f]

Minor criteria
1. Leukoerythroblastosis[g]
2. Increase in serum lactate dehydrogenase level[g]
3. Anemia[g]
4. Palpable splenomegaly[g]

---

[a]Diagnosis requires meeting all three major criteria and two minor criteria.
[b]Small to large megakaryocytes with an aberrant nuclear/cytoplasmic ratio and hyperchromatic, bulbous, or irregularly folded nuclei and dense clustering.
[c]Requires the failure of iron replacement therapy to increase the hemoglobin level to the polycythemia vera range in the presence of decreased serum ferritin. Exclusion of polycythemia vera is based on hemoglobin and hematocrit levels. A red cell mass measurement is not required.
[d]Requires the absence of BCR-ABL.
[e]Requires the absence of dyserythropoiesis and dysgranulopoiesis.
[f]Secondary to infection, autoimmune disorder or other chronic inflammatory condition, hairy cell leukemia or other lymphoid neoplasm, metastatic malignancy, or toxic (chronic) myelopathies. It should be noted that patients with conditions associated with reactive myelofibrosis are not immune to primary myelofibrosis and the diagnosis should be considered in such cases if other criteria are met.
[g]Degree of abnormality could be borderline or marked.

DIAGNOSTIC ALGORITHMS IN PV, ET, AND PMF

In most instances, PV is suspected because of the perception of an "increased" hemoglobin or hematocrit. Therefore, it is important to be familiar with the three standard deviation upper limit for hemoglobin level for adults: $\sim$18.2 g/dL in males and 16.7 g/dL in females for non-Hispanic whites and Mexican-Americans and $\sim$17.9 g/dL and 16.3 g/dL for non-Hispanic blacks (46,47). At the same time, it should also be recognized that the right tail of the Gaussian distribution for the general population includes readings that are outside of this range (thus giving the false perception of an abnormal result) and that the left tail of the Gaussian distribution for PV patients includes readings that lie in the "normal" reference range (thus giving the false perception of a normal result). Therefore, an apparently "increased" hemoglobin does not always imply a true increase in RCM (i.e., true polycythemia) and vice versa (i.e., inapparent PV). Similarly, the distinction among the three *BCR-ABL*–negative MPDs (i.e., PV, ET, and PMF) is not always apparent from the hemoglobin or hematocrit reading.

The PVSG advocated the use of RCM measurement to address the aforementioned shortcomings in the diagnosis of PV. The WHO criteria emphasized, instead, the value of histology in that regard. The discovery of the *JAK2* mutation in association with virtually all patients with PV has erased any residual interest in the use of RCM measurement for the diagnosis of MPDs. As previously mentioned, *JAK2*V617F occurs in approximately 95% of PV patients (14–17). Among the remaining ∼5% of *JAK2*V617 F-negative PV patients, the majority carry *JAK2* exon 12 mutations (18). Therefore, peripheral blood *JAK2* mutation screening is the currently preferred initial test for evaluating a patient with suspected PV (Fig. 2) (44). In order to minimize the consequences of false-positive or false-negative test results as well as to capture the few cases that are *JAK2*V617 F-negative PV, a concomitant measurement of serum Epo level, which is abnormally low in more than 90% of patients with PV, is recommended (Fig. 2) (48).

Neither *JAK2*V617 F nor *JAK2* exon 12 mutations are seen in lymphoid disorders (33–36), solid tumor (37–39), or secondary myeloproliferation (40,41). However, *JAK2*V617 F occurs in approximately 50% of patients with either ET or PMF, and at a lesser frequency in other myeloid neoplasms (31,32). Therefore, it is reasonable to include *JAK2*V617 F mutation screening in the diagnostic work-up of both thrombocytosis and bone marrow fibrosis, and the presence of the mutation in this instance excludes reactive myeloproliferation (Figs. 3 and 4). However, it should be noted that the absence of the mutation does not exclude the possibility of a MPD diagnosis and its presence cannot distinguish one MPD from another; input from bone marrow examination is required in this regard (Figs. 2–4).

Once clonal erythrocytosis or thrombocytosis is excluded through *JAK2* mutation analysis and bone marrow examination, the possibility of congenital polycythemia (CP) or congenital thrombocythemia should be addressed. When CP is suspected, initial laboratory testing should include the measurement of the oxygen tension at which hemoglobin is 50% saturated (p50) (Fig. 2). Decreased p50 suggests the presence of either high-oxygen-affinity hemoglobinopathy (autosomal dominant) (49) or 2,3-bisphosphoglycerate (2,3-BPG) deficiency, usually a consequence of BPG mutase mutation (autosomal recessive) (50). If the p50 is normal, then the possibility of mutations involving either the von Hippel-Lindau (*VHL*) tumor suppressor gene or Epo receptor (EPOR) should be considered (Fig. 2) (51,52). CP has also been rarely associated with mutations involving the hypoxia-inducible factor 1α (*HIF-1α*) prolyl hydroxylase genes (53,54).

In the presence of adequate cellular oxygen, the VHL protein directly interacts with HIF-1α and such interaction requires oxygen-dependent enzymatic hydroxylation of HIF-1α proline residues, which is mediated by prolyl hydroxylases. VHL-HIF-1α binding results in ubiquitinylation and subsequent proteasomal degradation of HIF-1α. These oxygen-dependent reactions help maintain low intracellular levels of HIF-1α. Hypoxia undermines the aforementioned

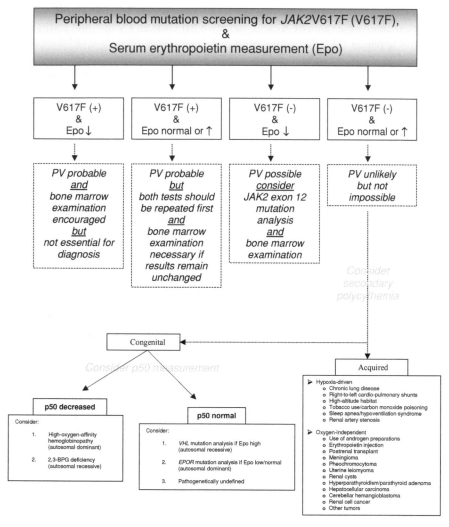

Figure 2 Genetic tests–based diagnostic algorithm for the evaluation of "increased" hemoglobin. PV, polycythemia vera; p50, oxygen tension at which hemoglobin is 50% saturated; VHL, von Hippel-Lindau; EPOR, erythropoietin receptor; BPG, 2,3-bisphosphoglycerate. *Source*: From Ref. 65.

regulatory system and instead stabilizes HIF-1α with subsequent upregulation of HIF-1α–dependent gene expression (e.g., EPO, etc.). The same abnormal effect could result under normoxic conditions, in the presence of defective VHL or prolyl hydroxylases (53,54).

It is now well recognized that a substantial proportion of patients with CP associated with increased Epo carry a *VHL* mutation (chromosome locus

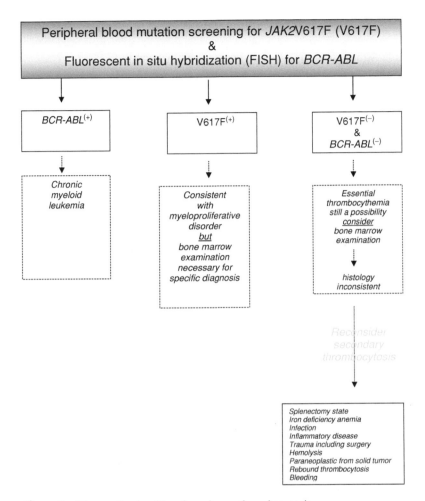

Figure 3   Diagnostic algorithm for primary thrombocytosis.

3p26-p25) that is either sporadic (55–58) or endemic (i.e., Chuvash polycythemia) (53). In Chuvash polycythemia, an autosomal recessive phenotype, a homozygous 598 C>T *VHL* mutation (R200 W) results in impaired HIF-1α degradation. Chuvash-type (homozygous 598 C>T) and other homozygous, compound heterozygous, or simple heterozygous *VHL* mutations have also been described in sporadic CP with increased Epo levels (56,59,60). Similarly, *EPOR* mutation–associated CP has been reported in several families (e.g., exons 7 and 8; 6002G>A, 5974insG, del5985–5991, and 5967insT, etc.) and is characterized by an autosomal-dominant inheritance pattern and decreased or normal serum Epo level (51,52,61–64). Most *EPOR* mutations are heterozygous and result in a C-terminal–truncated receptor that is more efficient in signal transduction (52).

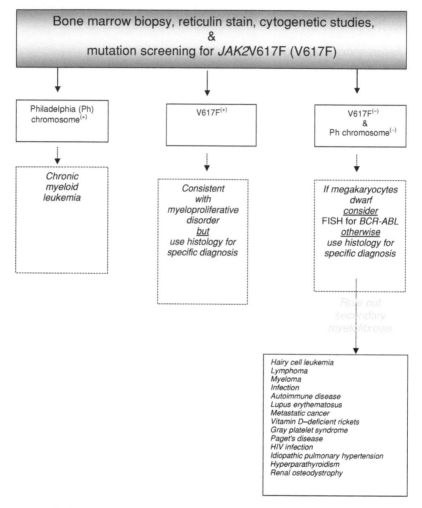

Figure 4   Diagnostic algorithm for suspected primary myelofibrosis.

Most recently, an autosomal-dominant CP associated with a heterozygous 950 C>G prolyl hydroxylase mutation was described in a single family; the mutant protein displayed weak binding to HIF-1α and decreased enzymatic activity (54).

REFERENCES

1. Dameshek W. Some speculations on the myeloproliferative syndromes. Blood 1951;6:372–375.
2. Tefferi A, Gilliland DG. Oncogenes in myeloproliferative disorders. Cell Cycle 2007;6:550–566.

3. Tefferi A, Gilliland DG. Classification of myeloproliferative disorders: From Dameshek towards a semi-molecular system. Best Pract Res Clin Haematol 2006;19:361–364.
4. Vardiman JW, Harris NL, Brunning RD. The World Health Organization (WHO) classification of the myeloid neoplasms. Blood 2002;100:2292–2302.
5. Steer EJ, Cross NC. Myeloproliferative disorders with translocations of chromosome 5q31–35: Role of the platelet-derived growth factor receptor beta. Acta Haematol 2002;107:113–122.
6. Pardanani A, Brockman SR, Paternoster SF, et al. FIP1L1-PDGFRA fusion: Prevalence and clinicopathologic correlates in 89 consecutive patients with moderate to severe eosinophilia. Blood 2004;104:3038–3045.
7. Robyn J, Lemery S, McCoy JP, et al. Multilineage involvement of the fusion gene in patients with FIP1L1/PDGFRA-positive hypereosinophilic syndrome. Br J Haematol 2006;132:286–292.
8. Tefferi A, Pardanani A. Clinical, genetic, and therapeutic insights into systemic mast cell disease. Curr Opin Hematol 2004;11:58–64.
9. Daley GQ, Van Etten RA, Baltimore D. Induction of chronic myelogenous leukemia in mice by the P210bcr/abl gene of the Philadelphia chromosome. Science 1990;247:824–830.
10. Kelliher MA, McLaughlin J, Witte ON, Rosenberg N. Induction of a chronic myelogenous leukemia-like syndrome in mice with v-abl and BCR/ABL. Proc Natl Acad Sci USA 1990;87:6649–6653.
11. Virchow R. Weisses blut. Froiep's Notzien 1845;36:151.
12. Nowell PC, Hungerford DA. A minute chromosome in human chronic granulocytic leukemia. J Natl Cancer Inst 1960;25:85.
13. Rowley JD. Letter: A new consistent chromosomal abnormality in chronic myelogenous leukaemia identified by quinacrine fluorescence and Giemsa staining. Nature 1973;243:290–293.
14. Baxter EJ, Scott LM, Campbell PJ, et al. Acquired mutation of the tyrosine kinase JAK2 in human myeloproliferative disorders. Lancet 2005;365:1054–1061.
15. Levine RL, Wadleigh M, Cools J, et al. Activating mutation in the tyrosine kinase JAK2 in polycythemia vera, essential thrombocythemia, and myeloid metaplasia with myelofibrosis. Cancer Cell 2005;7:387–397.
16. Kralovics R, Passamonti F, Buser AS, et al. A gain of function mutation in Jak2 is frequently found in patients with myeloproliferative disorders. N Engl J Med 2005;352:1779–1790.
17. James C, Ugo V, Le Couedic JP, et al. A unique clonal JAK2 mutation leading to constitutive signalling causes polycythaemia vera. Nature 2005;434:1144–1148.
18. Scott LM, Tong W, Levine R, et al. JAK2 exon 12 mutations in polycythemia vera and idiopathic erythrocytosis. N Engl J Med 2007;356:459–468.
19. Pikman Y, Lee BH, Mercher T, et al. MPLW515 L is a novel somatic activating mutation in myelofibrosis with myeloid metaplasia. PLoS Med 2006;3:e270.
20. Pardanani AD, Levine RL, Lasho T, et al. MPL515 mutations in myeloproliferative and other myeloid disorders: A study of 1182 patients. Blood 2006;108:3472–3476.
21. Cools J, DeAngelo DJ, Gotlib J, et al. A tyrosine kinase created by fusion of the PDGFRA and FIP1L1 genes as a therapeutic target of imatinib in idiopathic hypereosinophilic syndrome. N Engl J Med 2003;348:1201–1214.

22. Golub TR, Barker GF, Lovett M, Gilliland DG. Fusion of PDGF receptor beta to a novel ets-like gene, tel, in chronic myelomonocytic leukemia with t(5;12) chromosomal translocation. Cell 1994;77:307–316.

23. Xiao S, Nalabolu SR, Aster JC, et al. FGFR1 is fused with a novel zinc-finger gene, ZNF198, in the t(8;13) leukaemia/lymphoma syndrome. Nat Genet 1998;18:84–87.

24. Nagata H, Worobec AS, Oh CK, et al. Identification of a point mutation in the catalytic domain of the protooncogene c-kit in peripheral blood mononuclear cells of patients who have mastocytosis with an associated hematologic disorder. Proc Natl Acad Sci USA 1995;92:10560–10564.

25. Loh ML, Vattikuti S, Schubbert S, et al. Mutations in PTPN11 implicate the SHP-2 phosphatase in leukemogenesis. Blood 2004;103:2325–2331.

26. Shannon KM, O'Connell P, Martin GA, et al. Loss of the normal NF1 allele from the bone marrow of children with type 1 neurofibromatosis and malignant myeloid disorders. N Engl J Med 1994;330:597–601.

27. Lauchle JO, Braun BS, Loh ML, et al. Inherited predispositions and hyperactive Ras in myeloid leukemogenesis. Pediatr Blood Cancer 2006;46:579–585.

28. Wasserman LR. The treatment of polycythemia. A panel discussion. Blood 1968;32:483–487.

29. Tefferi A, Lasho TL, Schwager SM, et al. The JAK2 tyrosine kinase mutation in myelofibrosis with myeloid metaplasia: Lineage specificity and clinical correlates. Br J Haematol 2005;131:320–328.

30. Wolanskyj AP, Lasho TL, Schwager SM, et al. JAK2 mutation in essential thrombocythaemia: Clinical associations and long-term prognostic relevance. Br J Haematol 2005;131:208–213.

31. Steensma DP, Dewald GW, Lasho TL, et al. The JAK2 V617F activating tyrosine kinase mutation is an infrequent event in both "atypical" myeloproliferative disorders and myelodysplastic syndromes. Blood 2005;106:1207–1209.

32. Jones AV, Kreil S, Zoi K, et al. Widespread occurrence of the JAK2 V617F mutation in chronic myeloproliferative disorders. Blood 2005;106:2162–2168.

33. Melzner I, Weniger MA, Menz CK, et al. Absence of the JAK2 V617F activating mutation in classical Hodgkin lymphoma and primary mediastinal B-cell lymphoma. Leukemia 2006;20:157–158.

34. Lee JW, Soung YH, Kim SY, et al. JAK2 V617F mutation is uncommon in non-Hodgkin lymphomas. Leuk Lymphoma 2006;47:313–314.

35. Sulong S, Case M, Minto L, et al. The V617F mutation in Jak2 is not found in childhood acute lymphoblastic leukaemia. Br J Haematol 2005;130:964–965.

36. Levine RL, Loriaux M, Huntly BJ, et al. The JAK2V617F activating mutation occurs in chronic myelomonocytic leukemia and acute myeloid leukemia, but not in acute lymphoblastic leukemia or chronic lymphocytic leukemia. Blood 2005;106:3377–3379.

37. Lee JW, Soung YH, Kim SY, et al. Absence of JAK2 V617F mutation in gastric cancers. Acta Oncol 2006;45:222–223.

38. Lee JW, Kim YG, Soung YH, et al. The JAK2 V617F mutation in de novo acute myelogenous leukemias. Oncogene 2006;25:1434–1436.

39. Scott LM, Campbell PJ, Baxter EJ, et al. The V617F JAK2 mutation is uncommon in cancers and in myeloid malignancies other than the classic myeloproliferative disorders. Blood 2005;106:2920–2921.

40. Tefferi A, Sirhan S, Lasho TL, et al. Concomitant neutrophil JAK2 mutation screening and PRV-1 expression analysis in myeloproliferative disorders and secondary polycythaemia. Br J Haematol 2005;131:166–171.

41. Kralovics R, Teo SS, Buser AS, et al. Altered gene expression in myeloproliferative disorders correlates with activation of signaling by the V617F mutation of Jak2. Blood 2005;106:3374–3376.

42. Tefferi A, Vardiman JW. The diagnostic interface between histology and molecular tests in myeloproliferative disorders. Curr Opin Hematol 2007;14:115–122.

43. Di Nisio M, Barbui T, Di Gennaro L, et al. The haematocrit and platelet target in polycythemia vera. BJH 2007;6:550–566.

44. Tefferi A, Gilliland DG. The JAK2V617 F tyrosine kinase mutation in myeloproliferative disorders: Status report and immediate implications for disease classification and diagnosis. Mayo Clin Proc 2005;80:947–958.

45. Thiele J, Kvasnicka HM. Clinicopathological criteria for differential diagnosis of thrombocythemias in various myeloproliferative disorders. Semin Thromb Hemost 2006;32:219–230.

46. Hollowell JG, van Assendelft OW, Gunter EW, et al. Hematological and iron-related analytes–reference data for persons aged 1 year and over: United States, 1988–1994. Vital Health Stat 2005;11:1–156.

47. Beutler E, Waalen J. The definition of anemia: What is the lower limit of normal of the blood hemoglobin concentration? Blood 2006;107:1747–1750.

48. Mossuz P, Girodon F, Donnard M, et al. Diagnostic value of serum erythropoietin level in patients with absolute erythrocytosis. Haematologica 2004;89:1194–1198.

49. Jones RT, Shih TB. Hemoglobin variants with altered oxygen affinity. Hemoglobin 1980;4:243–261.

50. Hoyer JD, Allen SL, Beutler E, et al. Erythrocytosis due to bisphosphoglycerate mutase deficiency with concurrent glucose-6-phosphate dehydrogenase (G-6-PD) deficiency. Am J Hematol 2004;75:205–208.

51. Sokol L, Luhovy M, Guan Y, et al. Primary familial polycythemia: A frameshift mutation in the erythropoietin receptor gene and increased sensitivity of erythroid progenitors to erythropoietin. Blood 1995;86:15–22.

52. de la Chapelle A, Traskelin AL, Juvonen E. Truncated erythropoietin receptor causes dominantly inherited benign human erythrocytosis. Proc Natl Acad Sci USA 1993;90:4495–4499.

53. Ang SO, Chen H, Hirota K, et al. Disruption of oxygen homeostasis underlies congenital Chuvash polycythemia. Nat Genet 2002;32:614–621.

54. Percy MJ, Zhao Q, Flores A, et al. A family with erythrocytosis establishes a role for prolyl hydroxylase domain protein 2 in oxygen homeostasis. Proc Natl Acad Sci USA 2006;103:654–659.

55. Pastore YD, Jelinek J, Ang S, et al. Mutations in the VHL gene in sporadic apparently congenital polycythemia. Blood 2003;101:1591–1595.

56. Cario H, Schwarz K, Jorch N, et al. Mutations in the von Hippel-Lindau (VHL) tumor suppressor gene and VHL-haplotype analysis in patients with presumable congenital erythrocytosis. Haematologica 2005;90:19–24.

57. Percy MJ, McMullin MF, Jowitt SN, et al. Chuvash-type congenital polycythemia in 4 families of Asian and Western European ancestry. Blood 2003;102: 1097–1099.

58. Pastore Y, Jedlickova K, Guan Y, et al. Mutations of von Hippel-Lindau tumor-suppressor gene and congenital polycythemia. Am J Hum Genet 2003;73:412–419.
59. Bento MC, Chang KT, Guan Y, et al. Congenital polycythemia with homozygous and heterozygous mutations of von Hippel-Lindau gene: Five new Caucasian patients. Haematologica 2005;90:128–129.
60. Randi ML, Murgia A, Putti MC, et al. Low frequency of VHL gene mutations in young individuals with polycythemia and high serum erythropoietin. Haematologica 2005;90:689–691.
61. Yoshimura A, Longmore G, Lodish HF. Point mutation in the exoplasmic domain of the erythropoietin receptor resulting in hormone-independent activation and tumorigenicity. Nature 1990;348:647–649.
62. Arcasoy MO, Degar BA, Harris KW, et al. Familial erythrocytosis associated with a short deletion in the erythropoietin receptor gene. Blood 1997;89:4628–4635.
63. Arcasoy MO, Harris KW, Forget BG. A human erythropoietin receptor gene mutant causing familial erythrocytosis is associated with deregulation of the rates of Jak2 and Stat5 inactivation. Exp Hematol 1999;27:63–74.
64. Kralovics R, Indrak K, Stopka T, et al. Two new EPO receptor mutations: Truncated EPO receptors are most frequently associated with primary familial and congenital polycythemias. Blood 1997;90:2057–2061.
65. Tefferi A, Pardanani A. Evaluation of "increased" hemoglobin in the JAK2 mutations era: A diagnostic algorithm based on genetic tests. Mayo Clin Proc 2007;82:599–604.

2

Diagnostic Utility of Bone Marrow Pathology in Chronic Myeloproliferative Disorders

Juergen Thiele

Institute for Pathology, University of Cologne, Cologne, Germany

Attilio Orazi

Department of Pathology, Indiana University, School of Medicine, Indianapolis, Indiana, U.S.A.

Hans Michael Kvasnicka

Institute for Pathology, University of Cologne, Cologne, Germany

INTRODUCTION

Following the recent discovery of an activating JAK2V617F mutation in patients with Philadelphia chromosome–negative (Ph^{1-}) chronic myeloproliferative disorders or neoplasms (MPNs—according to the forthcoming WHO nomenclature), currently a conflict of opinion exists on whether and to which extent conventional methods of diagnosis and classification, such as bone marrow (BM) morphology, are still needed (1). In this context, it is important to note that the mutation has been reported to occur at a strikingly different incidence (2–4) among the various types of clinicopathologically defined conditions. Detection of the JAK2V617F mutation has been described in up to 95% of polycythemia vera (PV) cases and in 30–50% cases of essential thrombocythemia (ET) and primary myelofibrosis (PMF; chronic idiopathic myelofibrosis). The mutation has also been found, although at a much lower frequency, in a minority (5–10%) of cases of chronic myelomonocytic leukemia, chronic myeloid leukemia, myelodysplastic syndromes, and acute myeloid leukemia, as well as in other atypical myeloproliferative disorders (3–6).

In spite of the enthusiasm raised by the discovery of the JAK2 mutation and the potential value of a molecular-genetic–based classification of MPNs (1), a number of problems remain. Among these, important questions relate to the role of BM morphology, traditionally one of the yardsticks for the diagnosis of MPNs. In particular, the following issues have to be detailed and clarified:

(1) Identification of characteristic BM features in the major MPN entities (e.g., PV, ET, and PMF), with special focus on those of value in identifying the early (prodromal) disease stages.
(2) Standardization of their evaluation to facilitate reproducibility by experienced hematopathologists.
(3) Relevant correlations between BM histopathology and clinical data (e.g., in regard to evolution of disease, including myelofibrotic or acute transformation, and survival).

HISTOPATHOLOGY—BONE MARROW FEATURES

Polycythemia Vera

With regard to the BM histopathology and its contribution to the diagnosis of PV, we are facing a somewhat unfavorable situation. In the original and updated criteria of the Polycythemia Vera Study Group (PVSG), BM findings are not even mentioned (7), and in the current WHO classification, they are considered as a minor criterion for substantiating the diagnosis (8). The major reason why BM morphology has been neglected as a useful tool is that the disease has been traditionally defined by clinical, laboratory, and biologic parameters, which are generally assumed to be sufficient for the establishment of diagnosis (9). In the era of JAK2V617F, it should be emphasized that about 95% of PV patients carry this mutation (1–4) and for this reason, in addition to the relevant laboratory and clinical markers, BM morphology seems to be a minor issue in the total setting of diagnostic procedures. On the other hand, in correlation to clinical findings, a clear pattern of histopathologic features emerges and can be used to confirm the diagnosis in cases without clear-cut hematological and molecular genetic data. One should be aware that PV reveals a dynamically evolving disease process, and it is not surprising that in the beginning a number of patients do not fulfill all of the required diagnostic criteria, particularly with regard to the red cell mass or hemoglobin/hematocrit values (7,10–12). These patients have often been reported to exhibit "latent PV" or "benign erythrocytosis" and are regarded as a heterogeneous group that may eventually develop overt polycythemic PV (13,14). Importantly, some patients have an initial/early prodromal phase of

PV that is accentuated by thromboembolic episodes as the first manifestation of the disease (15), but in whom a diagnosis is not possible by conventional criteria. In these instances, demonstration of the characteristic histologic BM features, in association with a low erythropoietin level and assessment of the JAK2V617F mutation, could lead to early diagnosis and appropriate therapy. The BM biopsy performed at diagnosis is also important to establish a "baseline picture" against which sequential specimens can be compared. This is important since histopathology provides the best means to detect various stages of PV or post-PV, therapy–induced effects, and/or post-PV complications (16–19).

The histopathology of prepolycythemic and full-blown PV is characterized by a hypercellular BM due to a trilineage proliferation (panmyelosis) of erythroid and granulocytic precursors in variable proportions, associated with megakaryocytic proliferation of cells displaying distinctive morphologic features (12,20–29). Some of these findings are more significant than others in establishing the diagnosis of PV and in distinguishing it from reactive or secondary polycythemia (SP) as well as from the other types of MPNs (24,27,30,31). For example, although hypercellularity in relation to age-matched hematopoiesis is a characteristic feature of PV, the data of the PVSG display that 13% of patients with PV revealed a normal or only slight increase in marrow cellularity (16,32,33). On the other hand, hypercellularity may occasionally also be encountered in cases of SP that usually present with a mild to moderate increase in hematopoiesis (24,27,29). Additionally, in PV the usually small and rounded islets of nucleated erythroid precursors show a conspicuous enlargement and a tendency to merge into sheets. Although these changes are significantly more pronounced in PV, they may be also expressed in a few cases with severe SP and therefore this feature may not serve as a reliable diagnostic parameter, especially in the early stage of the disease (29,34). A similar situation may be observed regarding the neutrophil cell lineage because an increase in pro- and metamyelocytes (left-shifting) is frequently displayed in PV and may be also prominent in SP.

However, the characteristic features of the megakaryocytic proliferation in PV have been acknowledged to enable a differentiation between PV, the other subtypes of MPNs, as well as SP (24,27–31). Previous studies reported by the PVSG showed that 95% of biopsies from patients with PV have an increase in the number of megakaryocytes (32,33). In this context, several groups have observed that aside from the increase, their cytological appearance exerts a discriminating impact. It has been repeatedly emphasized that megakaryopoiesis in early as well as full-blown PV is characterized by pleomorphic forms, that is, megakaryocytes displaying marked differences in size with small, medium-sized, large, and giant megakaryocytes that are either dispersed or loosely clustered (21,22,24,26,27, 34–36). In particular, the large megakaryocytic forms show hyperlobulated nuclei, but usually fail to exhibit any other gross abnormality (e.g., a severe deviation from a normal nuclear–cytoplasmic maturation ratio) or display a significant number of abnormal bulky nuclei like in PMF. The identification of these forms may thus serve as a diagnostic hallmark, since they are in contrast to the small to medium-sized

Table 1   Relative Incidence of Borderline to Marked Reticulin
and/or Collagen Myelofibrosis (MF) in Initially Performed Bone
Marrow Biopsies Derived from about 1300 Specimens with MPNs
Diagnosed According to the WHO Classification (45)[a]

	MF-0 (%)	MF-1 (%)	MF-2 (%)	MF-3 (%)
PV	84	15	1	0
ET	99	1	0	0
PMF	27	38	17	18

[a]For further details concerning fiber grading, see Table 2.

megakaryocytes usually found in SP (27,29,34). This histological pattern of an
increased and left-shifted erythroid and granulocytic proliferation associated with
a pleomorphous megakaryopoiesis (24,25,37), typically seen in PV, is in contrast
to that seen in ET, which lacks a significant proliferation of the other cell lineages
(35–39).

Previous reports have indicated that occasionally patients with the clinical
features of ET may later (i.e., 2–5 years) develop overt erythrocytosis and therefore
manifest the features of PV (40,41). In the PVSG trial, 3 of the 91 patients with
presumptive ET transformed to PV during the observation period (42). It seems
reasonable to question whether these patients had ET at all. In fact, the PVSG
criteria have been shown to be unable to diagnose the initial (latent, occult) state
of PV (7,9,18). The initial (latent) PV with excess of platelets, although it may
mimic ET, should be recognized properly and not be considered as one of the
so-called overlapping cases (12).

At the time of the initial diagnosis, it has been found that about 10–20%
of the patients already have a mild to moderate (reticulin) fibrosis (16,24–26,
28,29,43,44) (also found in our study; Table 1). It is noteworthy that the relevant
PVSG data describe a significantly higher incidence of 36% in 226 patients with
pretreatment biopsies (16,33). This higher frequency, particularly the finding of
marked (collagen) fibrosis, may be indicative of a later stage of the disease (as
we mentioned earlier, early disease cases had been missed by the PVSG criteria).
Finally, it has to be stated that usually SP does not demonstrate any significant
increase in fibers (27,29–31).

Essential Thrombocythemia

Persuasive evidence has been gathered by several groups on the relevant impact
of BM morphology in the differential diagnosis of the various subtypes of MPNs
characterized by thrombocytosis, and, more specifically, to define more clearly the
histological patterns essential for a correct diagnosis of ET (24,26,35–37,46–50).
For many years, the recognized "gold standard" criteria for diagnosing ET have
been those outlined by the PVSG group, which are based on the separation of ET
from other thrombocythemic MPNs, particularly chronic myelogenous leukemia

and overt PV or PMF (42,51–53). A critical reevaluation of these diagnostic guidelines, which up to now have been incorporated into all relevant clinical trials, reveals that they do not allow for a clear-cut distinction of ET from prodromal stages of PMF or PV, which are often associated with thrombocytosis (12,39). As a consequence of the inclusion of histopathology in the current WHO classification (49,50,54), serious diagnostic discrepancies are encountered when BM specimens derived from patients with the clinical diagnosis of ET based on the PVSG criteria (42) are evaluated by hematopathologists (37,46–50,55).

In contrast to prefibrotic PMF with accompanying thrombocythemia (i.e., "false" ET), in true ET, according to the WHO classification (54), neither a relevant increase in cellularity nor a significant left-shifted neutrophil granulopoiesis is observed. Any case with a mild to moderate granulocytic and erythroid growth pattern (panmyelosis) and an erythropoietin level below the reference range is suspicious for occult (prepolycythemic) PV mimicking ET (12). Regarding megakaryopoiesis in ET, gross disturbances of the histologic topography (significant abnormal localization and/or extensive dense clustering of these cells) are not seen. These cells show a more or less random distribution within the BM, with scattered forms or a few loose clusters. In (true) ET, a predominance of large to giant mature megakaryocytes with extensively folded (staghorn-like) nuclei (24,26,35–39,46–50,56), surrounded by a correspondingly mature cytoplasma, is found. These features are clearly distinguishable from prefibrotic early PMF by displaying extensive dense clustering of hypolobulated (cloud-like) and hyperchromatic nuclei of megakaryocytes, with their striking nuclear maturation defects (24,37–39,46–50) that result in a marked anomaly of their nuclear–cytoplasmic ratio.

Finally, at presentation, there is no substantial increase in reticulin fibers and collagen fibrosis is not observable in true ET (Table 1)—a finding that contrasts with the allowance of some degree of fibrosis according to the criteria of the PVSG (42). The lack of significant reticulin fibrosis has been reported in a large series of patients where minimal to slight reticulin fibrosis was described in only 3% of cases (24,57) corresponding with our data (58).

Discrimination from reactive thrombocytosis may be easily accomplished (59) because there is no predominance of large to giant megakaryocytes with nuclear hyperlobulation detectable, and often a granulocytic proliferation associated with various degrees of inflammatory marrow reactions may be present (35,36,39). In case of molecular markers, an incidence of the JAK2V617F mutation is dependent on whether the PVSG (42) or WHO (54) criteria are applied; however, the reported frequencies range between 30% and 50% (2–4,60–63). Therefore, this marker exerts a minor diagnostic importance because only a positive finding will help to exclude reactive thrombocytosis.

Primary Myelofibrosis

There has been a general consensus, based on the PVSG (64) and also the Italian guidelines (65), that criteria applied for the diagnosis of the so-called chronic idiopathic myelofibrosis should include a leukoerythroblastic blood smear morphology with teardrop poikilocytosis, splenomegaly due to extramedullary hematopoiesis (myeloid metaplasia), and anemia of varying degree, all in the presence of relevant fibrosis of the BM (66,67). However, some investigators have recognized that in many patients, a striking variability in the hematological findings may be observed at the time of initial presentation (28,66,68–70). These wide ranges of clinical data are paralleled by a significant heterogeneity of BM features, occasionally revealing only a minimal or mild increase in reticulin fibers—the so-called hypercellular phase (23,69,70). Only in the two last decades has the evolution of this condition been elucidated, primarily due to clinicopathological investigations based on a careful analysis of sequential BM biopsy specimens (71,72). In this context, the overt fibrotic (classical) stage, in which extramedullary hematopoiesis, splenomegaly associated with BM collagen fibrosis, and variable osteosclerosis may be present, that is, agnogenic myeloid metaplasia (AMM) or myelofibrosis with myeloid metaplasia (MMM) (64–67,70), is now regarded as an advanced stage that has evolved from an initial hypercellular-prefibrotic or prodromal phase. Recently, an international working group on myelofibrosis research and treatment has recognized this important issue and proposed the term chronic primary myelofibrosis (PMF) and clearly discriminated this condition from myelofibrosis developing in the setting of PV or ET (73).

PMF initially presents with a hypercellular BM characterized by a prominent granulocytic and megakaryocytic myeloproliferation with a concomitant reduction and maturation arrest of the nucleated erythroid precursors, in the absence of BM reticulin fibrosis (Table 1) or with only a borderline to mild degree of reticulin fibrosis, i.e., grades 0 and 1 according to the guidelines of a recently established consensus scoring system for BM fibrosis (45). Most conspicuous is the abnormal megakaryopoiesis, which is characterized not only by a disturbance of BM histologic topography (extensive clustering of megakaryocytes, with loose to dense clusters, with abnormal localization of these toward the endosteal borders), but also by the striking abnormalities in their morphology and maturation. Significant anomalies of megakaryocyte include a high degree of cellular pleomorphism with variations in size that range from small to giant forms, and in particular of abnormal nuclear foldings and an aberration of the nuclear–cytoplasmic ratio created by large bulbous and hyperchromatic cloud-like shaped nuclei. Furthermore, apart from their disorganized nuclear lobulation, there are many naked (bare) megakaryocytic nuclei detectable (21,24,37,44,69,74–76). Overall, the megakaryocytes in PMF are regularly characterized by a more pronounced degree of cytological atypia (e.g., megakaryocytic dysplasia, dysmegakaryopoiesis) than that seen in any other subtype of the MPNs, ET in particular (35–39,47–50,59). Megakaryocytic dysplasia is thus one of the most important features discriminating prefibrotic–early-stage PMF (i.e., false ET) from true ET, a concept also stressed by the WHO classification system (54). Although progression of PMF is unpredictable, increasing megakaryocytic maturation defects seem to be associated with a more rapid transition from the prefibrotic into overt fibrosclerotic stages. As has been elucidated in different studies (57,71,77,78), there is a more than 65% probability of progression from a prefibrotic early stage to a full-blown disease associated with clinical signs and symptoms of myeloid metaplasia conforming with the classical diagnostic criteria (64–67,79).

In contrast to the initial prefibrotic or early (reticulin fibrotic) stages of PMF, the more advanced fibro-osteosclerotic phases of disease (conforming with classical MMM/AMM) are characterized by a significant amount of reticulin deposition and the appearance of coarse bundles of collagen fibers in the BM. According to a previously quoted semiquantitative fiber scoring system (45), these stromal changes are consistent with grades 2 and 3 of myelofibrosis (Table 1). Additional features indicating an advanced to terminal stage include plaque to budd-like osteosclerosis (endophytic bone formation) that is often associated with patchy hematopoiesis replaced by adipose tissue, that is, progressive hypoplasia (21,23,24,26,69,76–78). Similar to the prodromal stages, atypical megakaryopoiesis remains the most prominent feature including the presence of numerous naked nuclei of megakaryocytes. Dilated marrow sinuses (69,80,81) with intraluminal hematopoiesis, especially megakaryocytes, are also among the prominent marrow findings.

In regard to the presence of the JAK2V617F mutation, prefibrotic hypercellular stages express a positivity of less than 30% (60), whereas advanced classical stages corresponding mostly with MMM/AMM (64–67) show approximately a 50% incidence (1–4,60). It is noteworthy that the progression of myelofibrosis is significantly associated with a relevant set of target genes (matrix modeling genes) capable of regulating fibrillogenesis, but is generally not influenced by the JAK2V617F mutation status (82).

STANDARDIZED EVALUATION OF BONE MARROW FEATURES

The ongoing discussion and controversy, particularly among clinicians and hematopathologists, concerns the reproducibility of the morphological features proposed by the WHO criteria for the distinction of the subtypes of MPNs (20). Generally, one should be aware that the assessment of laboratory data (with accepted threshold values) is significantly different from the interpretation of histopathological patterns. There is always a certain range of subjectivity associated with evaluating BM tissue. However, to ameliorate this bias, a set of various methods may be applied to achieve a consensus among different observers. Morphometric analysis employing different techniques (25,35,76,83), including even automatic image analysis (84), can be applied to BM biopsy and has been shown to be useful in classifying MPNs. These elaborate methods are, however, poorly suited for diagnostic laboratories. For this reason, a semiquantitative grading system with standardization of relevant features is badly needed for clinical practice and efforts in this direction have already begun (38,50,69,45).

In regard to BM cellularity, in accordance with previous evaluations by several groups of investigators, ample evidence has been provided that this feature (expansion of hematopoiesis) is age dependent (85–88). Grading of the BM

Table 2 Consensus on the Grading of Myelofibrosis (MF) as Adapted from the Literature (45,89–91)

Grading	Description[a]
MF-0	Scattered linear reticulin with no intersections (cross-overs) corresponding to normal bone marrow
MF-1	Loose network of reticulin with many intersections, especially in perivascular areas
MF-2	Diffuse and dense increase in reticulin with extensive intersections, occasionally with only focal bundles of collagen and/or focal osteosclerosis
MF-3	Diffuse and dense increase in reticulin with extensive intersections with coarse bundles of collagen, often associated with significant osteosclerosis

[a]Fiber density should be assessed in hematopoietic (cellular) areas.

fiber content (i.e., myelofibrosis) was formerly performed by using different semiquantitative staging systems (89–93). In this context, it is important to differentiate between reticulin and collagen and to restrict the evaluation of fiber density to the areas of hematopoiesis (areas with cellularity). This was achieved by developing a consensus grading system (45), which is outlined in Table 2.

In contrast to the relatively easily reproducible assessment of cellularity and degree of myelofibrosis, other parameters, such as proliferative patterns of granulopoiesis and erythropoiesis, and above all, the special morphological features of megakaryopoiesis, may cause significant difficulties. These are more dependent on "descriptive" definitions and their lack of standardization is prone to generate significant dissent. Major difficulties are frequently encountered in MPNs with marked thrombocytosis. These include, especially, the differentiation of ET (39,54) from prefibrotic early stages of PMF associated with thrombocytosis (48–50,74) as well as PV with an elevated platelet count (38,59).

Thus, to avoid disagreement among various observers, a more systematic approach to reading BM biopsies is warranted (shown in Fig. 1). A proper hematopathological description should include the arrangement of the megakaryocytes within the marrow space (histologic topography) and the presence/absence of certain nuclear and cellular abnormalities, in particular those that underline maturation defects. Although these alteration have been precisely described in numerous well-illustrated previous studies (21,23,29,36,37,48,72), a conflict of opinion still exists, whether an untrained pathologist or even clinician would be able to recognize these features on routinely processed BM biopsy material (such as a H&E-stained BM section). In keeping with previous data (38,39,59), a form sheet for the identification and evaluation of histological features of diagnostic impact was developed. This focuses on the most critical morphological parameters, including certain components of hematopoiesis and stroma (Table 3). According to our experience, there is little disagreement regarding the distinctive BM features of

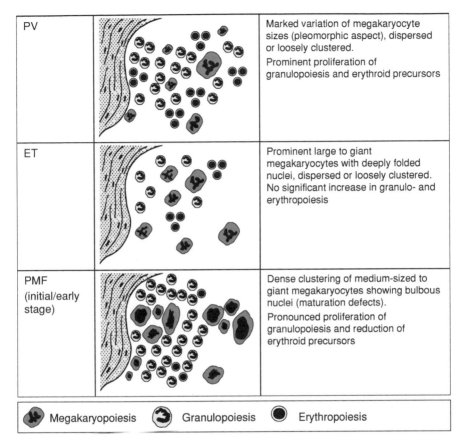

PV		Marked variation of megakaryocyte sizes (pleomorphic aspect), dispersed or loosely clustered. Prominent proliferation of granulopoiesis and erythroid precursors
ET		Prominent large to giant megakaryocytes with deeply folded nuclei, dispersed or loosely clustered. No significant increase in granulo- and erythropoiesis
PMF (initial/early stage)		Dense clustering of medium-sized to giant megakaryocytes showing bulbous nuclei (maturation defects). Pronounced proliferation of granulopoiesis and reduction of erythroid precursors

Megakaryopoiesis   Granulopoiesis   Erythropoiesis

Figure 1 Schematic presentation of BM features with alterations of the three major cell lineages characterizing MPNs.

advanced-stage PMF with the entities shown in Table 3 (see also Fig. 1 for further details).

In accordance with the issues of the WHO classification (20), the different subtypes of MPNs are characterized by specific histological patterns due to the combination of distinctive features usually present at disease diagnosis (Table 4). In this context, it should be emphasized that a single abnormality is not sufficient on its own to achieve a correct differentiation between these disease entities. Consequently, one should try to gather as many parameters as possible. This facilitates the recognition of the most characteristic "overall" histological pattern, the yardstick for diagnosis and subtyping.

Finally, any given histological classification cannot hope to capture or sub-type all biological true cases of MPNs with a 100% guarantee of accuracy. Thus,

Table 3 Discriminating Features Generating Histological Patterns in Initially
Performed Bone Marrow Biopsy Sections (Modified Cologne Evaluation Form)

	ET	PMF-0 (prefibrotic stage)	PMF-1 (early – reticulin fibrotic stage)	PV
I. Cellularity (age-matched)	0	+++	+++	+++
II. Fibers:				
1. Increased reticulin	0	0	+++	–[a]
2. Collagen	0	0	0	0
III. Megakaryopoiesis				
1. Increased quantity	+++	++	++	++
2. Size:				
Small	0	+	+	+
Medium	+	+	+	+
Large	+	+	+	+
Giant	+	+	+	+
3. Histotopography:				
Endosteal translocation	+	+	+	+
Cluster formation:				
Size:				
Small (at least 3 cells)	+	0	0	+
Large (more than 7 cells)	0	+	+	0
Quality:				
Dense	0	+	++	0
Loose	+	+	+	+
4. Nuclear features:				
Hypolobation (bulbous/cloud-like)	0	++	++	0
Hyperlobation (staghorn-like)	++	0	0	++
5. Maturation defects	0	++	++	0
6. Naked nuclei	+	+++	+++	0
IV. Neutrophil granulopoiesis				
1. Increased quantity	0	++	++	+++
2. Left-shifting	0	+	+	++
V. Erythropoiesis				
1. Increased quantity	0	0	0	+++
2. Left-shifting	0	+	0	+++
VI. Lymphoid nodules	0	0	0	+
VII. Iron deposits	0	0	0	0

Semiquantitative evaluation (relative incidence): 0, usually absent to 10%; +, 10–50%; ++, 50–80%;
+++, 80–100%.
[a]In PV between 10–20% of initial bone marrow biopsies reveal an increase in reticulin fibers.

Table 4 Semiquantitative Differentiation of Prominent Features in Initial Bone Marrow Biopsy Sections Including Formation of Characteristic Histological Patterns

	ET	PMF-0 (prefibrotic stage)	PMF-1 (early – reticulin fibrotic stage)	PV
Cellularity (age-matched)	0	+++	+++	+++
Megakaryopoiesis				
Size:				
Small	0	+++	+++	+++
Giant	+++	+++	+++	+++
Hypolobation (bulbous/cloud-like)	0	+++	+++	0
Hyperlobation (staghorn-like)	+++	0	0	+++
Dense clusters	0	+++	+++	0
Maturation defects	0	+++	+++	0
Neutrophil granulopoiesis				
Increased quantity	0	+++	+++	+++
Erythropoiesis				
Increased quantity	0	0	0	+++
Fibers (reticulin)	0	0	+++	[a]

Incidence of features that are detectable in bone marrow biopsies in these patients: 0, ≤ 10%; +++, ≥ 80%.
[a] In PV, between 10% and 20% of initial bone marrow biopsies reveal an increase in reticulin fibers.

the ideal approach to this problem is the combination with clinical and, if possible, molecular biological findings such as JAK2V617F.

CLINICOPATHOLOGICAL CORRELATIONS

Unfortunately, until now, relationships between hematological and morphological data, risk groups and disease evolution, the effects of therapy on disease evolution as opposed to the natural course of the disease, disease- or therapy-related complications, and various prospective factors have been evaluated mainly by observational and retrospective studies that included multiple sequential BM biopsies. It is reasonable to assume that these investigations may substitute, to a large extent, for the deficiency of randomized prospective clinical trials that often lacked systematically performed BM examinations.

Prodromal Stages

In the case of prodromal stages, scant knowledge has been gathered in the past decade, especially in PV (12,14,29,94,95) and PMF (57,59,74,77,78). Within this scenario of precursor manifestations, early-stage ET should be also mentioned. In these patients with platelet counts lower than those required to fulfill the diagnostic criteria of the PVSG (42) or the WHO (54) classifications, relevant complications

Table 5 Clinical Findings at Presentation of 68 Patients (37 Male, 31 Female; Median Age 53/64 Years) with Sustained or Gradually Increasing Borderline to Mild Erythrocytosis (17–18.5 g/dL in Men/15–16.5 g/dL in Women)

	Mean ± STD
Hemoglobin (g/dL)	
men	18.2 ± 1.2
women	17.4 ± 2.5
Leukocytes ($\times 10^9$/L)	14.1 ± 8.9
Thrombocytes ($\times 10^9$/L)	524 ± 290
LAP score	176 ± 110
LDH (U/L)	340 ± 203
Palpable spleen (cm below costal margin)	2.1 ± 2.9
Erythropoietin level ($\leq$ 8 U/L)	92%
Thrombocyte count[a] ($> 600 \times 10^9$/L)	52%

All patients developed overt polycythemic PV about 6 months to 2 years later.
[a]These 35 patients were, at the beginning, clinically mimicking ET according to the PVSG criteria (42).

have been described to occur (28,96–99). In a cohort of patients with prodromal stages of PV that eventually evolved to overt disease but did not fulfill the required diagnostic criteria at the beginning (Table 5), about 50% would have been initially diagnosed as ET according to the PVSG criteria (42). It has been long noted that when BM fiber content increases to a relevant degree in quantity and modifies its quality (reticulin fibrosis and/or collagen fibrosis), the phenomenon is normally associated with relevant hematological abnormalities (100), as is typically seen in fibrotic-stage PMF (101). To postulate a precursor stage of PMF poses some difficulties because until now, this entity has been diagnosed based on the presenting findings of the so-called myeloid metaplasia, that is, an abnormal extramedullary localization of clonally transformed (neoplastic) hematopoietic cells (64–67).

It should not be overlooked that a concern has been expressed regarding the use of the term prefibrotic-stage PMF (in the majority of cases instead of ET), since it was argued that this diagnosis is prone to instill considerable fear in the patients, since PMF means a life-threatening disease with a survival ranging between 5 and 7 years (66,67). However, the latter is true only for the grossly fibrotic stages of the disease. Similar to a diagnosis of carcinoma in situ of the uterine cervix or of a variety of mucosal layers, the clinicians should inform their patients that this is a prodromal condition characterized by an unpredictable progression that usually takes a considerable amount of time (69,102,103). A stepwise evolution of the prefibrotic disease that is accompanied by abnormal hematological data nevertheless is experienced by many of these patients. These prodromal, prefibrotic stages usually do not display the classical clinical features

Table 6 Clinical Data Associated with Stage of Disease (Prefibrotic versus Overt Fibrotic) in PMF (see Table 2)

	Prefibrotic PMF (fiber score 0 and 1)	Overt fibrotic PMF (fiber score 2 and 3)
No. of patients	470	242
Hemoglobin (g/dL)		
Men	13.7 ± 2.5	11.6 ± 2.7
Women	13.1 ± 2.1	11.4 ± 2.5
Leukocytes ($\times 10^9$/L)	13.2 ± 9.2	13.8 ± 12.3
Thrombocytes ($\times 10^9$/L)	984 ± 575[a]	582 ± 421
LDH (U/L)	338 ± 374	559 ± 380
Spleen size (cm below costal margin)	1.2 ± 2.1	4.1 ± 4.7
Peripheral myeloblasts (%)	0.6 ± 0.3	0.9 ± 2.4
Peripheral erythroblasts (%)	0.1 ± 1.2	1.8 ± 5.2

[a] About 80% of this cohort reveal a platelet count in excess of 600×10^9/L and therefore may mimick ET when considering the relevant PVSG criteria (42).

of extramedullary hematopoiesis (Table 6) consistent with MMM, but frequently an elevated platelet count that may be easily confused with ET when applying the PVSG criteria (39,42,48).

Dynamics of Myelofibrosis and Therapeutic Effects

In case of myelofibrosis in MPNs, one has to clearly differentiate between the histological finding of an increase in the fiber content beyond normal (reticulin and/or collagen) and the clinical signs and symptoms of myeloid metaplasia, as shown for PMF in Figure 2. The latter includes the phenotypic manifestations of a leukoerythroblastic reaction and the presence of circulating teardrop cells in the peripheral blood smear seen in association with significant splenomegaly and anemia.

Controversial issues have been recorded concerning the progression of myelofibrosis in cases of PV. Only a few reports have attempted to assess the frequency of this phenomenon by comparing the results of the repeatedly performed trephine biopsies (16,24,26). When evaluating the dynamics of myelofibrosis in PV, it needs to be stressed that about 10–20% of patients are already present with a mild to moderate degree of (reticulin) fibrosis at onset (24,29,43,44). The development of marked (collagen) myelofibrosis was found to occur in less than 20% of patients and seems to be a very slowly advancing process compared to the relatively early development seen in PMF, but which still clearly exceeded in speed the myelofibrotic progression seen (rarely) in ET (Table 7) (16,24,43). Myelofibrosis and therefore post-PV secondary MF (73) displays not only a strong time-related correlation, but also unfortunately a positive relationship to prior treatments with cytostatic therapy (9,18,19,104,105). On the other

Table 7 Dynamics (Relative Incidence) of Myelofibrosis (MF), According to Grading of Reticulin and/or Collagen (45), in Sequential Trephine Biopsies (Intervals Ranging Between 3 and 5 Years) in about 500 Patients with Ph[1−] MPNs[a]

	\multicolumn{4}{c}{Grading of myelofibrosis}			
	MF-0	MF-1	MF-2	MF-3
PV	48% (stable)	12% (progression)	23% (progression)	17% (progression)
ET	96% (stable)	4% (progression)		
PMF				
stage				
0	10% (stable)	42% (progression)	20% (progression)	28% (progression)
1	5% (regression)	31% (stable)	32% (progression)	32% (progression)
2		9% (regression)	41% (stable)	50% (progression)

[a]For comparison, see Table 2.

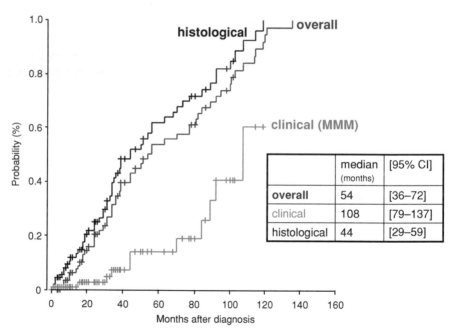

Figure 2 Risk of progression into myelofibrosis in initial/early-stage PMF (180 patients) with discrimination between histopathology (increase at least one grade; Table 2) and clinical findings of extramedullary hematopoiesis (MMM).

hand, acute leukemic transformation, a condition associated with excess of blasts in the BM, is a relatively rare event, according to sequential BM examinations, accounting for less than 10% (24,69,78). Recently published data emphasize the low risk of leukemic transformation in these patients with a 15-year risk rate of only 7% (19).

Unfortunately, many ET studies regarding disease progression and the development of relevant complications do not include a follow-up inclusion of repeatedly performed BM biopsy examinations. Moreover, it has to be taken into account that ET diagnosed according to the PVSG (42,51), as opposed to ET of the WHO classification (54), implies significantly more adverse events in the former (PVSG defined ET) than in the latter (WHO defined ET), in particular regarding complications such as fibrosis, therapeutic strategies, and the outcome (24,44,48,57,58). This is because, as outlined before, only a fraction of the PVSG ET cases (approximately 30–50%, depending on risk group) may be regarded as "true" ET (39,46, 48–50,54). For this reason, the relevant data reported for so-called PVSG ET have to be discussed very critically. In a retrospective cohort of 195 ET patients, evolution into overt myelofibrosis (i.e., AMM/MMM) occurred in 13 cases (6.7%) after a median of 8 years from diagnosis (106). A significant shortcoming of this study is the lack of clear-cut data concerning the systematic evaluation of BM biopsies at onset, and it seems likely that sequential trephines were performed only when patients already developed signs and symptoms of AMM/MMM (106). The risk of overt fibrosis and of blast crisis is extremely low in ET. When initial/early PMF is explicitly excluded, an increase in reticulin according to histopathology and a very rarely development of advanced myelofibrosis or MMM (Table 7) was found in less than 4% after a mean observation time of more than 3 years (24,44,57,58). In cases diagnosed according to the PVSG criteria (42), blastic crises, including transformation into acute megakaryocytic leukemia, were reported in 3–7% of patients with ET (107). In contrast, follow-up studies based on sequential examinations of BM biopsies have found that a significant increase in blasts (more than 30%) is an extremely rare event in true ET (24,26). These strikingly expressed discrepancies of myelofibrotic and blastic transformations are in keeping with the assumption that the cohort of patients diagnosed according to the PVSG criteria (42) also included a group having PMF with a high platelet count (48), which have a higher risk for these complications (Table 6).

Keeping in consideration the above-mentioned discrepancies between the two classification systems used to diagnose ET (48), the results of the UK-PT1 trial (108) on hydroxyurea (HU) versus anagrelide therapy in patients with ET, at a high risk for vascular events (age at least 60 years, current or previous platelet counts of $1,000 \times 10^9$/L or more, a history of ischemia, thrombosis, embolism, or hemorrhage), should be read carefully. In this randomized prospective study, overt myelofibrotic transformation (i.e., MMM) occurred after 39 months with an overall incidence of 2.6%, but significant differences between both treatment groups were reported. As a consequence of these data, the higher risk of myelofibrosis in the anagrelide group (3.95%) was attributed to a treatment effect (108). However, several important limitations impair the general validity of these observations (109,110). First of all, the prior cytoreductive treatment received by one-third of the patients probably precluded the evaluation of an "untreated" BM biopsy sample at the time of study enrollment (108). Moreover, there is no information about the incidence of nonrepresentative or unclassifiable BM biopsy specimens

Table 8   Risk of Myelofibrotic Transformation within 36 Months of Follow-Up in 539 High-Risk ET Patients Classified According to PVSG (42, 108) Compared to the WHO (54) Guidelines

Incidence of myelofibrotic transformation	PVSG ET	WHO classification	
		ET	Prefibrotic/early PMF
According to clinical definition			
%	2.2	0	2.8
95% CI			1.2–4.4
According to increase in bone marrow fibers[a]			
%	10.8	0	13.6
95% CI			10.3–16.7
Overall incidence			
%	2.8	0	3.5[b]
95% CI			1.8–5.2

[a]Manifest myelofibrosis (at least grade 2) or increase in one grade in less than 12 months of follow-up.
[b]$p = 0.002$ (two-sided exact significance) for ET versus prefibrotic/early stages of PMF according to WHO.
Abbreviation: CI, confidence interval.

at study entry or during follow-up of the patients, and no exact data are available about the time that had elapsed between original clinical diagnosis and study entry BM examination. Most of all, repeatedly performed BM biopsies were available in only 12 of the 21 cases with reported progression (108), and thus, myelofibrosis was assessed mainly by clinical diagnosis following the modified Italian criteria consistent with MMM (65,111). Because the rate of myelofibrotic transformation seemed to be relatively high in relation to the short-termed end point (39 months), particularly in the anagrelide group, we tried to verify these data by performing a multicenter study on 539 cases with high-risk ET in explicit accordance with the diagnostic requirements of the UK-PT1 trial (108). The latter was specifically concerned with the histopathological definition of manifest myelofibrosis (at least grade 2) (45) or increase in one grade in less than 12 months of follow-up (108). According to our data, when applying the PVSG guidelines (42), the overall incidence of myelofibrotic transformation after 36 months of follow-up examination was 2.8% (Table 8). It is noteworthy that, as already mentioned (Fig. 2), histological assessment of fiber increase (45) versus clinical definition of myelofibrosis exhibited disparate probabilities (10.8% vs. 2.2%). In significant contrast, when applying the WHO classification (20,54,110) on this cohort, there was no transformation into myelofibrosis either by clinical or morphological standards in (true) ET opposed to early-stage PMF (Table 8). In this context, it has to be emphasized that PMF with accompanying thrombocytosis (Table 6) was characterized by an enhanced probability to develop this complication, including MMM (Table 7).

Further statistical analysis of the data proved that the reported higher risk of myelofibrotic transformation seen in ET in the anagrelide group of the UK-PT1 trial (108) is not related to treatment effects, but rather to the already indicated heterogeneity of disease entities (Table 8) included in that study. In particular, when comparing the relative risks and odds ratios (112) for myelofibrotic progression between the UK-PT1 trial results and our own data, significant differences could be observed. The mean odds ratio for progression in the UK-PT1 trial (113) was 3.20 with a confidence interval ranging between 1.18 and 9.01, contrasting the Cologne data that discriminated and compared true ET (54,110) with prefibrotic early PMF (39,48–50). The latter evaluation showed a mean odds ratio of 4.03 and a significant higher variability of the confidence interval from 0.53 up to 30.24. Based on these results, it can be derived that overall randomization in the UK-PT1 trial does not overrule the effect of disease heterogeneity, that is, the underlying, significantly different myelofibrotic progression rates of true ET versus PMF with associated thrombocytosis (false ET). These findings are generally in keeping with the results of other studies. The latter report that the development of gross myelofibrosis or MMM according to clinical definition (65,111) after only a few years of follow-up was predominately detectable in patients with early to more advanced stages of PMF mimicking ET at onset (38,39,67,69).

In case of thromboreductive therapy in ET, anagrelide was shown to exert an inhibitory effect on the endoreduplicative activity of megakaryopoiesis with an arrest of maturation at lower ploidy levels, resulting in a predominance of immature megakaryocytes incapable of shedding platelets (114–118). Although a platelet-lowering effect may also be achieved by HU treatment, a comparative study on BM features between anagrelide and the latter agent revealed that both drugs generate a left-shifted megakaryopoiesis. A comparative study between anagrelide and hydroxyurea (HU), which is also effective at causing thromboreduction, showed that both drugs are capable of causing left-shifted megakaryopoiesis in the BM. However, HU causes more conspicuous maturation defects comparable to severe dysplastic changes (119), a finding that supports concerns about a possible leukemogenic potential of this drug (120–122).

In PMF, sequentially performed BM biopsy examinations within a long-term period of follow-up have proved to be essential in confirming the notion of a stepwise histopathological disease progression that parallels the worsening clinical parameters (57,68,77,78). In all studies, however, speed of progression was not predictable, particularly in the early stages, which revealed a wide range of results (Table 7). As already mentioned, concerning prodromal stages of PMF, one has to distinguish clearly between the histological features of (reticulin/collagen) fiber increase of one grade in the BM (45) and the clinical phenotype of MMM (66,111). These important differences for the understanding of the evolution of the disease process (69) are shown in Figure 2.

In a recently published review on MPNs, which is primarily based on a molecular genetic classification (*JAK2V617F*), prodromal stages of PMF are unfortunately not taken into account (1). According to this classification for

JAK2-positive and JAK2-negative myelofibrosis, "reticulin" fibrosis grade 3 or higher (on a 0–4 graded scale) (91), that is, overt collagen fibrosis, is required to establish the diagnosis. Thus, the authors' approach (1) still follows the diagnostic guidelines of the PVSG (42,48). Consequently, the ET category probably incorporates a large fraction of early-stage PMF patients who presented with thrombocytosis (see also Table 6) mimicking ET (31,38,69). Since histopathology (except for a significant increase in fibers) is not taken into account by this classification, the proposed approach is therefore of limited value in comparison with the well-established clinicopathological guidelines for the diagnosis of MPNs.

An additional important question is regarding the issue whether cytoreductive therapy (i.e., HU) is effective in decreasing BM fibrosis in PMF patients, particularly in cases previously treated with interferon (IFN). Several clinical trials testing this hypothesis have failed to show any relevant regression of the fiber content in cases of PMF (123,124). This has been further confirmed by follow-up studies based on repeated BM biopsies (77,78,125). Overall, a less than 10% rate of regression (usually only one grade of myelofibrosis; Table 2), mostly without clinical relevance, may be detected (Table 7) (78,126). In contrast, a total regression of myelofibrosis can be achieved only by allogenic, peripheral, hematopoietic stem cell transplantation. In transplanted patients, a significant fibrolytic effect is usually achieved, approximately by 6 months; the amount of osteosclerosis, however, did not change significantly during the same observation period (127,128). Even when using reduced intensity conditioning (low-dose myeloablative pretransplant therapy), (127,129), immunohistochemistry combined with morphometry revealed persistent maturation defects of megakaryocytes (e.g., the presence of dwarf forms with dysplastic aspects in the posttransplant period). These anomalies of megakarypoiesis may be responsible for posttransplantation thrombocytopenia (128). To further compound this issue, even without prior cytoreductive therapy, mild to moderate degrees of myelodysplastic changes may occur in PMF in the natural course of the disease (126). An increased amount of BM dysplasia may occasionally indicate an insidious transition into an accelerated or blastic phase.

Prognosis

In PV, data concerning the life expectancy of patients compared with the general population are limited and somewhat incongruent (130,131). Based on early reports, it was concluded that life expectancy of these patients was not different from that of the general population (131). The relatively short follow-up of the patients in these series, however, may have masked late complications that affect prognosis, such as development of leukemia or myelofibrosis (19,113,132). On the other hand, studies with longer follow-up times, but a small number of patients, have reported a shortened life expectancy (133,134). These observations are supported by our data (103), which disclosed an overall loss of life expectancy of about 20%, with a significantly higher disease impact in older patients. In a recently published study, the overall mortality rate was 2.94 deaths/100 persons per year with a significant impact of age, ranging from 8 years in patients older than 70 years to more than 15 years in younger patients (113). These findings may be explained by the longer follow-up (19,113), which highlights the negative effect of late vascular events and hematologic complications, such as transformation into acute leukemia (132) or progression to post-PV myelofibrosis (16,18). Overall, the median duration of survival is, in general, more than 15 years (18,113,135). According to our own findings (103), men had higher mortality rates than women in each age group. In regard to the cause of death in PV, an excess of lethal vascular complications with an average vascular event/malignancy ratio of 1/0.8 could be calculated (113), whereas patients under 50 years revealed an excess of death from malignancy with a vascular event/malignancy ratio of 1/2.5 (19). In this context, the long-term exposure to myelosuppressive agents could play a causative role in younger patients (105,132,136). Survival of young patients who progress to acute leukemia or post-PV myelofibrosis is similar to that of older patients undergoing the same complication (113).

In ET, diagnosed by the PVSG criteria (42), controversial data have been published in larger series of patients regarding clinical findings in relation to prognosis (99,113,130,131). No significant loss of life expectancy was reported in a Spanish study (131), which is at variance with other trials, such as the one from Olmsted county (130) or from Western Germany (25,45). However, most investigators agree that a history of thrombotic and hemorrhagic events and especially the occurrence of these complications during follow-up have a significant influence on survival (99,113,137,138). For this reason, in ET patients, therapeutic interventions are aimed at the prevention of both thrombosis and hemorrhagic complications, a strategy that has been found to be beneficial for improving survival (109,138,139). In a retrospective evaluation of 162 patients with (true) ET, conforming to the diagnostic guidelines of the WHO (54), loss of life expectancy was not significantly reduced in comparison with the normal population (56). According to our data, however, in patients with ET characterized by a history of thrombotic and/or hemorrhagic episodes, survival is worse in comparison with a low-risk group lacking these complications (103). These patients regularly reveal a significantly higher rate of clinical complications, which is responsible for the overall worsening of prognosis (113). As has been extensively discussed before, there are significant differences in the PVSG versus the WHO classification system concerning the diagnosis of ET (48). To elucidate the diagnostic power of the WHO concept, we reevaluated 476 patients who were initially classified as ET in accordance with the PVSG (42). The patients were followed for 3.782 person-years (median 8 years). According to the PVSG criteria, a median observed survival of 13.7 years and a 15-year relative (age-adjusted) survival rate of 74.9% (Table 9) could be calculated. On the other hand, classification by the WHO criteria (54), implying an inclusion of BM morphology at onset, allowed a discrimination into three groups with significantly different survival patterns: true ET with a 15-year age-adjusted relative survival rate of 83.9%, and contrasting prefibrotic (PMF-0), and early (PMF-1) stages of myelofibrosis with a 15-year survival of only 67.9%

Table 9 Observed and Relative (Age-Adjusted) Survival Rates in ET Patients
Classified According to PVSG (42) and WHO (54) Guidelines.

	PVSG	WHO classification		
	ET	ET	PMF-0	PMF-1
No. of patients	476	167	174	135
Observed survival (years)				
Median	13.7	16.1	11.9	9.3
95% CI	11.2–16.2	14.7–17.5	10.1–13.8	8.3–10.2
Relative survival rates (%)				
5 years	91.4 ± 4.6	100.0 ± 4.4	92.1 ± 7.1	83.0 ± 9.5
10 years	85.8 ± 6.7	99.1 ± 7.8	80.8 ± 11.7	67.3 ± 17.8
15 years	74.9 ± 14.7	83.9 ± 17.6	67.9 ± 23.7	55.4 ± 29.8

Abbreviations: CI, confidence interval.

and 55.4%, respectively (Table 9). Overall observed and age-adjusted relative
survival rates are shown in Figure 3. It seems reasonable to assume that the well-
known heterogeneity of survival in ET patients classified according to the PVSG
(42) is related to the presence of disease heterogeneity in these cases, with only
a proportion of them representing true ET (35,39). Thus, only by scrupulously
following the WHO guidelines (54) can the initial stages of myelofibrosis be
definitely excluded. These findings have to be emphasized particularly in regard
to therapeutic modalities and risk of leukemic transformation, since significant
different patterns of disease progression have to be expected (110).

In the case of PMF, an extremely heterogeneity of survival patterns has been
reported based on univariate (140–142) and multivariate (102,125,143–150) evaluation methods, which have been used to identify independent prognostic features.
However, the validity of these predictive data has been impaired by relatively small
study populations and different diagnostic criteria for patient enrollment (69). In
particular, patients with other causes of myelofibrosis, that is, post-PV myelofibrosis and acute panmyelosis with myelofibrosis (acute or malignant myelofibrosis)
(140,148,151), were not always strictly excluded. Moreover, only a few series considered the full spectrum of initial prefibrotic and early- to advanced classical disease stages (MMM) into prognostic classification (69,102,144,152). Despite these
inconsistencies, in most study cohorts, degree of anemia (69,102,125,140,144–
146,148–153), age at diagnosis (102,143,144,147–149), occurrence of peripheral
blood precursors (68,125,146,148,149), and platelet, as well as leukocyte, counts
(69,102,125,146,147,150) were found to exert a prognostic impact. Furthermore,
in some series, cytogenetic abnormalities were additional indicators for a worsening of prognosis (154,155).

Regarding the heterogeneity of survival patterns, it is reasonable to assume
that the prognosis of PMF may depend on the stage in which it is first recognized
(69,102). Consequently, early prefibrotic stages show a more favorable outcome

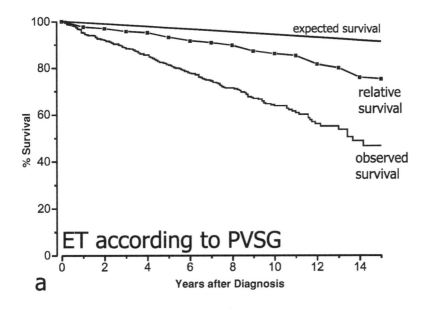

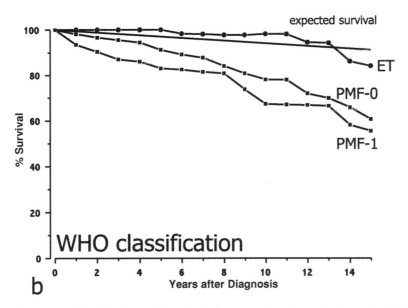

Figure 3 (A), (B): Observed and relative age-adjusted survival rates in ET patients (*n* = 476) classified according to PVSG (42) and WHO (54) criteria. ET shows no significant loss in life expectancy (relative survival) compared with prefibrotic PMF (PMF-0) and early fibrotic PMF (PMF-1) stages (*p* = 0.0001).

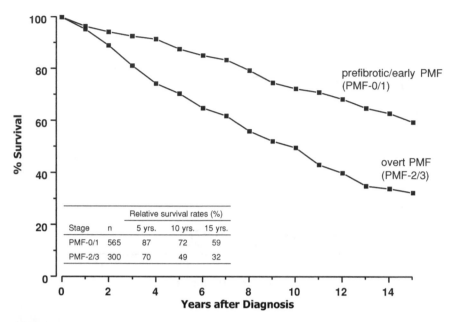

Figure 4 Survival rates according to stage fiber grading (Table 2) of PMF: patients ($n = 459$) with pre- and early-fibrotic stages (PMF-0/1) display significantly higher 5- and 10-year survival rates than the 267 patients with advanced (classical) stages (PMF-2/3) corresponding with MMM/AMM.

than the advanced stages of disease (Fig. 4). However, in multivariate risk classification, the extent of BM fibrosis (45) alone revealed no significant influence on survival (69,102,142–144). Similarly, in early disease stages, application of the well-known Lille score (150), which is based on the presence of two adverse hematological features (hemoglobin < 10g/dL, leukocytes < 4 or > 30 × 10⁹/L), fails to separate the three distinct prognostic groups (69) with low (0 factor), intermediate (1 factor), and high risk (2 factors). It might be speculated that the observed disproportional risk distribution with a proportion of high- and intermediate-risk patients lower than 1% and 12% is related to the fact that in this widely used classification (150), only cases with classical MMM (i.e., advanced stages of disease), were included in the generation of the cut-off values for adverse hematological features (69,102). In consideration of a recently published, multivariate-risk model for PMF (102), a simplified scoring system for stratification of prognosis can be constructed. This includes, as the most important prognostic parameters: age, degree of anemia, and leukocyte and platelet counts. Application of this easily manageable prognostic staging system provides a substantial improvement of prognostic efficiency for all stages of the disease process, in particular for patients in early-phase PMF (69). All these results are in keeping with the assumption that in multivariate-risk calculations, features indicating generalization of disease (i.e., expansion of extramedullary clonally transformed hematopoiesis) have the most important impact on prognosis in PMF (69,102,144).

In conclusion, more and more insight has been gained regarding the issue that the examination of BM specimens not only enhances diagnostic reliability in MPNs, but also elucidates the mutual relationships between clinical data and histopathology as well as the dynamics of the disease process, including pro-dromal stages. In this context, it is important to note that specimen processing and morphological evaluation should be performed by experienced pathologists trained to identify specific constellations of histological patterns that have been proven to exert a discriminatory impact regarding recognition of MPN subtypes. In the era of molecular genetic classification systems (1), it is especially most important to value clinical and morphological parameters that have been shown to exert a predominant impact on achieving a correct diagnosis that is truly predictive of disease prognosis. The latter has been very recently accomplished by a group of international experts (156).

REFERENCES

1. Campbell PJ, Green AR. The myeloproliferative disorders. N Engl J Med 2006;355(23):2452–2466.
2. Wadleigh M, Gilliland GD. The Jak2^{V617F} tyrosine kinase mutation in myeloprolif-erative disorders: Summary of published literature and a perspective. Curr Hematol Malig Rep 2006;1(2):75–80.
3. Tefferi A, Gilliland DG. The JAK2^{V617F} tyrosine kinase mutation in myeloprolifer-ative disorders: status report and immediate implications for disease classification and diagnosis. Mayo Clin Proc 2005;80(7):947–958.
4. Nelson ME, Steensma DP. JAK2 V617F in myeloid disorders: what do we know now, and where are we headed? Leuk Lymphoma 2006;47(2):177–194.
5. Jelinek J, Oki Y, Gharibyan V, et al. JAK2 mutation 1849G>T is rare in acute leukemias but can be found in CMML, Philadelphia chromosome-negative CML, and megakaryocytic leukemia. Blood 2005;106(10):3370–3373.
6. Steensma DP, McClure RF, Karp JE, et al. JAK2 V617F is a rare finding in de novo acute myeloid leukemia, but STAT3 activation is common and remains unexplained. Leukemia 2006;20(6):971–978.
7. Pearson TC. Evaluation of diagnostic criteria in polycythemia vera. Semin Hematol 2001;38(1):21–24.
8. Pierre R, Imbert M, Thiele J, et al. Polycythaemia vera. In: Jaffe ES, Harris NL, Stein H, Vardiman JW eds. WHO Classification of Tumours: Tumours of Haematopoietic and Lymphoid Tissues. Lyon: IARC Press, 2001:32–38.
9. Spivak JL. Polycythemia vera: myths, mechanisms, and management. Blood 2002;100(13):4272–4290.
10. Najean Y, Triebel F, Dresch C. Pure erythrocytosis: reappraisal of a study of 51 cases. Am J Hematol 1981;10(2):129–136.
11. Westwood N, Dudley JM, Sawyer B, et al. Primary polycythaemia: diagnosis by non-conventional positive criteria. Eur J Haematol 1993;51(4):228–232.

12. Thiele J, Kvasnicka HM, Diehl V. Initial (latent) polycythemia vera with thrombocytosis mimicking essential thrombocythemia. Acta Haematol 2005;113(4): 213–219.

13. Messinezy M, Sawyer B, Westwood NB, et al. Idiopathic erythrocytosis—additional new study techniques suggest a heterogeneous group. Eur J Haematol 1994;53(3):163–167.

14. Ruggeri M, Tosetto A, Frezzato M, et al. The rate of progression to polycythemia vera or essential thrombocythemia in patients with erythrocytosis or thrombocytosis. Ann Intern Med 2003;139(6):470–475.

15. Gruppo Italiano Studio Policitemia. Polycythemia vera: the natural history of 1213 patients followed for 20 years. Ann Intern Med 1995;123(9):656–664.

16. Ellis JT, Peterson P, Geller SA, et al. Studies of the bone marrow in polycythemia vera and the evolution of myelofibrosis and second hematologic malignancies. Semin Hematol 1986;23(2):144–155.

17. Najean Y, Dresch C, Rain JD. The very long-term course of polycythaemia: A complement to the previously published data of the Polycythaemia Vera Study Group. Br J Haematol 1994;86(1):233–235.

18. Bilgrami S, Greenberg BR. Polycythemia rubra vera. Semin Oncol 1995;22(4): 307–326.

19. Passamonti F, Malabarba L, Orlandi E, et al. Polycythemia vera in young patients: A study on the long-term risk of thrombosis, myelofibrosis, and leukemia. Haematologica 2003;88(1):13–18.

20. Vardiman JW, Pierre R, Thiele J, et al. Chronic myeloproliferative disorders. In: Jaffe ES, Harris NL, Stein H, Vardiman JW, eds. WHO Classification of Tumours: Tumours of Haematopoietic and Lymphoid Tissues. Lyon: IARC Press, 2001: 16–59.

21. Georgii A, Vykoupil KF, Buhr T, et al. Chronic myeloproliferative disorders in bone marrow biopsies. Pathol Res Pract 1990;186(1):3–27.

22. Bartl R, Frisch B, Wilmanns W. Potential of bone marrow biopsy in chronic myeloproliferative disorders (MPD). Eur J Haematol 1993;50(1):41–52.

23. Dickstein JI, Vardiman JW. Issues in the pathology and diagnosis of the chronic myeloproliferative disorders and the myelodysplastic syndromes. Am J Clin Pathol 1993;99(4):513–525.

24. Georgii A, Buesche G, Kreft A. The histopathology of chronic myeloproliferative diseases. Baillieres Clin Haematol 1998;11(4):721–749.

25. Thiele J, Kvasnicka HM, Fischer R. Histochemistry and morphometry on bone marrow biopsies in chronic myeloproliferative disorders—aids to diagnosis and classification. Ann Hematol 1999;78(11):495–506.

26. Georgii A, Buhr T, Buesche G, et al. Classification and staging of Ph-negative myeloproliferative disorders by histopathology from bone marrow biopsies. Leuk Lymphoma 1996;22:15–29.

27. Thiele J, Kvasnicka HM, Muehlhausen K, et al. Polycythemia rubra vera versus secondary polycythemias. A clinicopathological evaluation of distinctive features in 199 patients. Pathol Res Pract 2001;197(2):77–84.

28. Michiels JJ, Thiele J. Clinical and pathological criteria for the diagnosis of essential thrombocythemia, polycythemia vera, and idiopathic myelofibrosis (agnogenic myeloid metaplasia). Int J Hematol 2002;76(2):133–145.

29. Thiele J, Kvasnicka HM. Diagnostic impact of bone marrow histopathology in polycythemia vera (PV). Histol Histopathol 2005;20(1):317–328.
30. Thiele J, Kvasnicka HM, Diehl V. Bone marrow features of diagnostic impact in erythrocytosis. Ann Hematol 2005;84(6):362–367.
31. Thiele J, Kvasnicka HM. Is it justified to perform a bone marrow biopsy examination in sustained erythrocytosis? Curr Hematol Malig Rep 2006;1(2):87–92.
32. Ellis JT, Silver RT, Coleman M, et al. The bone marrow in polycythemia vera. Semin Hematol 1975;12(4):433–444.
33. Ellis JT, Peterson P. The bone marrow in polycythemia vera. Pathol Annu 1979;14(1):383–403.
34. Thiele J, Kvasnicka HM, Zankovich R, et al. The value of bone marrow histology in differentiating between early-stage polycythemia vera and secondary (reactive) polycythemias. Haematologica 2001;86(4):368–374.
35. Thiele J, Schneider G, Hoeppner B, et al. Histomorphometry of bone marrow biopsies in chronic myeloproliferative disorders with associated thrombocytosis— features of significance for the diagnosis of primary (essential) thrombocythaemia. Virchows Arch A Pathol Anat Histopathol 1988;413(5):407–417.
36. Buhr T, Georgii A, Schuppan O, et al. Histologic findings in bone marrow biopsies of patients with thrombocythemic cell counts. Ann Hematol 1992;64(6): 286–291.
37. Thiele J, Kvasnicka HM, Diehl V, et al. Clinicopathological diagnosis and differential criteria of thrombocythemias in various myeloproliferative disorders by histopathology, histochemistry, and immunostaining from bone marrow biopsies. Leuk Lymphoma 1999;33(3/4):207–218.
38. Thiele J, Kvasnicka HM, Orazi A. Bone marrow histopathology in myeloproliferative disorders—current diagnostic approach. Semin Hematol 2005;42(4): 184–195.
39. Thiele J, Kvasnicka HM. Clinicopathological criteria for differential diagnosis of thrombocythemias in various myeloproliferative disorders. Semin Thromb Hemost 2006;32(3):219–230.
40. Shih LY, Lee CT. Identification of masked polycythemia vera from patients with idiopathic marked thrombocytosis by endogenous erythroid colony assay. Blood 1994;83(3):744–748.
41. Jantunen R, Juvonen E, Ikkala E, et al. Development of erythrocytosis in the course of essential thrombocythemia. Ann Hematol 1999;78(5):219–222.
42. Murphy S, Peterson P, Iland H, et al. Experience of the Polycythemia Vera Study Group with essential thrombocythemia: a final report on diagnostic criteria, survival, and leukemic transition by treatment. Semin Hematol 1997;34(1):29–39.
43. Kreft A, Nolde C, Busche G, et al. Polycythaemia vera: bone marrow histopathology under treatment with interferon, hydroxyurea, and busulphan. Eur J Haematol 2000;64(1):32–41.
44. Buhr T, Georgii A, Choritz H. Myelofibrosis in chronic myeloproliferative disorders. Incidence among subtypes according to the Hannover Classification. Pathol Res Pract 1993;189(2):121–132.
45. Thiele J, Kvasnicka HM, Facchetti F, et al. European consensus for grading of bone marrow fibrosis — and assessment of cellularity. Haematologica 2005;90(8): 1128–1132.

46. Thiele J, Kvasnicka HM. Diagnostic differentiation of essential thrombocythaemia from thrombocythaemias associated with chronic idiopathic myelofibrosis by discriminate analysis of bone marrow features—a clinicopathological study on 272 patients. Histol Histopathol 2003;18(1):93–102.

47. Thiele J, Kvasnicka HM, Zankovich R, et al. Relevance of bone marrow features in the differential diagnosis between essential thrombocythemia and early-stage idiopathic myelofibrosis. Haematologica 2000;85(11):1126–1134.

48. Thiele J, Kvasnicka HM. Chronic myeloproliferative disorders with thrombocythemia: a comparative study of two classification systems (PVSG, WHO) on 839 patients. Ann Hematol 2003;82(3):148–152.

49. Florena AM, Tripodo C, Iannitto E, et al. Value of bone marrow biopsy in the diagnosis of essential thrombocythemia. Haematologica 2004;89(8):911–919.

50. Gianelli U, Vener C, Raviele PR, et al. Essential thrombocythemia or chronic idiopathic myelofibrosis? A single-center study based on hematopoietic bone marrow histology. Leuk Lymphoma 2006;47(9):1774–1781.

51. Pearson TC. Diagnosis and classification of erythrocytoses and thrombocytoses. Baillieres Clin Haematol 1998;11(4):695–720.

52. Tefferi A, Murphy S. Current opinion in essential thrombocythemia: pathogenesis, diagnosis, and management. Blood Rev 2001;15(3):121–131.

53. Murphy S. Diagnostic criteria and prognosis in polycythemia vera and essential thrombocythemia. Semin Hematol 1999;36(1):9–13.

54. Imbert M, Pierre R, Thiele J, et al. Essential thrombocythaemia. In: Jaffe ES, Harris NL, Stein H, Vardiman JW, eds. WHO Classification of Tumours: Tumours of Haematopoietic and Lymphoid Tissues. Lyon: IARC Press, 2001: 39–41.

55. Annaloro C, Lambertenghi Deliliers G, Oriani A, et al. Prognostic significance of bone marrow biopsy in essential thrombocythemia. Haematologica 1999;84(1): 17–21.

56. Thiele J, Kvasnicka HM, Vardiman J. Bone marrow histopathology in the diagnosis of chronic myeloproliferative disorders: a forgotten pearl. Best Pract Res Clin Haematol 2006;19(3):413–437.

57. Kreft A, Buche G, Ghalibafian M, et al. The incidence of myelofibrosis in essential thrombocythaemia, polycythaemia vera, and chronic idiopathic myelofibrosis: a retrospective evaluation of sequential bone marrow biopsies. Acta Haematol 2005;113(2):137–143.

58. Thiele J, Kvasnicka HM, Schmitt-Graeff A, et al. Follow-up examinations including sequential bone marrow biopsies in essential thrombocythemia (ET): A retrospective clinicopathological study of 120 patients. Am J Hematol 2002;70(4): 283–291.

59. Thiele J, Kvasnicka HM, Diehl V. Standardization of bone marrow features—Does it work in hematopathology for histological discrimination of different disease patterns? Histol Histopathol 2005;20(2):633–644.

60. Bock O, Busche G, Koop C, et al. Detection of the single hotspot mutation in the JH2 pseudokinase domain of Janus kinase 2 in bone marrow trephine biopsies derived from chronic myeloproliferative disorders. J Mol Diagn 2006;8(2): 170–177.

61. Kralovics R, Passamonti F, Buser AS, et al. A gain-of-function mutation of JAK2 in myeloproliferative disorders. N Engl J Med 2005;352(17):1779–1790.

62. Wolanskyj AP, Lasho TL, Schwager SM, et al. JAK2 mutation in essential thrombocythaemia: clinical associations and long-term prognostic relevance. Br J Haematol 2005;131(2):208–213.

63. Antonioli E, Guglielmelli P, Pancrazzi A, et al. Clinical implications of the JAK2 V617F mutation in essential thrombocythemia. Leukemia 2005;19(10): 1847–1849.

64. Laszlo J. Myeloproliferative disorders (MPD): myelofibrosis, myelosclerosis, extramedullary hematopoiesis, undifferentiated MPD, and hemorrhagic thrombocythemia. Semin Hematol 1975;12(4):409–432.

65. Barosi G. Myelofibrosis with myeloid metaplasia: diagnostic definition and prognostic classification for clinical studies and treatment guidelines. J Clin Oncol 1999;17(9):2954–2970.

66. Tefferi A. Myelofibrosis with myeloid metaplasia. N Engl J Med 2000;342(17): 1255–1265.

67. Dingli D, Mesa RA, Tefferi A. Myelofibrosis with myeloid metaplasia: new developments in pathogenesis and treatment. Intern Med 2004;43(7):540–547.

68. Thiele J, Zankovich R, Steinberg T, et al. Agnogenic myeloid metaplasia (AMM)—correlation of bone marrow lesions with laboratory data: a longitudinal clinicopathological study on 114 patients. Hematol Oncol 1989;7(5):327–343.

69. Thiele J, Kvasnicka HM. Hematopathologic findings in chronic idiopathic myelofibrosis. Semin Oncol 2005;32(4):380–394.

70. Dickstein JI, Vardiman JW. Hematopathologic findings in the myeloproliferative disorders. Semin Oncol 1995;22(4):355–373.

71. Thiele J, Kvasnicka HM, Boeltken B, et al. Initial (prefibrotic) stages of idiopathic (primary) myelofibrosis (IMF)—a clinicopathological study. Leukemia 1999;13(11):1741–1748.

72. Thiele J, Kvasnicka HM. Prefibrotic chronic idiopathic myelofibrosis—a diagnostic enigma? Acta Haematol 2004;111(3):155–159.

73. Mesa RA, Verstovsek S, Cervantes F, et al. Primary myelofibrosis (PMF), post–polycythemia vera myelofibrosis (post-PV MF), post–essential thrombocythemia myelofibrosis (post-ET MF), blast phase PMF (PMF-BP): Consensus on terminology by the international working group for myelofibrosis research and treatment (IWG-MRT). Leuk Res 2007;31(6):737–740.

74. Thiele J, Imbert M, Pierre R, et al. Chronic idiopathic myelofibrosis. In: Jaffe ES, Harris NL, Stein H, Vardiman JW, eds. WHO Classification of Tumours: Tumours of Haematopoietic and Lymphoid Tissues. Lyon: IARC Press, 2001: 35–38.

75. Thiele J, Kvasnicka HM, Zankovich R, et al. Clinical and morphological criteria for the diagnosis of prefibrotic idiopathic (primary) myelofibrosis. Ann Hematol 2001;80(3):160–165.

76. Thiele J, Hoeppner B, Zankovich R, et al. Histomorphometry of bone marrow biopsies in primary osteomyelofibrosis/sclerosis (agnogenic myeloid metaplasia)—correlations between clinical and morphological features. Virchows Arch A Pathol Anat Histopathol 1989;415(3):191–202.

77. Buhr T, Buesche G, Choritz H, et al. Evolution of myelofibrosis in chronic idiopathic myelofibrosis as evidenced in sequential bone marrow biopsy specimens. Am J Clin Pathol 2003;119(1):152–158.

78. Thiele J, Kvasnicka HM, Schmitt-Gräff A, et al. Dynamics of fibrosis in chronic idiopathic (primary) myelofibrosis during therapy: a follow-up study on 309 patients. Leuk Lymphoma 2003;44(6):549–553.

79. Cervantes F, Barosi G, Demory JL, et al. Myelofibrosis with myeloid metaplasia in young individuals: disease characteristics, prognostic factors, and identification of risk groups. Br J Haematol 1998;102(3):684–690.

80. Thiele J, Rompcik V, Wagner S, et al. Vascular architecture and collagen type IV in primary myelofibrosis and polycythaemia vera: an immunomorphometric study on trephine biopsies of the bone marrow. Br J Haematol 1992;80(2): 227–234.

81. Kvasnicka HM, Thiele J. Bone marrow angiogenesis: methods of quantification and changes evolving in chronic myeloproliferative disorders. Histol Histopathol 2004;19(4):1245–1260.

82. Bock O, Neuse J, Hussein K, et al. Aberrant collagenase expression in chronic idiopathic myelofibrosis is related to the stage of disease but not to the JAK2 mutation status. Am J Pathol 2006;169(2):471–481.

83. Buesche G, Hehlmann R, Hecker H, et al. Marrow fibrosis, indicator of therapy failure in chronic myeloid leukemia—prospective long-term results from a randomized-controlled trial. Leukemia 2003;17(12):2444–2453.

84. Tripodo C, Valenti C, Ballaro B, et al. Megakaryocytic features useful for the diagnosis of myeloproliferative disorders can be obtained by a novel unsupervised software analysis. Histol Histopathol 2006;21(8):813–821.

85. Gruppo RA, Lampkin BC, Granger S. Bone marrow cellularity determination: comparison of the biopsy, aspirate, and buffy coat. Blood 1977;49(1):29–31.

86. Hartsock RJ, Smith EB, Petty CS. Normal variations with aging of the amount of hematopoietic tissue in bone marrow from the anterior iliac crest. A study made from 177 cases of sudden death examined by necropsy. Am J Clin Pathol 1965;43: 326–331.

87. Fong TP, Okafor LA, Schmitz TH, et al. An evaluation of cellularity in various types of bone marrow specimens. Am J Clin Pathol 1979;72(5):812–816.

88. Paul M, Chandy M, Pulimood R, et al. Cellularity of bone marrow—a comparison of trephine biopsies and aspirate smears. Indian J Pathol Microbiol 1989;32(3): 186–189.

89. Thiele J, Kvasnicka HM, Werden C, et al. Idiopathic primary osteo-myelofibrosis: a clinico-pathological study on 208 patients with special emphasis on evolution of disease features, differentiation from essential thrombocythemia, and variables of prognostic impact. Leuk Lymphoma 1996;22(3/4):303–317.

90. Bauermeister DE. Quantitation of bone marrow reticulin—a normal range. Am J Clin Pathol 1971;56(1):24–31.

91. Manoharan A, Horsley R, Pitney WR. The reticulin content of bone marrow in acute leukaemia in adults. Br J Haematol 1979;43(2):185–190.

92. Pasquale D, Chikkappa G. Comparative evaluation of bone marrow aspirate particle smears, biopsy imprints, and biopsy sections. Am J Hematol 1986;22(4):381–389.

93. Beckman EN, Brown AW, Jr. Normal reticulin level in iliac bone marrow. Arch Pathol Lab Med 1990;114(12):1241–1243.

94. Berglund S, Zettervall O. Incidence of polycythemia vera in a defined population. Eur J Haematol 1992;48(1):20–26.

95. Pearson TC, Wetherley-Mein G. The course and complications of idiopathic erythrocytosis. Clin Lab Haematol 1979;1(3):189–196.
96. Michiels JJ, Juvonen E. Proposal for revised diagnostic criteria of essential thrombocythemia and polycythemia vera by the Thrombocythemia Vera Study Group. Semin Thromb Hemost 1997;23(4):339–347.
97. Sacchi S, Vinci G, Gugliotta L, et al. Diagnosis of essential thrombocythemia at platelet counts between 400 and 600 × 10(9)/L. Gruppo Italiano Malattie Mieloproliferative Cronichc(GIMMC). Haematologica 2000;85(5):492–495.
98. Regev A, Stark P, Blickstein D, et al. Thrombotic complications in essential thrombocythemia with relatively low platelet counts. Am J Hematol 1997;56(3): 168–172.
99. Lengfelder E, Hochhaus A, Kronawitter U, et al. Should a platelet limit of 600 × 10(9)/L be used as a diagnostic criterion in essential thrombocythaemia? An analysis of the natural course including early stages. Br J Haematol 1998;100(1): 15–23.
100. Thiele J, Kvasnicka HM. Myelofibrosis in chronic myeloproliferative disorders—dynamics and clinical impact. Histol Histopathol 2006;21(12):1367–1378.
101. Thiele J, Kvasnicka HM. Grade of bone marrow fibrosis is associated with relevant hematological findings—a clinicopathological study on 865 patients with chronic idiopathic myelofibrosis. Ann Hematol 2006;85(4):226–232.
102. Kvasnicka HM, Thiele J, Werden C, et al. Prognostic factors in idiopathic (primary) osteomyelofibrosis. Cancer 1997;80(4):708–719.
103. Kvasnicka HM, Thiele J. The impact of clinicopathological studies on staging and survival in essential thrombocythemia, chronic idiopathic myelofibrosis, and polycythemia rubra vera. Semin Thromb Hemost 2006;32(4):362–371.
104. Najean Y, Rain JD, Billotey C. Epidemiological data in polycythaemia vera: a study of 842 cases. Hematol Cell Ther 1998;40(4):159–165.
105. Finazzi G, Caruso V, Marchioli R, et al. Acute leukemia in polycythemia vera: an analysis of 1638 patients enrolled in a prospective observational study. Blood 2005;105(7):2664–2670.
106. Cervantes F, Alvarez-Larran A, Talarn C, et al. Myelofibrosis with myeloid metaplasia following essential thrombocythaemia: actuarial probability, presenting characteristics, and evolution in a series of 195 patients. Br J Haematol 2002;118(3): 786–790.
107. Radaelli F, Mazza R, Curioni E, et al. Acute megakaryocytic leukemia in essential thrombocythemia: an unusual evolution? Eur J Haematol 2002;69(2): 108–111.
108. Harrison CN, Campbell PJ, Buck G, et al. Hydroxyurea compared with anagrelide in high-risk essential thrombocythemia. N Engl J Med 2005;353(1): 33–45.
109. Barbui T, Finazzi G. When and how to treat essential thrombocythemia. N Engl J Med 2005;353(1):85–86.
110. Thiele J, Kvasnicka HM. A critical reappraisal of the WHO classification of the chronic myeloproliferative disorders. Leuk Lymphoma 2006;47(3):381–396.
111. Barosi G, Ambrosetti A, Finelli C, et al. The Italian Consensus Conference on Diagnostic Criteria for Myelofibrosis with Myeloid Metaplasia. Br J Haematol 1999;104(4):730–737.

112. Bland JM, Altman DG. Statistics notes. The odds ratio. BMJ 2000;320(7247):1468.
113. Passamonti F, Rumi E, Pungolino E, et al. Life expectancy and prognostic factors for survival in patients with polycythemia vera and essential thrombocythemia. Am J Med 2004;117(10):755–761.
114. Solberg LA, Jr., Tefferi A, Oles KJ, et al. The effects of anagrelide on human megakaryocytopoiesis. Br J Haematol 1997;99(1):174–180.
115. Yoon SY, Li CY, Mesa RA, et al. Bone marrow effects of anagrelide therapy in patients with myelofibrosis with myeloid metaplasia. Br J Haematol 1999;106(3):682–688.
116. Tomer A. Effects of anagrelide on in vivo megakaryocyte proliferation and maturation in essential thrombocythemia. Blood 2002;99(5):1602–1609.
117. Mazur EM, Rosmarin AG, Sohl PA, et al. Analysis of the mechanism of anagrelide-induced thrombocytopenia in humans. Blood 1992;79(8):1931–1937.
118. Thiele J, Kvasnicka HM, Fuchs N, et al. Anagrelide-induced bone marrow changes during therapy of chronic myeloproliferative disorders with thrombocytosis. An immunohistochemical and morphometric study of sequential trephine biopsies. Haematologica 2003;88(10):1130–1138.
119. Thiele J, Kvasnicka HM, Ollig S, et al. Anagrelide does not exert a myelodysplastic effect on megakaryopoiesis: a comparative immunohistochemical and morphometric study with hydroxyurea. Histol Histopathol 2005;20(4):1071–1076.
120. Sterkers Y, Preudhomme C, Lai JL, et al. Acute myeloid leukemia and myelodysplastic syndromes following essential thrombocythemia treated with hydroxyurea: high proportion of cases with 17p deletion. Blood 1998;91(2):616–622.
121. Barbui T. The leukemia controversy in myeloproliferative disorders: is it a natural progression of disease, a secondary sequela of therapy, or a combination of both? Semin Hematol 2004;41(2):15–17.
122. Finazzi G, Ruggeri M, Rodeghiero F, et al. Second malignancies in patients with essential thrombocythaemia treated with busulphan and hydroxyurea: long-term follow-up of a randomized clinical trial. Br J Haematol 2000;110(3):577–583.
123. Bachleitner-Hofmann T, Gisslinger H. The role of interferon-alpha in the treatment of idiopathic myelofibrosis. Ann Hematol 1999;78(12):533–538.
124. Sacchi S. The role of alpha-interferon in essential thrombocythaemia, polycythaemia vera, and myelofibrosis with myeloid metaplasia (MMM): a concise update. Leuk Lymphoma 1995;19(1/2):13–20.
125. Visani G, Finelli C, Castelli U, et al. Myelofibrosis with myeloid metaplasia: clinical and haematological parameters predicting survival in a series of 133 patients. Br J Haematol 1990;75(1):4–9.
126. Thiele J, Kvasnicka HM, Schmitt-Graeff A, et al. Bone marrow histopathology following cytoreductive therapy in chronic idiopathic myelofibrosis. Histopathology 2003;43(5):470–479.
127. Rondelli D, Barosi G, Bacigalupo A, et al. Allogeneic hematopoietic stem-cell transplantation with reduced-intensity conditioning in intermediate- or high-risk patients with myelofibrosis with myeloid metaplasia. Blood 2005;105(10): 4115–4119.
128. Thiele J, Kvasnicka HM, Dietrich H, et al. Dynamics of bone marrow changes in patients with chronic idiopathic myelofibrosis following allogeneic stem cell transplantation. Histol Histopathol 2005;20(3):879–889.

129. Kroger N, Zabelina T, Schieder H, et al. Pilot study of reduced-intensity conditioning followed by allogeneic stem cell transplantation from related and unrelated donors in patients with myelofibrosis. Br J Haematol 2005;128(5):690–697.

130. Mesa RA, Silverstein MN, Jacobsen SJ, et al. Population-based incidence and survival figures in essential thrombocythemia and agnogenic myeloid metaplasia: an Olmsted County Study, 1976–1995. Am J Hematol 1999;61(1):10–15.

131. Rozman C, Giralt M, Feliu E, et al. Life expectancy of patients with chronic non-leukemic myeloproliferative disorders. Cancer 1991;67(10):2658–2663.

132. Passamonti F, Rumi E, Arcaini L, et al. Leukemic transformation of polycythemia vera: a single center study of 23 patients. Cancer 2005;104(5):1032–1036.

133. Anger B, Haug U, Seidler R, et al. Polycythemia vera. A clinical study of 141 patients. Blut 1989;59(6):493–500.

134. Ania BJ, Suman VJ, Sobell JL, et al. Trends in the incidence of polycythemia vera among Olmsted County, Minnesota residents, 1935–1989. Am J Hematol 1994;47(2):89–93.

135. Brandt L, Anderson H. Survival and risk of leukaemia in polycythaemia vera and essential thrombocythaemia treated with oral radiophosphorus: are safer drugs available? Eur J Haematol 1995;54(1):21–26.

136. Marchioli R, Finazzi G, Landolfi R, et al. Vascular and neoplastic risk in a large cohort of patients with polycythemia vera. J Clin Oncol 2005;23(10):2224–2232.

137. Michiels JJ. Normal life expectancy and thrombosis-free survival in aspirin treated essential thrombocythemia. Clin Appl Thromb Hemost 1999;5(1):30–36.

138. Barbui T, Barosi G, Grossi A, et al. Practice guidelines for the therapy of essential thrombocythemia. A statement from the Italian Society of Hematology, the Italian Society of Experimental Hematology, and the Italian Group for Bone Marrow Transplantation. Haematologica 2004;89(2):215–232.

139. Barbui T, Finazzi G. Management of essential thrombocythemia. Crit Rev Oncol Hematol 1999;29(3):257–266.

140. Hasselbalch HC. Idiopathic myelofibrosis—an update with particular reference to clinical aspects and prognosis. Int J Clin Lab Res 1993;23(3):124–138.

141. Manoharan A, Smart RC, Pitney WR. Prognostic factors in myelofibrosis. Pathology 1982;14(4):455–461.

142. Anger B, Seidler R, Haug U, et al. Idiopathic myelofibrosis: a retrospective study of 103 patients. Haematologica 1990;75(3):228–234.

143. Varki A, Lottenberg R, Griffith R, et al. The syndrome of idiopathic myelofibrosis. A clinicopathologic review with emphasis on the prognostic variables predicting survival. Medicine (Baltimore) 1983;62(6):353–371.

144. Strasser-Weippl K, Steurer M, Kees M, et al. Age and hemoglobin level emerge as most important clinical prognostic parameters in patients with osteomyelofibrosis: introduction of a simplified prognostic score. Leuk Lymphoma 2006;47(3): 379–380.

145. Rupoli S, Da Lio L, Sisti S, et al. Primary myelofibrosis: a detailed statistical analysis of the clinicopathological variables influencing survival. Ann Hematol 1994;68(4):205–212.

146. Okamura T, Kinukawa N, Niho Y, et al. Primary chronic myelofibrosis: clinical and prognostic evaluation in 336 Japanese patients. Int J Hematol 2001;73(2): 194–198.

147. Reilly JT. Idiopathic myelofibrosis: pathogenesis, natural history, and management. Blood Rev 1997;11(4):233–242.
148. Barosi G, Berzuini C, Liberato LN, et al. A prognostic classification of myelofibrosis with myeloid metaplasia. Br J Haematol 1988;70(4):397–401.
149. Cervantes F, Pereira A, Esteve J, et al. Identification of 'short-lived' and 'long-lived' patients at presentation of idiopathic myelofibrosis. Br J Haematol 1997;97(3): 635–640.
150. Dupriez B, Morel P, Demory JL, et al. Prognostic factors in agnogenic myeloid metaplasia: a report on 195 cases with a new scoring system. Blood 1996;88(3): 1013–1018.
151. Njoku OS, Lewis SM, Catovsky D, et al. Anaemia in myelofibrosis: its value in prognosis. Br J Haematol 1983;54(1):79–89.
152. Kreft A, Weiss M, Wiese B, et al. Chronic idiopathic myelofibrosis: prognostic impact of myelofibrosis and clinical parameters on event-free survival in 122 patients who presented in prefibrotic and fibrotic stages. A retrospective study identifying subgroups of different prognoses by using the RECPAM method. Ann Hematol 2003;82(10):605–611.
153. Ozen S, Ferhanoglu B, Senocak M, et al. Idiopathic myelofibrosis (agnogenic myeloid metaplasia): clinicopathological analysis of 32 patients. Leuk Res 1997; 21(2):125–131.
154. Reilly JT, Snowden JA, Spearing RL, et al. Cytogenetic abnormalities and their prognostic significance in idiopathic myelofibrosis: a study of 106 cases. Br J Haematol 1997;98(1):96–102.
155. Demory JL, Dupriez B, Fenaux P, et al. Cytogenetic studies and their prognostic significance in agnogenic myeloid metaplasia: a report on 47 cases. Blood 1988;72(3):855–859.
156. Tefferi A, Thiele J, Orazi A, et al. Proposals and rationale for revision of the World Health Organization diagnostic criteria for polycythemia vera, essential thrombocythemia, and primary myclofibrosis: recommendations from an ad hoc international expert panel. Blood, epub ahead of print.

3

Conventional and Molecular Cytogenetics of Ph-Negative Chronic Myeloproliferative Disorders

Vesna Najfeld

Departments of Pathology and Medicine, The Mount Sinai School of Medicine, New York, New York, U.S.A.

INTRODUCTION

The Ph-negative myeloproliferative disorders (MPDs) are disorders arising in a single clone of multipotent precursor cells in which one or all myeloid lineages are abnormally amplified. Classic and more frequent Ph-negative MPDs include polycythemia vera (PV), primary myelofibrosis (PMF), and essential thrombocytopenia (ET), while less frequent are neutrophilic leukemia, hypereosinophilic syndrome or chronic eosinophilic leukemia, systemic mast cell proliferations, atypical chronic myelogenous leukemia, and unclassifiable myeloperoliferative disorders. PV is characterized not only by the overproduction of erythrocytes, but also to a varying degree, of granulocytes and platelets; ET, by the overproduction of megakaryocytes and platelets; and PMF, by the presence of extramedulary blast cells and overproduction of fibrotic tissue in the marrow. PV, ET, and PMF have overlapping clinical, biological, and cytogenetic features and a variable tendency to evolve into acute leukemia. Recently, these diseases have also been united by the presence of the same mutation, the constitutively active *JAK2V617F* in 92–97% of patients with PV, and approximately 50% of patients with PMF and ET (1–3).

CONTRIBUTION OF *JAK2V617F* SOMATIC MUTATION TO THE MPD PHENOTYPE

Janus associated kinase 2 (*JAK2*) is a tyrosine kinase located on chromosome 9, band region p24.1 (4). The full gene sequence of *JAK2* spans more than 140kb and contains 25 exons, yielding a transcript of 5.1kb and a protein of 130 kDa. *JAK2* is associated with cytokine receptors that lack kinase domain, such as interleukins, GM-CSF, stem cell factor, erythropoietin, and thrombopoietin, and is responsible for trans-autophosphorylation. Once *JAK2* is phosphorylated, it phosphorylates the recruited signal transducers and activators of transcription (STATs), then the STATs are released, after which they dimerize and translocate to the nucleus where they activate transcription of their target genes (5,6). Several lines of evidence indicate that the *JAK2V617F* somatic mutation is an important genetic contributor to the Ph-negative MPD phenotype. First, an acquired somatic mutation in the *JAK2* gene results in a valine to phenylalanine substitution at position 617 (*JAK2V617F*) in exon 14 and is responsible for the MPD phenotype in more than 90% of the patients with PV, more than 50% with ET, and more than 50% with PMF (7). The mutation occurs in the tyrosine kinase autoregulatory JH2 domain, causing the loss of the inhibitory effect of the JH2 domain of the kinase activity, resulting in the constitutive activation of *JAK2* and downstream signaling molecules such as STAT and ERK (8,9). Second, the V617F mutation is present in a multipotent progenitor cell committed to granulocytic, erythroid (3), and lymphoid (both T and B) (10) differentiation, consistent with the notion that Ph-negative, *JAK2V617F*-positive MPDs originate in an early stem cell capable of differentiating into both myeloid and lymphoid lineages. Third, erythroid progenitor cells harboring the *JAK2V617F* mutation are capable of forming erythropoietin-independent erythroid colonies, the hallmark of PV (1). Fourth, and probably the most important evidence, is that *JAK2V617* mutant cells when transfected into murine bone marrow cells, produce erythrocytosis, and subsequent myelofibrosis in the recipient animals (1,11,12), suggesting a putative causal role for the mutation.

MODERN CYTOGENETICS METHODS

Despite technological advances, the cytogenetics analysis of bone marrow cells from patients with Ph-negative MPDs, other than chronic myelogenous leukemia (CML), remains a laborious and time-consuming process. It requires highly skilled and trained observers to interpret "fuzzy" looking chromosomes, which may have suboptimal morphology and/or banding, in order to detect microdeletions and translocations. In addition, between 5% and 20% of marrow samples may have either a low mitotic yield or are otherwise uninformative due to "dry tap" or poor specimen collection (13).

Currently used conventional and molecular cytogenetics methods for the detection of chromosomal and genetic lesions include: G-banding of metaphase chromosomes, interphase fluorescence in situ hybridization (FISH), hypermetaphase FISH, fiber FISH, multicolor karyotyping with 24 different colors, comparative genomic hybridization (CGH), and array CGH. The goal of these modern cytogenetics methods is an increase in the resolution at which chromosomal rearrangements can be identified. While in conventional cytogenetics the target is a whole chromosome in a metaphase spread at the resolution of $\sim$ 5 Mb, the molecular cytogenetic methods may utilize analysis of interphase nuclei at the resolution of 50 kb to 2 Mb, or fiber-FISH analysis of chromatin strands at the 5- to 500-kb resolution. Moreover, the current resolution of array CGH is restricted only by the clone size and by the density of clones on the array, some of which may contain a resolution at the level of a single nucleotide. The use of a single cytogenetic method for detection of the underlying genomic defect(s) in Ph-negative MPDs is not adequate anymore because detailed analysis requires multiple methods to identify genetic and epigenetic mechanisms in disease processes.

BONE MARROW VERSUS PERIPHERAL BLOOD

In contrast to the *BCR-ABL* fusion–positive CML, which shows a very tight correlation between *BCR-ABL* fusion–positive interphase cells in the bone marrow and peripheral blood cells at diagnosis (14), such studies are difficult to conduct in Ph-negative MPDs for the following four reasons: (1) there is a great diversity of chromosomal abnormalities and for some chromosomal rearrangements, commercial probes are not available; (2) MPD-derived peripheral blood (PB) granulocytes, similar to Ph-positive CML, do not divide spontaneously in peripheral blood (exceptions are CD34-positive myelofibrosis–derived cells); (3) the abnormal MPD clone may be present in the bone marrow at the very low frequency but not in PB granulocytes; and (4) del(20q)-bearing cells represent a subclone that is only retained in bone marrow and not present in clonal peripheral blood granulocytes (15), providing evidence that blood granulocytes are not a reliable surrogate for bone marrow in detecting karyotype abnormalities of myeloid cells using conventional cytogenetics methods.

CHROMOSOME ABNORMALITIES AT DIAGNOSIS

By using conventional cytogenetics for the diagnosis of over 600 patients with PV, 1000 patients with PMF, and over 300 patients with ET, chromosome abnormalities are detected at the rate of 20–25%, 45–50%, and 8%, respectively (Table 1). In the Mount Sinai series of 333 patients with PV that were evaluated between 1984 and 2007, an abnormal karyotype was detected at diagnosis in 25.5% of the patients [(16) and unpublished updated observations]. With the addition of the more sensitive FISH technology, the frequency of the five most recurrent chromosomal abnormalities may be increased to 29% in bone marrow specimens (16) and become detectable in 23% of peripheral blood granulocyte samples (17). Similar chromosomal abnormalities are found in all Ph-negative MPDs; however, their frequencies differ in each of these disorders (Fig. 1). Based on the published cytogenetics results on over 2000 patients, it may be said that the current unifying concept of genetic instability in the Ph-negative MPDs is a loss or gain of the genetic material.

Table 1 Number and Frequency of Abnormal Karyotype in PV, PMF, and ET

| Disorder | No. of patients | Abnormal | | References |
		Karyotype no. (%)	FISH mean (%)	
PV	631	130 (20.6)	23.2	16,17,20,45,77,81,82,83
IMF	1,030	458 (44)	45.3	22,33,37,38,46,54,58,77,83,84,85
ET	338	27 (8)	12	48,77,82,83,86

Chromosomal/FISH Abnormality	PV	PMF	ET
		% Abnormal	
+1q	4–6	7–19	16
del(5)(q21q34)	7–10	4–5	1–2
del(7)(7q31)	3–9	5–15	?
+8	13–20	11–15	15
+9/+i(9)(p10) (P21=red)	16–27	13–21	~1
12q translocations	rare	6–15	rare
del(13)(q31)/ del(D13S319 (red) and del(LAMP1) (aqua)	5–13	13–42	10
del(20)(q11q13)	16–25	6–20	30

Figure 1 Type and frequency of chromosomal abnormalities in PV, PMF, and ET. (The frequency data were compiled from references shown in Table 1.)

The most frequent anomaly in PV is the gain of the short arms of chromosome 9 present in the Mount Sinai series of 333 patients in 27% of the abnormal cases. This may be an underestimation as many complex translocations, when reevaluated with FISH, may include part of the short arms of chromosome 9 (see later in the chapter). On the other hand, del(13q) is rarely present in PV but is present in over 30% of the patients with PMF and an abnormal karyotype (18). Both the presence of an abnormal karyotype and *JAK2V617F* mutation is a poor prognostic indicator in PMF (19), but is not yet known for PV and ET.

TRISOMY 9 AND GAIN OF 9p

The initial observation in 1988 (20) that chromosome 9 anomaly (Fig. 1) is the most frequent in PV was not only confirmed with molecular cytogenetics methods in 2002 (16), but it turns out to be a very important and insightful observation for three reasons. First, trisomy of chromosome 9 and gain of the short arms of chromosome 9 as a result of either partial deletion, unbalanced translocations, or through the formation of isochromosome of the 9p (resulting in tetrasomy 9p) was not only the most frequent in our series, but the addition of FISH method resulted in 50% of the abnormal PV patients showing 9p abnormalities (16). Preliminary array CGH results confirmed that the gain of 9p is the most frequent chromosomal gain in PV [(21), see later]. Moreover, using the CGH method, a gain of 9p was also reported to occur in 48% of the 25 patients with PMF (22). Different chromosomal rearrangements may contribute to trisomy, tetrasomy, or amplification of 9p, as shown in Table 2, of which unbalanced der(9)t(1;9), resulting in trisomy of both 1q and 9p, appears to be the most frequent and relatively specific for PV with at least 15 reported cases (16,23,24). Detailed FISH analysis demonstrated that der(9)t(1;9) is generated by heterochromatic juxtaposition of the satellite II family of 1q to the satellite III family of 9q, thus providing preliminary evidence that heterochromatin recombinations may favor a gene dosage effect (23). The prognostic clinical value of +9/+9p is still elusive but appears to occur exclusively in *JAK2V617F*-positive patients (Table 3). Second, duplication, triplication, or amplification of the mutated *JAK2* allele on 9p24.1 chromosomal region as a result of +9/+9p may have an increased level of constitutive signaling (1) (Fig. 2). Third, loss of 9p heterozygosity has been detected in 30% of the PV patients as a result of uniparental disomy (25).

REARRANGEMENTS OF *JAK2*

JAK2 has been shown to form fusion proteins with three different genes: *TEL/ETV6* (26), *BCR* (27), and *PCM1* (28) in atypical Ph-negative MPDs and lymphoid neoplasms (29). We therefore hypothesized that patients with 9p24 chromosomal abnormalities may have additional *JAK2* structural rearrangements. Consequently, we retrospectively investigated, using highly sensitive FISH technology, whether patients with 9p24 chromosomal abnormalities showed *JAK2* rearrangements.

Table 2   Recurrent Chromosome 9 Abnormalities
Resulting in Trisomy or Tetrasomy of Chromosome
9 Short Arms (9p in Ph-negative MPD)

Chromosomal abnormality	No. of 9p copies
trisomy 9	3
+ del(9q)	3
+der(9)t(1;9)(q12;q10)	3
i(9p)(p10)	4
i(9p)(p10),i(9q)(q10)	2[a]
der(13)t(9;13)(p12;p11)	3
der(15)(p13;p13)	4
der(9;18)(p10;q10)	3
der(9;21)t(9;21)(p13;p13)	4
9p amplification	3–20

[a]Rearranged 9p.

Table 3   Cytogenetics Abnormalities in V617F[+]
and V617F[-] patients with Ph-negative MPD[a]

	V617F[+]	V617F[-]
del(20q) total	46	3
PV	30	2
IMF	10	1
ET	6	0
del(13q) total	3	9
IMF	2	9
ET	1	0
Translocations total	3	10
IMF	2	5
ET	1	5
Trisomy 9 total	15	0
PV	7	0
IMF	3	0
ET	5	0
trisomy 8 total	6	2
PV	3	0
IMF	2	1
ET	1	1
−5/del(5q) total	2	1
ET	2	1
Total	75	25

[a]Compiled data from Refs. 75 and 77.

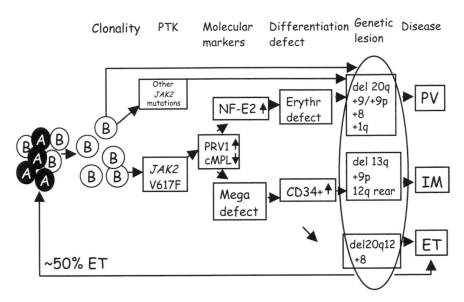

Figure 2 Hypothetical multistep pathogenesis of Ph-negative MPDs. Current understanding of the pathogenesis of Ph-negative MPDs might be explained by this model whereby the majority of PV patients and 50% of PMF and ET patients have clonal origin of the disease, JAK2V167F mutation, and chromosomal rearrangements. Approximately 50% of the patients may have other *JAK2* mutations and/or rearrangements as well as recurrent chromosomal abnormalities. The model will not explain rare patients without *JAK2* rearrangement and normal karyotype.

JAK2 FISH studies of PV patients with normal karyotype and PMF patients with an abnormal karyotype [del(20q) and del(13q)] did not show any *JAK2* rearrangements. In contrast, PV patients that exhibited chromosome 9p abnormalities showed a high affinity, 87%, for the gain of *JAK2* (30). We also identified *JAK2* rearrangements with chromosome 12 in 3 patients with the following results: A novel *JAK2-NF-E2* fusion was observed in the first patient; a previously described *JAK2-ETV16* fusion was confirmed in the second patient; and a chromosomal exchange between *JAK2* and *NF-E2* was identified in the third patient. These preliminary studies provide additional support that *JAK2* rearrangements, other than the *JAK2V617F* somatic mutation, may contribute to the MPD, myelodysplastic (MDS), as well as to the lymphoid leukemic phenotype.

DELETION 20q12

Until 1992, the majority of cytogenetics studies described del(20q) as a terminal deletion with the breakpoint at q11 band region. Subsequent FISH mapping studies demonstrated that del(20q) represents an interstitial deletion, and molecular heterogeneity of the breakpoint sites was established because both centromeric and telomeric breakpoints were observed (31). The more recent fine mappings identify two minimally deleted regions: a 2.7 Mb for the MPD, spanning D20S108 (proximal) and D20S481 (distal), and a 2.6 Mb for other myeloid malignancies spanning R52161 (proximal) and WI-12515 (distal) region (32). There is a common overlapping region of 1.6 kb, and as such, may constitute the major mechanism for the loss of heterozygosity.

Deletion of the long arms of chromosome 20 is a recurrent, nonrandom clonal chromosomal abnormality in Ph-negative MPDs, MDS, and acute myeloid leukemia (AML) (Fig. 1). Among 333 patients with PV studied at Mount Sinai, del(20q) was present in 16% with an abnormal karyotype, but the frequency of up to 30% have been reported (33,34). An interstitial deletion of chromosome 20 is present in all hematopoietic elements, except T cells, consistent with the notion that it has arisen in a pluripotent stem cell. As mentioned above, the presence of del(20q) in bone marrow cells, but not in clonally derived peripheral blood granulocytes (15), is consistent with the current hypothesis that PV, and probably other Ph-negative MPDs, may have a similar multistep pathogenesis (Fig. 2) as has been already established for the Ph-positive, *BCR-ABL* fusion–positive CML as well as for the Ph chromosome–negative CML (35,36). Moreover, this study confirms the previous notion that an interphase-FISH (I-FISH) analysis of peripheral blood may not always reflect the size of the chromosomally abnormal clone present in the bone marrow of patients with Ph-negative MPD.

In myeloproliferative disorders, sole del(20q) does not appear to adversely affect survival (37–39), and in MDS it is associated with favorable outcome (40). I-FISH may greatly enhance the detection of del(20q) in these disorders, up to 24% (38), but the abnormality, at least in PV, may be dormant for many years before del(20q) cells gain a proliferative advantage (16). Molecular cytogenetics utilizing metaphase-FISH (M-FISH), CGH, and genome wide screening, failed to detect cryptic or occult 20q aberrations within the 20q11.2-q13.1 region in 14 patients with PV and a normal karyotype (41). This finding does not exclude the possibility that genetic imbalances, smaller than 5 Mb, may be present in this region of chromosome 20. In treated PV patients, the application of M-FISH may identify rare cryptic translocations involving chromosome 20, such as t(1;20)(p36;q13) and t(18;20)(p11;q13) (42).

Deletion 20q is identified primarily in JAK2V167F-positive patients, but rare PV and ET patients with del(20q) were observed to be JAK2V167F mutation-negative (Table 3), raising the possibility that cooperating genes may be responsible, in some patients, for the Ph-negative MPD phenotype. In a PV and an ET patient, granulocytes with the 20q deletion outnumbered *V617F*-positive granulocytes, suggesting that the del(20q) occurred before the *JAK2* mutation (43), also consistent with the stepwise pathogenesis.

TRISOMY 8

Gain of chromosome 8 is a nonrandom recurrent abnormality in Ph-negative MPD; it is also one of the three most frequent abnormalities in MDS and is present in

10% of the patients with malignant hematopoietic disorders of both myeloid and lymphoid lineages. In PV, trisomy 8 was demonstrated in myeloid cells characterized by CD11c and CD14 but not in lymphoid cells expressing CD33 and CD22 antigens (44). Interestingly, CD34$^+$ cells, which are the precursors of myeloid as well as lymphoid cells, also had trisomy 8. The prognostic significance in PV is unknown but its indolent clinical impact may be evidenced by the observations that some patients with PV have trisomy 8 for over 20 years (45). In contrast, recent evidence suggested that in myelofibrosis, gain of chromosome 8 may be associated with poor prognosis (46). Such a negative prognostic impact of trisomy 8 could not be demonstrated in 107 patients who were retrospectively evaluated using FISH methodology on paraphin-embedded bone marrow sections (38). A unique observation for PV is the simultaneous presence of both +8 and +9. It is very rarely seen in any other hematological malignancies and it is a recurrent finding in PV, with the frequency of approximately 3–4%.

TRISOMY 1q

Duplication of the long arms of chromosome 1 is found in approximately 15% of patients with Ph-negative MPDs and 13% of patients with MDS with an abnormal karyotype (47). The unbalanced translocations resulting in trisomy 1q is demonstrated in 11% of PV, 22% of PMF, and 14% of ET patients and represents the third most frequent abnormality in PV. As mentioned above, der(9)t(1;9)(q12;q10) is relatively specific for PV. While in PMF and ET der(1;7)(p10;p10) is a recurrent anomaly; in ET, it is associated with unfavorable prognosis and leukemic transformation (48). Interestingly, 70% of the patients with myelofibrosis following PV (PPMF) showed trisomy 1q as a result of unbalanced translocations. In all cases, a common trisomic region spanning 1q21q22 to 1q32 has been identified (49). PPMF is considered cytogenetically different from both primary myelofibrosis and PV. It is unclear presently whether trisomy 1q may be a secondary event as a result of disease progression and/or treatment. However, the observations that 85% of the patients had chromosome 1 rearrangements at the presentation of PV and that it was the sole defect in 47% of the patients suggests that genes located in the trisomic region either initiate or contribute toward the pathogenesis of these disorders (47).

DELETION 13q13.3-q14.3

Deletions of 13q are more frequent in PMF (25–30% of abnormal karyotype) (18) than in PV (9–13%), but are also found as recurrent abnormalities in MDS and lymphoid malignancies (different breakpoints). In the Mount Sinai series of 91 patients with PMF, del(13q) was detected in 33% of the 48 PMF patients with an abnormal karyotype (unpublished personal observations). Among the patients with del(13q), 91% have breakpoints in the region of 13q12–14 to q21–22. Fine FISH mapping have defined commonly deleted region to 13q13.3-q14.3 encompassing RB1, D13S319, and D13S25 loci (50). Cryptic 13q deletions do occur, but are rare and are easily identified with the FISH method in both bone marrow and peripheral blood. Trisomy 13 may be a rare, nonrandom abnormality associated with PMF that may be an indicator of an early blast transformation (18). Most of the patients with del(13q) are negative for *JAK2V617F* mutation (Table 3).

MONOSOMY 7 OR DELETION 7q

Monosomy 7 or deletion 7q is cytogenetically detected in 6–8% of the patients with PV and PMF (16,46). They are rarely found in patients with ET. Monosomy or deletion of chromosome 7, together with -5/del(5q), are the most frequent findings in therapy-related MDS or AML as well as frequent observations in de novo MDS and other myeloid malignancies (51). Monosomy 7/del(7q) in PMF is associated with unfavorable prognosis in one study (25 vs. 99 months for patients with normal karyotype, $p < 0.001$) (52), and with leukemic transformation in another study (53). One reported ET patient, with monosomy 7, was negative for *JAK2V617F* mutation.

12q ABNORMALITIES

Balanced translocations of the long arms of chromosome 12 are recurrent in patients with PMF (7–11% among abnormal), rare in patients with PV, and not reported in patients with ET (54). There are at least 15 reported 12q translocations in PMF [t(1;12)(p31;q21) and (p12;q24), t(4;12)(q26;q15) and (q33;q21), t(5;12)(q13;q24) and (p14;q21), t(7;12)(p11;q24), t(8;12)(p23;q21), t(12;13)(q24;q14), t(12;17)(q25;q11), inv(12)(p12q24) and add(12)(q21;q24), t(2;12)(p13;q14), der(12)inv(12)(p12p14)t(10;12)(q24;p13)] implicating 12q13–21 region in the pathogenesis of PMF [(54–59), and author's unpublished observations]. The exact role of 12q rearrangements as a trigger in deregulation of normal hematopoiesis and its prognostic role in PMF remains to be elucidated. One reported patient with t(12;12)(p12;q13) was negative for *JAK2V617F* mutation. As noted above, structural rearrangements between *JAK2* were most frequent with chromosome 12 (30). Teferri (58) identified del(12p) as one of the abnormalities associated with inferior survival, but this observation has not been confirmed by other studies.

RECURRENT BALANCED TRANSLOCATIONS

Rare recurrent balanced abnormalities in atypical Ph-negative MPD are shown in Table 4. They generally involve *PDGFRB* gene at 5q33, *FGFR1* gene on 8p11 (these disorders are referred to as myeloproliferative syndrome or stem cell leukemia syndrome), and *PDGFRA* gene on 4q12. The number of reported cases affecting 5q33, 8p11, and 4q12 chromosomal regions among 18,000 specimens from patients with hematological malignancies, evaluated between 1985 and 2003 at the Mount Sinai Medical Center, is very small and their frequency is approximately between 0.1% and 0.02%. The most frequently reported

Table 4 Chromosomal Translocations in Ph-negative MPD[a]

Chromosomal abnormality	Genes involved	MPD entity
t(9;12)(q34;p13)	*ETV6-ABL*	CML-like, T-ALL
5q33	*PDGFRB*	
t(5;12)(q33;p13)	*ETV6-PDGFRB*	CEL, CMML
t(5;7)(q33;q11)	*HIP1-PDGFRB*	CMML-like
t(5;10)(q33;q21)	*CCDC6-PDGFRB*	Ph-negatibe MPD
t(5;14)(q33;q32)	*KIA1509-PDGFRB*	Atypical MPD
t(5;14)(q33;q32)	*TRIP11-PDGFRB*	AML
t(5;14)(q33;q22)	*NIN-PDGFRB*	Atypical MPD
t(5;15)(q33;q15)	*TP53BP1-PDGFRB*	CEL
t(5;17)(q33;p11)	*SPECC1-PDGFRB*	Juvenile CMML
t(5;17)(q33;p13)	*RABEP1-PDGFRB*	CMML1
8p11	*FGFR1*	CMML
t(8;13)(p11;q12)	*ZNF198-FGFR1*	MPD syndrome, leukemia, lymphoma
t(7;8)(q32;p11)	*TRIM24-FGFR1*	MPD syndrome
t(6;8)(q27;p11)	*FGFR1OP-FGFR1*	Stem cell MPD
ins(12;8)(p11;p11p22)	*FGFR1 OP2-FGFR1*	MPD syndrome
t(8;17)(p11;q11)	*MYO18 A-FGFR1*	MPD syndrome
t(8;22)(p11;q11.2)	*BCR-FGFR1*	Lympho-proliferative disorder
4q12	*PDGFRA*	
del(4)(q12q12)	*FIP1L1-PDGFRA*	CEL
t(4;22)(q12;q11.2)	*BCR-FGFR1*	Atypical CML
4q12	*KIT*	SM
9p24	*JAK2*	
t(9;22)(p24;q11.2)	BCR-*JAK2*	CML-like
t(9;12)(p24;p13)	*JAK2-ETV6*	CML-like
der(9)t(9;12)(p24;q13)	*JAK-NF-E2*	MDS
t(8;9)(p22;p24)	PCM1-*JAK2*	CMPD, AL
der(9;18)t(p13;p11)	Not reported	PV, PV- > IMF
der(9;18)(p10;q10)	Not reported	PV, PV- > IMF, ET- > AML
der(9)t(1;9)(q12;q12)	Not reported	PV, MF
der(1;7)(q10;p10)	Not reported	ET
t(12)(q21 or q21)	Not reported	MF

[a]Slighltly modified from Ref. 63.

are t(5;12)(q33;p13) resulting in *ETV6-PDGFRB* fusion protein (60) and t(8;13) (p11;q12) resulting in the *ZNF198-FGFR1* fusion gene (61). The most specific abnormality is the cryptic deletion on 4q12 as a result of *FIP1L1-PDGFRA* fusion gene detected in 20–50% of the patients with chronic eosinophilic leukemia or hypereosinophilic syndrome (62). Most of these patients have a normal karyotype because the cryptic deletion on 4q12 is only 800 kb in size, but the more sensitive FISH technology will detect the majority of cases with this deletion at diagnosis. The most recent commercially available tricolor FISH probe will not only detect deletion 4q12 as a result of *FIP1L1-PDGFRA*, but will also identify a rare *BCR-PDGFRA* fusion resulting from the t(4;22)(q12;q11.2) rearrangement.

The above-mentioned conventional and molecular cytogenetic results in atypical Ph-negative MPDs as well as the presence of JAK2V617 F mutation in typical Ph-negative MPDs provide support that abnormalities in tyrosine kinase genes are central to the molecular pathogenesis of these disorders (63).

ARRAY STUDIES IN PV

Gene expression profiling as well as array CGH can identify candidate disease-specific gene(s) and molecular signature to aid in the diagnosis in addition to the pathophysiology of disease development. Some glimpses into the genes involved in the pathogenesis of PV were provided by microarray studies on isolated mature granulocytes or isolated CD34$^+$ cells from over 70 PV patients using different platforms (64,65). Although different groups of genes were found upregulated and downregulated, so far the best analysis include nine genes that can distinguish PV patients from normal controls and they include: *RNASE6*, *IRF8*, *MCL1*, *INHBC*, *SNRPE*, *KLF4*, *KLF2*, *ILF2*, *TRGV9*, and *LY86* (66). Many of these genes have functions that support their involvement in the pathogenesis of the disease. In another gene expression profiling of 64 PV patients, two 40-fold overexpression of *NF-E2* gene in PV led to the development of erythropoetin-independent erythroid colonies (67). Interestingly, the *NF-E2* gene is localized on 12q14, and, as mentioned above, 12q12-q21 rearrangements are relatively specific for PMF. The most recent application of high-resolution mapping, by using 250K SNP arrays with an average probe spacing of 12 kb, on 24 patients with PV, ET, and PMF positive for *JAK2V617F* mutation, corroborated previous conventional cytogenetics observations (21). Moreover, the SNP studies confirmed previous chromosomal findings that amplification of 9p in a region harboring the *JAK2* locus along with 17q12.3 were the most common shared alterations in the MPDs while del 20q was only observed in ET patients ($p < 0.05$ vs. PV and PMF). Recurrent large alterations included del(1)(p23.1) (3 of 24 patients), +3 (q21.3-.q22.1) (3 of 24 patients), +9(p24) (6 of 24 patients), +10(q.3-q23.1) (3 of 24 patients), and +11 (p15.p21.3) (4 of 24 patients). SNP analysis of the CD34$^+$ cells from 9 patients with PV positive for *JAK2V617F* mutation demonstrated 21 genes in recurrently amplified chromosomal regions with significantly elevated expression levels, including *NFIB* on 9p24, and 7 genes in recurrently deleted regions had significantly depressed expression level, including *TOP1* on 20q.

JAK2 MUTATION IS NOT THE INITIAL GENETIC EVENT IN THE MOLECULAR PATHOGENESIS OF MPD

Molecular detection of the *JAK2V617F* mutation in patients with clonal hematopoiesis is diagnostic for Ph-negative MPD but will not differentiate between PV, ET, PMF, or rare cases of AML and MDS. There is no doubt that the *JAK2V617F* somatic mutation is a major genetic contributor for the Ph-negative

MPD phenotype. However, in this rapidly evolving field, there are currently six lines of evidence that *JAK2V617F* somatic mutation is neither the initiating event nor the only genetic event resulting in the Ph-negative phenotype. First, there are rare, 3–7%, *JAK2V617F*-negative PV patients as well as ~50% PMF and ET patients that do not harbor JAK2V617 mutation (7). In PMF, bone marrow fibrosis is not part of the malignant clone, consistent with the previous observation that stromal cells and hematopoietic cells were not derived from a common stem cell precursor (68). Patients with JAK2V167F-positive ET never harbor a homozygous mutation, providing evidence that *JAK2*$^+$ patients should be considered as a biological continuum with PV (69). Second, other novel *JAK2* mutations were described in a smaller proportion, ~5–15%, of Ph-negative, *JAK2V617F*-negative MPD patients (70–72). At least one *JAK2* exon 12 mutation, when transfected into a murine model, resulted in a myeloproliferative phenotype, including erythrocytosis (73). Two other mutations, JAK2T7875 N activating mutation resulted in MPD with features of megakaryoblastic leukemia (70) and *JAK2Δ*IREED mutation, involving a 5-amino acid deletion within the JH2 pseudokinase domain, identified in a Down syndrome patient, produced B cell precursor acute lymphoblastic leukemia (73), indicating that other *JAK2* mutations may also contribute to the lymphoid leukemic phenotype. Third, as mentioned above, chromosomal translocations that fuse *JAK2* to another protein (Table 4) are also capable of inducing both myeloproliferative and lymphoid disease (27–29). Fourth, wild-type *JAK2* was identified in EPO-independent erythroid colonies in a proportion of PV patients with clonal hematopoiesis (74). Fifth, transformation of MPD to AML was documented to occur in JAK2V617-negative clone from patients that had *JAK2V617F*-positive disease (75,76). Finally, recurrent chromosomal abnormalities, such as del(20q), trisomy 8, and 12q translocations, were detected in at least 25 patients with PV, ET, and PMF who had *JAK2V617F*-negative disease (75,77) (Table 3). Figure 2 shows a hypothetical model in Ph-negative MPD.

THE ROLE OF MODERN CYTOGENETICS IN THE JAK2V167F ERA

The clinical and experimental results presented here indicate that we are at the threshold of understanding molecular events that lead to the development of these disorders. A specific diagnostic marker, such as *BCR-ABL* fusion, is still elusive for the Ph-negative MPDs. However, conventional chromosomal studies can aid in the diagnosis of patients who are *JAK2*-negative, as recommended by Campbell and Green (78), and may provide clues to the as yet unknown pathogenesis of *JAK2V617F*-negative, Ph-negative–MPD patients. Moreover, International Working Group consensus criteria for PMF recommended the baseline and follow-up bone marrow or peripheral blood cytogenetics for patients with PMF (79). The WHO diagnostic criteria for ET include no evidence of the Ph chromosome and no *BCR-ABL* fusion as well as no evidence of del(5q), t(3;3)(q21;q26), and inv(3)(q21q26). Consequently, their recommendation is that conventional cytogenetics is the sine qua non for the diagnosis of ET (80). The addition of modern molecular cytogenetics methods will certainly contribute in identifying chromosomal regions that may aid not only in diagnosis, but in distinguishing PV from PMF, ET, and other rare and atypical MPDs. Identification of these underlying genetic defects will eventually make it possible to easily assess the efficacy of treatment as has already been established for the *BCR-ABL* quantitation in patients with CML treated with imatinib.

REFERENCES

1. James C, Ugo V, Le Couedic JP, et al. A unique clonal *JAK2* mutation leading to constitutive signaling causes polycythemia vera. Nature 2005;434:1144–11482.
2. Levine RL, Wadleigh M, Cools J, et al. Activating mutation in the tyrosine kinase JAK2 in polycythemia vera, essential thrombocythemia, and myeloid metaplasia with myelofibrosis. Cancer Cell 2005;7:387–397.
3. Baxter EJ, Scott LM, Campbell PJ, et al. Acquired mutation of the tyrosine kinase JAK2 in human myeloproliferative disorders. Lancet 2005;365:1054–1061.
4. Sandberg EM, Wallace TA, Godeny MD, et al. JAK2 tyrosine kinase: a true *JAK* for all trades? Cell Biochem Biophys 2004;41:207–232.
5. Valentino L, Pierre J. JAK/STAT signal transduction: regulators and implication in hematological malignancies. Biochem Pharmacol 2006;71(6):713–721.
6. Freener EP, Rosario F, Dunn SL, et al. Tyrosine phosphorylation of JAK2 in the JH domain inhibits cytokine signaling. Mol Cell Biol 2004;24:4968–4978.
7. Skoda R, Prchal JT. Chronic myeloproliferative disorders–introduction. Semin Hematol 2005;42:181–182.
8. O'Shea JJ, Gadina M, Schreiber RD. Cytokine signaling in 2002: new surprises in the JAK/STAT pathway. Cell 2002;109(suppl.):S2121–S2131.
9. Saharinen P, Vihinen M, Silvennoinen O. Autoinhibition of JAK2 tyrosine kinase is dependent on specific regions in its pseudokinase domain. Mol Biol Cell 2003;14:1448–1459.
10. Larsen TS, Christensen JH, Hasselbalch HC, et al. The JAK2 V617 mutation involves B- and T-lymphocytes lineages in a subgroup of patients with Philadelphia-chromosome negative chronic myeloproliferative disorders. Br J Haematol 2007;136:745–751.
11. Wernig G, Mercher T, Okabe R, et al. Expression of JAK2V617F causes a polycythemia vera-like disease with associated myelofibrosis in a murine bone marrow transplant model. Blood 2006;107:4274–4281.
12. Lacout C, Pisani DF, Tuliez M, et al. JAK2V617F expression in murine hematopoietic cells leads to MPD mimicking human PV with secondary myelofibrosis. Blood 2006;108(5):1652–1660.
13. Najfeld V. FISHing among myeloproliferative disorders. Semin Hematol 1997;34(1):55–63.
14. Schoch C, Schnittger S, Bursch S, et al. Comparison of chromosome banding analysis, interphase and hypermetaphase-FISH, qualitative and quantitative PCR for diagnosis and for follow-up in chronic myeloid leukemia: a study on 350 cases. Leukemia 2003;16:53–59.
15. Asimakopolous FA, Holloway TL, Nacheva EP, et al. Detection of chromosome 20q deletions in bone marrow metaphases but not peripheral blood granulocytes in

patients with myeloproliferative disorders and myelodysplastic syndromes. Blood 1994;87:1561–1570.

16. Najfeld V, Montella L, Scalise A, et al. Exploring polycythemia vera with fluorescence in situ hybridization: Additional cryptic 9p is the most frequent abnormality detected. Br J Haematol 2002;119:558–566.

17. Westwood NB, Gruszka-Westwood AM, Pearson CE, et al. The incidence of trisomy 8, trisomy 9, and D20S109 deletion in polycythemia vera: An analysis of blood granulocytes using interphase fluorescence in situ hybridization. Br J Haematol 2000;110:839–846.

18. Reilly JT. Cytogenetic and molecular genetic abnormalities in agnogenic myeloid metaplasia. Semin Oncol 2005;32:359–364.

19. Campbell PJ, Griesshammer M, Dohner K, et al. V617F mutation in JAK2 is associated with poorer survival in idiopathic myelofibrosis. Blood 2006;107:2098–2100.

20. Swolin B, Weinfeld A, Westin J. A prospective long-term cytogenetics study in Polycythemia vera in relation to treatment and clinical course. Blood 1988;72: 386–395.

21. Zhang W, Berkofsky-Fessler W, Levine R, et al. High-resolution SNP arrays and correlation with expression arrays identify novel genomic aberrations and potential disease genes in polycythemia vera and other myeloproliferative disorders. Blood 2006;108(11):111a (Abstract 359).

22. Al-Assar O, Ul-Hassan A, Browm R, et al. Gains of 9p are common genomic aberrations in idiopathic myelofibrosis: a comparative genomic hybridization study. Br J Haematol 2005;129:66–71.

23. Sambani C, La Starza R, Pierini V, et al. Leukemic recombinations involving heterochromatin in myeloproliferative disorders with t(1;9). Cancer Genet Cytogenet 2005;162:45–49.

24. Chen Z, Notohamiprodjom M, Guan X-Y, et al. Gain of 9p in the pathogenesis of polycythemia vera. Genes Chromosomes Cancer 1998;22:321–324.

25. Kralovics R, Guan Y, Prchal JT. Acquired uniparental disomy of chromosome 9p is a frequent stem cell defect in polycythemia vera. Exp Hematol 2002;30:229–236.

26. Lacronique V, Boureux A, Valle VD, et al. A TEL-JAK2 fusion protein with constitutive kinase activity in human leukemia. Science 1997;278(5341):1309–1312.

27. Griesinger F, Henning H, Hillmer F, et al. A BCR-JAK2 fusion gene as a result of a t(9;22)(p24;q2) translocation in a patient with a clinically typical chronic myelogenous leukemia. Genes Chromosomes Cancer 2005;44:329–333.

28. Reiter A, Walz C, Watmore A, et al. The t(8;9)(p22;p24) is a recurrent abnormality in chronic and acute leukemia that fuses PCM1 to JAK. Cancer Res 2005;65(7): 2662–2667.

29. Adelaide J, Perot C, Gelsi-Bojer V, et al. A t(8;9) translocation with PCM1-JAK2 fusion in a patient with T-cell lymphoma. Leukemia 2006;3:536–537.

30. Najfeld V, Berkofsky-Fessler W, Cozza A. FISH studies provide evidence that JAK2, via a myriad of mechanisms not limited to point mutations, has gain of function in polycythemia vera (PV) and myelodysplasia (MDS). Blood 2006;108(11): 763a (Abstract 2637).

31. Roulston D, Espinoza R, III, Stoffel M, et al. Molecular genetics of myeloid leukemia: Identification of the commonly deleted segment of chromosome 20 Blood 1993;82:3424–3429.

32. Bench AJ, Nacheva EP, Hood TL, et al. Chromosome 20 deletions in myeloid malignancies: reduction of the common deleted region, generation of a PAC/BAC contig and identification of candidate genes. Oncogene 2000;19:3902–3913.

33. Bench AJ, Cross NCP, Nacheva EP, et al. Myeloproliferative disorders. Best Pract Res Clin Haematol 2001;14:531–551.

34. Andrieux J, Demory JL. Karyotype and molecular cytogenetics studies in polycythemia vera. Curr Hematol Rep 2005;4:224–229.

35. Raskind WH, Steinmann L, Najfeld V. Clonal development of myeloproliferative disorders: Clues to hematopoietic differentiation and multistep pathogenesis of cancer. Leukemia 1998;12:108–116.

36. Kaye FJ, Najfeld V, Singer J, et al. Confirming evidence for the clonal development and stem cell origin of Philadelphia chromosome-negative chronic myelogenous leukemia. Am J Hematol 1984;17:93–96.

37. Tefferi A, Dingli D, Li C-Y, et al. Prognostic diversity among cytogenetics abnormalities in myelofibrosis with myeloid metaplasia. Cancer 2005;104:1656–1660.

38. Strasser-Weippl K, Steurer M, Kees M, et al. Prognostic relevance of cytogenetics determined by fluorescent in situ hybridization in patients having myelofibrosis with myeloid metaplasia. Cancer 2006;107:2801–2806.

39. Campbell LJ, Garson OM. The prognostic significance of deletion of the long arm of chromosome 20 in myeloid disorders. Leukemia 1994;8:67–71.

40. Greenberg P, Cox C, LeBeau MM, et al. International Scoring System for evaluating prognosis in myelodysplastic syndromes. Blood 1997;89:2079–2088.

41. Gribble SM, Reid AG, Bench AJ, et al. Molecular cytogenetics of polycythemia vera: Lack of occult rearrangements detectable by 20q LSP screening, CGH, and M-FISH. Leukemia 2003;17:1419–1421.

42. Busson M, Romana S, Khac FN, et al. Cryptic translocations involving chromosome 20 in polycythemia vera. Ann Genet 2004;47:365–371.

43. Kralovics R, Teo SS, Li S, et al. Acquisition of the V617F mutation of JAK2 is a late genetic event in a subset of patients with myeloproliferative disorders. Blood 2006;108:1377–1380.

44. Price CM, Kufer EJ, Colman SM, et al. Simultaneous genotypic and immunophenotyping analysis of interphase cells using dual color fluorescence: A demonstration of lineage involvement in polycythemia vera. Blood 1992;80:1033–1038.

45. Diez Martin JL, Graham DL, Petitt RM, et al. Chromosome studies in 104 patients with polycythemia vera. Mayo Clin Proc 1991;66:287–299.

46. Tefferi A, Messa RA, Schroeder G, et al. Cytogenetic findings and their clinical relevance in myelofibrosis with myeloid metaplasia. Br J Haematol 2001;113:763–771.

47. Najfeld V, Scalise A, Kalir D, et al. Trisomy of gene(s) on chromosome 1 are frequently involved in recurrent rearrangements among patients with Ph-negative myeloproliferative and myelodysplastic disorders. Blood 2003;102(11):660a (Abstract 2445).

48. Hsiao H-H, Ito Y, Sashida G, et al. De novo appearance of der(1;7)(q10;p10) is associated with leukemic transformation and unfavorable prognosis in essential thrombocythemia. Leuk Res 2005;29:1247–1252.

49. Andreaux J, Demory JL, Caulier ML, et al. Karyotypic abnormalities in myelofibrosis following polycythemia vera. Cancer Genet Cytogenet 2003;140:118–123.

50. Tanaka K, Arif M, Eguchi M, et al. Frequent allelic loss of the RB,D13S319 and D13S25 locus in myeloid malignancies with deletion/translocation of 13q14 of chromosome 13 but not in lymphoid malignancies. Leukemia 1999;13:1367–1373.
51. http://atlasgeneticsoncology.org/Anomalies/del7qID1093.html
52. Strasser-Weippl K, Steurer M, Kees M, et al. Chromosome 7 deletions are associated with unfavorable prognosis in myelofibrosis with myeloid metaplasia. Blood 2005;105:41–116.
53. Messa RA, Li C-Y, Ketterling RP, et al. Leukemic transformation in myelofibrosis with myeloid metaplasia: a single-institution experience with 91 cases. Blood 2005;105(3):973–977.
54. Andrieux J, Demory JL, Morel P, et al. Frequency of structural abnormalities of the long arms of chromosome 12 in myelofibrosis with myeloid metaplasia. Cancer Genet Cytogenet 2002;137:68–71.
55. Przepiorka D, Bryant E, Kidd P. Idiopathic myelofibrosis in blast transformation with 4;12 and 5;12 translocation and 7q deletion. Cancer Genet Cytogenet 1988;30(1): 139–144.
56. Borrego S, Antinolo G, Martin–Noya K, et al. Translocation (8;12) in a patient with agnogenic myeloid metaplasia. Cancer Genet Cytogenet 1993;71(2):183–184.
57. Huret JL, Brizard A, Briualt S, et al. Two additional cases of inversion 12 in human malignancies. Cancer Genet Cytogenet 1988;32(2):309–311.
58. Teferii A, Meyer RG, Wyatt WA, et al. Comparison of peripheral blood interphase cytogenetics with bone marrow karyotype analysis in myelofibrosis with myeloid metaplasia. Br J Haematol 2001;115:316–319.
59. Djordjevic V, Dencic-Fekete M, Jovanovic J, et al. Cytogenetics of agnogenic myeloid metaplasia: a study of 61 patients. Cancer Genet Cytogenet 2007;173:57–62.
60. Golub TR, Barker GF, Lovett M, et al. Fusion of PDGF receptor beta to a novel ets-like gene, tel, in chronic myelomonocytic leukemia with t (5;12) chromosomal translocation. Cell 1994;77:307–316.
61. Xiao S, Nalabolu SR, Aster JC, et al. FGFR1 is fused with a novel zinc-finger gene ZNF198 in the t(8;13) leukemia/lymphoma syndrome. Nat Genet 1998;18:84–87.
62. Cools J, Deangelo DJ, Gotlib J, et al. A tyrosine kinase created by a fusion of the PDGFRA and FIP1L! genes as a therapeutic target of imatinib in idiopathic hypereosinophilic syndrome. N Engl J Med 2003;348:1201–1214.
63. De Keersmaecker K, Cools J. Chronic myeloproliferative disorders: a tyrosine kinase tale. Leukemia 2006;20:200–205.
64. Pellagatti A, Vetrie D, Langford CF, et al. Gene expression profiling in polycythemia vera using cDNA microarray technology. Cancer Res 2003;63(14):3940–3944.
65. Steidl U, Schroeder T, Steidel C, et al. Distinct gene expression pattern of malignant hematopoietic stem and progenitor cells in polycythemia vera. Ann NY Acad Sci 2005;1044:94–108.
66. Berkofsky-Fessler WD. Transcriptional Profiling in Polycythemia Vera, V617 JAK2 Expressing Hematopoietic Progenitor Cells, and Other Hematological Malignancies. Ph.D. dissertation, Mount Sinai School of Medicine, 2006.
67. Goertler PS, Kreutz C, Donauer J, et al. Gene expression profiling in polycythemia vera: overexpression of transcription factorNF-E. Br J Haematol 2005;129: 138–150.
68. Di Ianni M, Moretti L, Del Papa B, et al. Chronic myeloproliferative disorders: the bone marrow stromal component is not involved in the malignant clone. Leukemia 2007;21:377–378.

69. Campbell PJ, Scott LM, Buck G, et al. Definition of subtypes of essential thrombocythaemia and relation to polycythemia vera based on JAK2V617F mutation status: a prospective study. Lancet 2005;306:1945–1953.
70. Mercher T, Weing G, Moore SA, et al. JAK2T875N is a novel activating mutation that results in myeloproliferative disease with features of megakaryoblastic leukemia in a murine bone marrow transplantation model. Blood 2006;108:2770–2779.
71. Ihle JN, Gilliland DG. *JAK2*: normal function and role in hematopoietic disorders. Curr Opin Genet Dev 2007;17:8–14.
72. Scott LM, Tong W, Levine RL, et al. *JAK2* exon 12 mutations in polycythemia vera and idiopathic erythrocytosis. N Engl J Med 2007;356:459–468.
73. Malinge S, Ben-Abdelali R, Settegrana C, et al. Novel activating JAK2 mutation in a patient with Down syndrome and B-cell precursor acute lymphoblastic leukemia. Blood 2007;109:2202–2204.
74. Nussenzveig RH, Swierczek SI, Jelinek J, et al. Polycythemia vera is not initiated by *JAK2^{V617F}* mutation. Experimental Hematology 2007;35:32–38.
75. Campbell PJ, Baxter EJ, Beer PA, et al. Mutation of *JAK2* in the myeloproliferative disorders: timing, clonality studies, cytogenetic associations, and role in leukemic transformation. Blood 2006;108:3548–3555.
76. Theocharides A, Boissinot M, Girdon F, et al. Leukemic blasts in transformed *JAK2-V617F* positive myeloproliferative disorders are frequently negative for the *JAK2-V617F* mutation. Blood 2007;110:375–379.
77. Vizmanos JL, Ormazabal C, Larrayoz MJ, et al. *JAK2* V617F mutation in classic chronic myeloproliferative diseases: a report on a series of 349 patients. Leukemia 2006;20:534–535.
78. Campbell PJ, Green AR. The myeloproliferative disorders. N Engl J Med 2006; 355:2452–2466.
79. Tefferi A, Barosi G, Messa RA, et al. International working group (IWG) consensus criteria for treatment response in myelofibrosis with myeloid metaplasia, for the IWG for myelofibrosis research and treatment IIWG-MRT). Blood 2006;108:1497–1503.
80. Finazzi G, Harrison C. Essential thrombocythemia. Semin Hematol 2005;42(4): 230–238.
81. Rege-Cambrin G, Mecucci C, Tricot G, et al. A chromosomal profile in polycythemia vera. Cancer Genet Cytogenet 1987;24:233–245.
82. Zamora L, Espinet B, Florensa L, et al. Is fluoresnce in situ hybridization a useful method in diagnosis of polycythemia vera patients? Cancer Genet Cytogenet 2004;151:139–145.
83. Bacher U, Haferlach T, Kern W, et al. Conventional cytogenetics of myeloproliferative diseases other than CML contributes valid information. Ann Hematol 2005;84: 250–257.
84. Dupriez B, Morel P, Demory JL, et al. Prognostic factors in agnogenic myeloid metaplasia: A report of 195 cases with a new scoring system. Blood 1996;88: 1013–1018.
85. Reilly JT. Idiopathic myelofibrosis; pathogenesis, natural history, and management. Blood Rev 1997;11:233–242.
86. Swolin B, Safai-Kutti S, Angehm E, et al. No increased frequency of trisomies 8 and 9 by fluorescence in situ hybridization in untreated patients with essenthial thrombocythemia. Cancer Genet Cytogenet 2001;126:56–59.

4

Congenital Causes of Erythrocytosis/Polycythemias and Thrombocytosis

Josef T. Prchal

University of Utah, Hematology Division, Salt Lake City, Utah, U.S.A.

Radek C. Skoda

University Hospital Basel, Department of Research, Experimental Hematology, Basel, Switzerland

OVERVIEW

Our understanding of the regulation of erythropoiesis and thrombopoiesis has continuously improved during the last years. The elucidation of the molecular basis of congenital polycythemias (erythrocytoses) and thrombocytoses demonstrates that the pathophysiology of these disorders can provide new information on the molecular control of platelet and red cell production and has clinical relevance as it leads to precise diagnosis, appropriate clinical management, and more efficient therapies.

In this chapter, we will review the pathophysiology of erythropoiesis and thrombopoiesis and define those clinical congenital disorders wherein the molecular basis has been defined. In addition, there is growing evidence that acquired myeloproliferative disorders (i.e., polycythemia vera and essential thrombocytemia, which are caused by somatic mutations, often have a familiar predisposition). This suggests the existence of germline mutations that either facilitate the somatic mutation(s) or contribute to somatic acquired mutations to result in a familiar clustering of myeloproliferative disorders. The molecular basis of these interactions remains yet to be defined.

REGULATION OF ERYTHROPOIESIS AS IT RELATES
TO POLYCYTHEMIAS: OVERVIEW

The erythrocyte production, erythropoiesis, is a tightly regulated system; however, all aspects of its regulation are still not fully elucidated. Much has, and remains to be learned from, uncovering the molecular basis of congenital and acquired mutations that disrupts its control.

The erythropoiesis can be viewed as composed of three stages: an initial stage, wherein the commitment of pluripotent hematopoietic progenitors to committed erythroid precursors takes place; the second stage, which is characterized by an expansion of erythroid progenitors that is largely regulated by erythropoietin (Epo), which is made effective by the appearance of its receptor (EpoR) expression that peaks on the surface of early erythroblasts and then declines; and the terminal stage composed of enucleation and removal of nucleotides and other remnants of organelles that may be toxic to mature circulating erythrocytes. We know more about mutations leading to anemias, as these appear more numerous and more clinically symptomatic. These occur in all stages of erythropoiesis, including its early stage. This is exemplified by the loss-of-function regulator of the early stage of erythropoiesis commitment, i.e., GATA 1 mutation, which perturbs multiple erythroid regulatory events as well as thrombopoiesis regulation and results in porphyria, thrombocytopenia, anemia with elevated fetal hemoglobin, and the thalassemic phenotype (1). However, in this review, we will concentrate only on those defects that have been demonstrated to lead to, or potentially could lead to, increased red cell mass (i.e., polycythemia). We should note here that polycythemia is often and inconsistently referred to by an alternate term (i.e. erythrocytosis) and since no consensus on usage has been reached, we will refer to the individual entities by a term used in the original description.

Erythropoiesis defects leading to polycythemia invariably occur at the second stage of erythropoiesis and include the *appropriate polycythemias* (2) that are defined by physiologically intact upregulation of Epo production to meet the tissue oxygen demand, which then drives augmented erythropoiesis (i.e., *secondary polycythemias*). The *inappropriate polycythemias* (2) are caused by inappropriate increases of erythropoietin signaling such as seen in two *primary polycythemias* (defects within the progenitors that lead to Epo hypersensitivity or independence), which drive the polycythemia phenotype. These are characterized by a low Epo level.

1. The congenital gain-of-function mutations of the *EPOR* gene leading to primary familial and congenital polycythemia (PFCP) wherein the Epo signal is augmented by the mutation.

2. The somatic (acquired) mutation located downstream to EpoR, that is, *JAK2V617F* mutation in polycythemia vera (PV).

In addition, there is a growing understanding of the regulation of Epo. Some of the congenital defects of this regulation lead to dysregulation of Epo production and can be inherited or acquired, and since they are Epo-driven, these are secondary polycythemic disorders. However, in some instances, their associated pathophysiology is also reflected in aberrant erythroid proliferation inappropriate to the circulating level of Epo, and thus have features of both primary and secondary polycythemia (i.e., Chuvash polycythemia).

However, as reflected by an entity of postrenal transplant erythrocytosis wherein the elevated red cell mass is non–Epo-mediated, some polycythemic states can also result from the dysregulation of angiotensin II signaling (3,4).

Regulation of Erythropoietin Production

Clearly, Epo is the principal regulator of erythropoietin signaling by its modulation of erythroid proliferation, prevention of apoptosis, and promoting the erythroid differentiation [reviewed by Krantz (5)]. Regulation of Epo production can be (a) hypoxia mediated and (b) hypoxia independent.

Molecular Basis of Hypoxia Sensing

HIF-1 Transcription Factor

Hypoxia is an important process in organismal development, energy metabolism, vasculogenesis, iron metabolism, tumor promotion, and erythropoiesis [reviewed by Hirota (6) and (7)]. The transcription factor HIF-1 is induced in hypoxic cells and binds to the *cis*-acting nucleotide sequence referred to as *hypoxia-responsive element* (HRE), first identified in the 3′-flanking region of the human *EPO* gene (8). Many hypoxia-inducible genes have been found to be directly regulated by HIF-1. However, this number is clearly an underestimate, as Semenza's laboratory showed that ∼3% of all genes expressed in endothelial tissue are HIF-1 regulated (9). HIF-1 is a heterodimeric transcription factor composed of an HIF-1α subunit and an HIF-1β subunit (Fig. 1). The HIF-1β subunit belongs to the basic helix-loop-helix (bHLH)-containing PER-ARNT-SIM (PAS)-domain family of transcription factors. However, only the HIF-1α (and HIF-2α, see below) are hypoxia regulated and exists only in HIF and thus are the key subunits, determining the hypoxia-modulated amount and activity of HIF-1 and HIF 2 and transcription of the hypoxia-inducible genes. Under normoxic conditions, the half-life of HIF-1 in the cell is only minutes HIF-1α is rapidly degraded by the von Hippel-Lindau (VHL) protein ubiquitin–proteasome pathway (10). This is initiated by a posttranslational hydroxylation event at residue P564 of the HIF-1α molecule by one of the several iron-containing proline hydroxylases that facilitates its binding to VHL protein and subsequent ubiquitination and

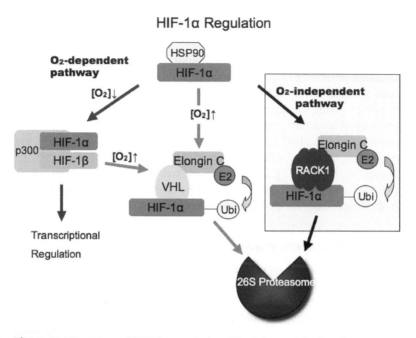

Figure 1 Overview of HIF-1α regulation. The left panel depicts the oxygen-dependent pathway. In the middle of the cartoon, in the presence of oxygen, HIF-1α is proline-hydroxylated, which allows interaction with Elongins C and E2, and VHL protein leading to the ubiquitinization and destruction of HIF-1α in proteasome. The left portion of the cartoon depicts the lack of HIF-1α degradation in hypoxia, formation of HIF-1α, and HIF-1β dimer, resulting in transcriptional regulation of HIF controlled genes. The right panel depicts the oxygen-independent pathway wherein RACK1 interacting with Elongins C and E2 promote ubiquitinization and destruction of HIF-1α in proteasome.

proteasomal degradation. Under hypoxic conditions, the HIF-1α protein is stabilized and translocated to the cell nucleus. It dimerizes with HIF-1β to form the HIF-1 and activates the transcription through HIF-1 binding to specific HREs. Another regulatory step involves O_2-dependent asparaginyl-hydroxylation of N803 in HIF-1α that requires the enzyme FIH-1 (factor inhibiting HIF-1). Hydroxylation of N803 during normoxia blocks the binding to another transcription factors p300 and CBP to HIF-1, resulting in inhibition of HIF-1-mediated gene transcription. Under hypoxic conditions, HIF-1α is not hydroxylated. The unmodified protein escapes the VHL binding, ubiquitination, and degradation. When N803 of HIF-1α is not asparaginyl-hydroxylated, p300 and CBP can bind to HIF-1 dimer, allowing transcriptional activation of HIF-1 target genes. This targeting and subsequent polyubiquitination of HIF-1α requires VHL, iron, O_2, and proline hydroxylase activity, and, as depicted in Figure 1, this complex constitutes the oxygen sensor (11,12).

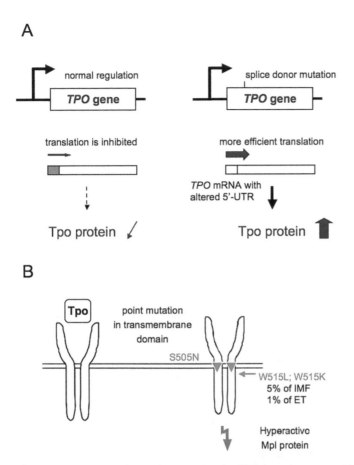

Figure 2 Summary of mutations causing familial thrombocytoses. (**A**) Translational control of Tpo protein production. *TPO* mRNA is transcribed at a constant rate, but translation of *TPO* mRNA is inhibited by the presence of upstream open reading frames (dark box) in the 5′-untranslated region (5′-UTR) of the normal *TPO* mRNA (left panel). A splice donor mutation in the *TPO* gene in patients with familial thrombocytosis (right panel) removes the inhibitory upstream open reading frames from the 5′-UTR and the *TPO* mRNA with altered 5′-UTR (white box) is more efficiently translated into Tpo protein. (**B**) Mutations in MPL. A point mutation located in the transmembrane domain of the Mpl protein (position 505) in patients with familial thrombocytosis results in hyperactive Mpl that transmits signals independent of ligand binding. The activating mutation in the juxtamembrane domain (position 515) found in patients with sporadic essential thrombocythemia and idiopathic myelofibrosis is indicated by an arrow.

HIF-2 Transcription Factor

HIF-1α and HIF-2α exhibit high sequence homology but have different mRNA expression patterns; HIF-1α is expressed ubiquitously whereas HIF-2α expression is restricted to certain tissues (6,13). Both HIF-1α and HIF-2α are regulated by an identical mechanism by hypoxia and form a dimer with the same HIF-1β subunit. Kidney is the main site of Epo production (i.e., renal interstitial cells) wherein HIF-1 is the principal regulator of *EPO* transcription (6), while in other tissues, such as brain (14) and liver (15) (that generates ∼20% of circulating Epo), *EPO* gene transcription is HIF-2 regulated (13). The recent discovery of an iron-responsive element in the 5′ untranslated region of *HIF-2α* reveals a novel regulatory link between iron availability and *HIF-2α* expression (16) that may impact control of erythropoiesis. Thus, when iron supply is limited, HIF-2α would decrease, and when iron is abundant, the liver HIF-2α would increase, thus increasing liver-synthesized Epo production and promoting erythropoiesis by connecting to hepcidine function (17).

Hypoxia Independent Regulation of HIF

O_2-dependent regulation of the HIF-1α subunit is mediated by prolyl hydroxylases, VHL protein, and proteosomal complex. Another regulation of HIF-independent of hypoxia has been recently described. This novel mechanism involves the receptor of activated protein kinase C (RACK1) as an HIF-1α-interacting protein that promotes prolyl hydroxylase/VHL-independent proteasomal degradation of HIF-1α. RACK1 competes with heat shock protein 90 (HSP90) for binding to the PAS-A domain of HIF-1α. HIF-1α degradation is abolished by RACK1 loss-of-function. RACK1 binds to proteasomal subunit, Elongin-C, and promotes ubiquitination of HIF-1α (Fig. 1). Thus, RACK1 is an essential component of an O_2/PHD/VHL independent mechanism for regulating HIF-1α (18).

REGULATION OF THROMBOPOIESIS

Platelet production is primarily controlled by thrombopoietin (Tpo), a secreted glycoprotein of 332 amino acids produced by liver (19,20). Tpo is also made in smaller quantities in the kidneys and by bone marrow stromal cells. The N-terminal amino acid sequence of Tpo (residues 1–153) shows similarities to Epo and is followed by a unique C-terminal carbohydrate-rich domain (amino acids 154–332) (21–23), which increases the stability and half-life of the Tpo protein. The *TPO* gene (official gene name: *THPO*) is located on human chromosome 3q27 (24). The Tpo receptor, called "myeloproliferative leukemia" (Mpl), is a member of the hematopoietic cytokine receptor superfamily (25–28). Mpl binds Tpo with a very high affinity and specificity and signals by activating the cytoplasmic tyrosine kinases Jak2 and Tyk2. Functionally, the activation of Jak2 is essential and cannot be substituted by Tyk2. Tpo signaling stimulates early megakaryocyte progenitors and promotes megakaryocytic maturation. However,

Tpo is not required for the terminal stages of megakaryocytic development and platelet shedding. The signaling cascades mediating the effects of Tpo have been studied extensively. Key players are the signal transducers and activators of transcription (Stat) proteins, particularly Stat5, but also the MAPK pathway and small Src-like kinases, e.g., Lyn (29). In addition to controlling the platelet count, Tpo also stimulates hematopoietic stem cells (HSC). Loss of *TPO* or *MPL* results in decreased HSC and progenitor numbers (30).

The production of *TPO* mRNA occurs at a constant rate and is not upregulated in situations with increased demand for platelet production, for example, thrombocytopenia induced by radiation or antibody lysis (31). Consistently, mice heterozygous for the *TPO* knockout allele have platelet counts intermediary to the homozygous knockout and wild type, demonstrating that the thrombocytopenia does not lead to a compensatory increase of transcription from the remaining wild-type locus (32). The production of Tpo protein is inhibited by a translational mechanism involving seven upstream open reading frames (uORFs) present in the 5'-untranslated region (5'-UTR) of the *TPO* mRNA (33). This mechanism prevents that pathologically high Tpo concentrations are reached under physiological conditions. Particularly, one uORF, designated uORF7, prevents the ribosomes from reaching the physiological start site for translation (33).

The concentration of Tpo in plasma is controlled by an autoregulatory feedback loop involving binding of circulating Tpo by Mpl on platelets followed by internalization and degradation of the ligand (31,34). Thus, an increase in platelet numbers will result in lower Tpo concentrations in the bone marrow and a decrease in platelet production. The megakaryocyte mass also contributes to the negative feedback mechanism (35,36), but not endothelial cells that also express *MPL* (37). Although small amounts of *TPO* mRNA are also detectable in bone marrow stromal cells (38,39), it has never been directly demonstrated that Tpo protein is actually made by stromal cells and the levels of Tpo in conditioned media from bone marrow cells remained below the detection limit (40). It is therefore questionable whether changes in *TPO* mRNA observed in bone marrow stromal cells are relevant to platelet production.

Although Tpo is the most potent regulator of megakaryopoiesis and platelet production, other cytokines and growth factors have also been described to have stimulatory effects. Interleukin-11 (IL-11) is a pleiotropic cytokine originally isolated from bone marrow stromal cells, which promotes megakaryocyte differentiation in vitro and results in increased platelet counts in vivo (41). IL-11 has been shown to shorten thrombocytopenia in patients undergoing chemotherapy and has been approved for this indication (42,43). Other cytokines with megakaryocyte stimulatory activity that have been tested for clinical applications are IL-3 and IL-6 (44). However, due to limited effectiveness and considerable side effects, these cytokines are not used for clinical purposes. Clinical trials with Tpo for the treatment of thrombocytopenia have been stopped because of the occurrence of neutralizing antibodies that caused severe thrombocytopenia (45,46). Recently, AMG531, a Tpo peptide agonist engineered into a recombinant immunoglobulin protein, has been shown to increase platelet levels in patients with idiopathic thrombocytopenia without causing significant adverse effects (47). This and other Tpo-mimetic compounds under development hold promise to become available for the treatment of patients with thrombocytopenia (48).

The transcriptional control of megakaryopoiesis and thrombopoiesis has been studied extensively in mouse models and cell lines (49–51). A number of transcriptional targets of Tpo signaling, including HOX transcription factors and hypoxia-induced transcription factors, have been identified that mediate the effects of Tpo on stem cell maintenance (50). Mutations in Myb have been shown to complement and correct thrombocytopenia in Mpl knockout mice (52), and altered expression levels of Gata1 and Fli1 can affect the numbers of megakaryocytes and platelets (53). Mutations in several of these transcription factors have been found in patients with hereditary platelet disorders.

FAMILIAL POLYCYTHEMIAS

Primary Familial and Congenital Polycythemia

Primary familial and congenital polycythemia (PFCP) is characterized by an auto-somal dominant mode of inheritance, and less frequently, by the occurrence of spo-radic cases (54,55). This can be contrasted with Chuvash polycythemia where the inheritance is autosomal recessive. The clinical features of PFCP include the presence of isolated erythrocytosis, absence of predisposition to development of acute leukemia or other myeloproliferative disorders, absence of splenomegaly, normal white blood cell and platelet counts, low plasma Epo levels, normal hemoglobin–oxygen dissociation curve (indicated by a normal P50), and hypersensitivity of erythroid progenitors to exogenous erythropoietin in vitro (56–59). PFCP is generally thought to be a benign condition, but it has been reported to be associated with predisposition to cardiovascular problems, such as hypertension, coronary artery disease, and cerebrovascular events, that are not clearly related to an elevated hematocrit (60–62). Association with cardiovascular disease, however, has not been described in all series.

The distal cytoplasmic region of the erythropoietin receptor (EpoR), in association with SHP-1, is required for down-regulation of Epo-mediated activation of JAK2/STAT5 proteins (63,64). Thus far, nine mutations of the Epo receptor (*EPOR*) have been convincingly linked with PFCP [reviewed by Gordeuk (65)]. All of these mutations result in truncation of the EPOR cytoplasmic carboxyl terminal, leading to loss of its negative regulatory domain, resulting in a gain-of-function of the EPOR. Three additional missense *EPOR* mutations have been described in families with PFCP, but they have not been linked to PFCP or any other disease phenotype (66). The absence of polycythemic phenotype in some patients with *EPOR* mutation is suggestive of a role played by gene modifiers or epigenetic factors in phenotypic penetrance (67).

Secondary Familiar Polycythemias

High Oxygen Affinity Hemoglobin Mutants

Affinity of Hb with oxygen is expressed as the P50, which is the partial pressure of oxygen in blood at which 50% of the Hb is saturated with oxygen. An abnormally low P50 reflects an increased affinity of hemoglobin for oxygen. During oxygenation and deoxygenation, there is considerable movement along the $\alpha1/\beta2$ interface (68). Several hemoglobin mutants have substitutions affecting this interface. Other Hb variants have amino acid substitutions involving the C-terminal residues of the β chain or of the 2,3-biphosphoglycerate (2,3-BPG) binding sites. All these substitutions can affect the cooperative nature of oxygen binding with heme, the change from T to R state and vice versa, and in turn, can change the affinity of Hb for oxygen. The majority of mutations affecting oxygen affinity give high affinity Hb variants, which results in relative tissue hypoxia leading to compensatory secondary appropriate polycythemia. There are about 100 Hb variants, listed on the globin server, known to be associated with high affinity for oxygen [http://globin.bx.psu.edu/hbvar/menu.html (last accessed on March 07, 2007)]. Thus, an autosomal dominant polycythemia with normal to elevated Epo level is suggestive of a mutant Hb with high affinity for oxygen (68). The therapy of this compensatory polycythemia by phlebotomies is ill-advised.

2,3-BPG Deficiency

Congenitally low erythrocyte 2,3-BPG level can occur because of deficiency of the red cell enzyme 2,3-BPG mutase (69,70). This is an extremely rare autosomal recessive condition. This disorder should be suspected in the case of isolated polycythemia (without any feature of myeloproliferative disorders, such as a progressive increase of RBC mass, high platelet and granulocyte count, and splenomegaly), absence of a family history, and low P50 (signifying high oxygen affinity). Mutant Hb still needs to be ruled out first. In these cases, the red cells will have high oxygen affinity; however, unlike high affinity Hb, the oxygen affinity of the hemolysate is normal and the level of 2,3-BPG is very low.

Congenital Methemoglobinemias

There are three types of hereditary methemoglobinemias [reviewed by Gregg and Prchal (71)]. Two are inherited as autosomal recessive traits: cytochrome b5R deficiency and cytochrome b5 deficiency. The third type is an autosomal dominant disorder, hemoglobin M (Hb M) disease, in which there is a mutation of one of the globin genes. All congenital methemoglobinemias are associated with suboptimal delivery of oxygen per red cell and this may result in compensatory secondary appropriate polycythemia. The resulting polycythemia is typically mild and its treatment is ill-advised, as it would only decrease tissue oxygen delivery and lead to tissue hypoxia.

DISORDERS OF HYPOXIA SENSING

Chuvash Polycythemia

This disorder is the first hereditary condition of augmented hypoxia-sensing to be recognized. Chuvash polycythemia (CP), the only known congenital endemic polycythemia, is an autosomal recessive hereditary polycythemia. The Chuvash people reside in the mid-Volga River region in Russia wherein CP affects hundreds of Chuvash people, making it the most common congenital polycythemia (72). Outside of Chuvashia, CP has also been found sporadically in diverse ethnic and racial groups (73–75), but recently a high prevalence of this disorder was reported in the Italian island of Ischia (76). In a study of five multiplex Chuvash families with CP, a mutation of VHL (598 C>T) was found in the affected individuals (77). This mutation impairs the interaction of pVHL with HIF-1α, thus reducing the rate of ubiquitin-mediated destruction of HIF-1α. As a result, the level of the HIF-1 heterodimer increases and leads to increased expression of target genes, including *EPO*, *VEGF*, and plasminogen activator inhibitor (*PAI*), among others (77,78). Chuvash polycythemia is a unique VHL syndrome characterized by homozygous germline mutation of VHL leading to predisposition to development of thrombosis, bleeding, cerebral vascular events, and increased mortality. It is characterized by an intact response to hypoxia despite increased basal expression of a broad range of hypoxia-regulated genes in normoxia. Unexpectedly, their erythroid progenitors are hypersensitive to Epo; thus, CP shares the features of both primary and secondary polycythemia. Despite an increased expression of HIF-1α and VEGF in normoxia, CP patients do not display predisposition to tumor formation. Imaging studies of 33 CP patients revealed unsuspected cerebral ischemic lesions in 45% but no tumors characteristic of VHL syndrome (79).

Homozygosity for the VHL 598 C>T has been reported to occur sporadically also in Caucasians in the United States and Europe and in the people of Southeast Asian (Indian subcontinent) ancestry (73,75). Thrombotic complications have been reported in some of these individuals. To address the question of whether the VHL 598 C>T substitution occurred in a single founder or resulted from recurrent mutational events, haplotype analysis was performed on subjects bearing the VHL 598 C>T mutation and normal unrelated individuals from Chuvash, Asian, Caucasian, Hispanic, and African-American ethnic groups (80). These studies indicated that in most individuals, the VHL 598 C>T mutation arose in a single ancestor between 12,000 and 51,000 years ago. However, a Turkish polycythemic family in Germany had a different haplotype, indicating that the VHL 598 C>T mutation in this family occurred independently (81).

In contrast, autosomal dominant mutations of the *VHL* gene cause *VHL syndrome* (82). Heterozygotes for dominant VHL mutations are at increased risk of developing hemangioblastomas, renal cell carcinoma, pheochromocytoma, pancreatic endocrine tumors, and endolymphatic sac tumors when they acquire a somatic mutation in the normal *VHL* allele (83,84). Some patients with VHL syndrome also develop acquired polycythemia (82). The development of hemangioblastoma and renal cell carcinoma associated with VHL tumor predisposition syndrome has been proposed to be related to the increased expression of HIF (85,86) and possibly VEGF (87). The absence of predisposition to tumorigenesis in CP patients implies that deregulation of HIF-1 and VEGF may not be sufficient to cause predisposition toward tumor formation in VHL syndrome.

Non–Chuvash Germline VHL Mutations

Non–Chuvash Germline VHL Mutations also cause polycythemia. Some patients with congenital polycythemia have proven to be compound heterozygotes for the Chuvash mutation, VHL 598 C>T, and other VHL mutations, including 562 C>G, 574 C>T, 388 C>G, and 311G>T (74,81,88). A Croatian boy was homozygous for VHL 571 C>G, the first example of a homozygous VHL germline mutation other than VHL 598 C>T causing polycythemia (74). Additionally, a Portuguese girl was a compound heterozygote for VHL 562 C>G and VHL 253 C>T (88,89). A few cases of congenital polycythemia, known to have mutations of only one *VHL* allele, confound an obvious pathophysiological explanation. Two Ukrainian children with polycythemia were heterozygotes for VHL 376G>T, but the father with the same mutation was not polycythemic (73). Peripheral blood erythroid progenitors from the children and father were hyperresponsive to recombinant Epo in in-vitro clonogenic assays in a way similar to what is seen in CP patients. An English patient was a heterozygote for VHL 598 C>T (75), although the inheritance of a deletion of a VHL allele or a null *VHL* allele in a trans position was not excluded in this patient. Subsequently, two VHL heterozygous patients with polycythemia were described in whom a null VHL allele was more rigorously excluded; (81,88) one of these patients also had ataxia-telangiectasia (88).

Proline Hydroxylase Deficiency

A family with proline hydroxylase mutation was recently described wherein heterozygotes for this mutation had a mild or borderline polycythemia that authors referred to as erythrocytosis (90); however, their erythroid progenitors were not tested. Because of the small family size, the possible nonerythroid phenotype could not be ascertained. However, this work underscores the importance of the hypoxia control of HIF signaling in genesis of polycythemic disorders.

Congenital Polycythemias with Elevated or Inappropriately Normal Levels of Erythropoietin of Yet Unidentified Defect

In our experience, the majority of patients with congenital polycythemias with normal or elevated Epo levels do not have *VHL* mutations, and the molecular basis of polycythemia in these cases remains to be elucidated. A proline hydroxylase mutation has been excluded in some, but not in all, of these patients. It is not clear why in some families the polycythemia is dominantly inherited (91), in others recessively, and in some it is sporadic, and why in families with the same mutation the phenotype can be different (89,92). Lesions in genes linked to the hypoxia-independent regulation of HIF as well as oxygen-dependent gene regulation pathways are leading candidates for mutation screening in polycythemic patients with normal or elevated Epo without *VHL* or proline hydroxylase mutations.

FAMILIAL THROMBOCYTHEMIAS

Hereditary syndromes with abnormal platelet production resulting in thrombocytopenia are more common than those manifesting with thrombocytosis. The thrombocytopenias have been reviewed recently and will not be discussed here (93–95). Familial thrombocytosis (also called hereditary thrombocythemia) can present either as single lineage diseases with solely increased megakaryopoiesis or as multilineage diseases in conjunction with increased granulopoiesis and/or erythropoiesis, resembling sporadic MPD. Due to their lineage-selective effects, activating mutations in *TPO* and *MPL* were strong candidates for causing familial thrombocytosis. Indeed, activating mutations in the *TPO* gene causing overproduction of Tpo protein by a mechanism of increased translational efficiency for the mutant *TPO* mRNA have been found in four families (96–100) (see Fig. 2). Thrombocytosis is inherited as an autosomal dominant trait with high penetrance and the clinical findings consist of thrombocytosis, normal hematocrit, normal leukocytes, and elevated serum Tpo levels. The clinical course is mild with occasional thrombotic complications or bleeding, but without leukemic transformation. *TPO* mutations have not been found in patients with sporadic ET (101). A mutation in the transmembrane domain of *Mpl* exchanging a serine in position 505 with an asparagine (S505 N) was reported in a family with autosomal dominant thrombocytosis (102) (see Fig. 2). The mutation was also found in a mutational screening using retroviruses in mice (103), but not in sporadic ET. In contrast, mutations in position 515 of Mpl that exchange a tryptophane with leucine (W515 L) or lysine (W515 K) are present in 1% of patients with ET and 5% of patients with IMF (see chap. 6). In other families with familial thrombocythemias, *TPO* and *MPL* were excluded as the diseases-causing gene through the absence of linkage and/or sequencing (104–107), indicating that in the majority of familial thrombocytosis the disease-causing gene still remains unknown.

We conclude that much has already been learned from the elucidation of the familial thrombocythemias and polycythemias, and this knowledge has contributed to better understanding of pathophysiology, molecular genetics, thrombopoiesis, and erythropoiesis. Ultimately, this knowledge should benefit our patients and also clinical hematologists and pathologists, allowing an evidence-based diagnosis and accurate management of these diseases.

REFERENCES

1. Phillips JD, Steensma DP, Pulsipher MA, et al. Congenital erythropoietic porphyria due to a mutation in GATA1: the first trans-acting mutation causative for a human porphyria. Blood 2007;109(6):2618–2621.

2. Erslev A. Secondary polycythemia (erythrocytosis). In: Beutler E, Lichtman MA, Coller BS, Kipps TJ, eds. William's Hematology, 5th ed. New York: McGraw-Hill, 2002, pp. 714–726.

3. Mrug M, Julian BA, Prchal JT. Angiotensin II receptor type 1 expression in erythroid progenitors: implications for the pathogenesis of postrenal transplant erythrocytosis. Semin Nephrol 2004;24(2):120–130.

4. Mrug M, Stopka T, Julian BA, et al. Angiotensin II stimulates proliferation of normal early erythroid progenitors. J Clin Invest 1997;100(9):2310–2314.

5. Krantz SB. Erythropoietin. Blood 1991;77(3):419–434.

6. Hirota K, Semenza GL. Regulation of angiogenesis by hypoxia-inducible factor 1. Crit Rev Oncol Hematol 2006;59(1):15–26.

7. Yoon D, Pastore YD, Divoky V, et al. Hypoxia-inducible factor-1 deficiency results in dysregulated erythropoiesis signaling and iron homeostasis in mouse development. J Biol Chem 2006;281(35):25703–25711.

8. Beck I, Ramirez S, Weinmann R, et al. Enhancer element at the $3'$-flanking region controls transcriptional response to hypoxia in the human erythropoietin gene. J Biol Chem 1991;266(24):15563–15566.

9. Manalo DJ, Rowan A, Lavoie T, et al. Transcriptional regulation of vascular endothelial cell responses to hypoxia by HIF-1. Blood 2005;105(2):659–669.

10. Maxwell P, Wiesener MS, Chang GW, et al. The tumour suppressor protein VHL targets hypoxia-inducible factors for oxygen-dependent proteolysis. Nature 1999;399:271–275.

11. Jaakkola P, Mole DR, Tian YM, et al. Targeting of HIF-alpha to the von Hippel-Lindau ubiquitylation complex by O_2-regulated prolyl hydroxylation. Science 2001;292:468–472.

12. Ivan M, Kondo K, Yang H, et al. HIF alpha targeted for VHL-mediated destruction by proline hydroxylation: implications for O_2 sensing. Science 2001;292:464–468.

13. Gruber M, Hu CJ, Johnson RS, et al. Acute postnatal ablation of HIF-2alpha results in anemia. Proc Natl Acad Sci U S A 2007;104(7):2301–2306.

14. Chavez JC, Baranova O, Lin J, et al. The transcriptional activator hypoxia inducible factor 2 (HIF-2/EPAS-1) regulates the oxygen-dependent expression of erythropoietin in cortical astrocytes. J Neurosci 2006;26(37):9471–9481.

15. Rankin EB, Biju MP, Liu Q, et al. Hypoxia-inducible factor-2 (HIF-2) regulates hepatic erythropoietin in vivo. J Clin Invest 2007;117(4):1068–1077.

16. Sanchez M, Galy B, Muckenthaler MU, et al. Iron-regulatory proteins limit hypoxia-inducible factor-2alpha expression in iron deficiency. Nat Struct Mol Biol 2007;14(5):420–426.

17. Dallalio G, Law E, Means RT, Jr. Hepcidin inhibits in vitro erythroid colony formation at reduced erythropoietin concentrations. Blood 2006;107(7):2702–2704.

18. Liu YV, Baek JH, Zhang H, et al. RACK1 competes with HSP90 for binding to HIF-1alpha and is required for O(2)-independent and HSP90 inhibitor-induced degradation of HIF-1alpha. Mol Cell 2007;25(2):207–217.

19. Kaushansky K. Thrombopoietin. N Engl J Med 1998;339(11):746–754.

20. Kaushansky K. Lineage-specific hematopoietic growth factors. N Engl J Med 2006;354(19):2034–2045.

21. de Sauvage FJ, Hass PE, Spencer SD, et al. Stimulation of megakaryocytopoiesis and thrombopoiesis by the c-mpl ligand. Nature 1994;369(6481):533–538.

22. Lok S, Kaushansky K, Holly RD, et al. Cloning and expression of murine thrombopoietin cDNA and stimulation of platelet production in vivo. Nature 1994;369(6481):565–568.

23. Bartley TD, Bogenberger J, Hunt P, et al. Identification and cloning of a megakaryocyte growth and development factor that is a ligand for the cytokine receptor Mpl. Cell 1994;77(7):1117–1124.

24. Gurney AL, Kuang WJ, Xie MH, et al. Genomic structure, chromosomal localization, and conserved alternative splice forms of thrombopoietin. Blood 1995;85(4): 981–988.

25. Souyri M, Vigon I, Penciolelli JF, et al. A putative truncated cytokine receptor gene transduced by the myeloproliferative leukemia virus immortalizes hematopoietic progenitors. Cell 1990;63(6):1137–1147.

26. Vigon I, Mornon JP, Cocault L, et al. Molecular cloning and characterization of MPL, the human homolog of the v-mpl oncogene: identification of a member of the hematopoietic growth factor receptor superfamily. Proc Natl Acad Sci U S A 1992;89(12):5640–5644.

27. Skoda RC, Seldin DC, Chiang MK, et al. Murine c-mpl: a member of the hematopoietic growth factor receptor superfamily that transduces a proliferative signal. Embo J 1993;12(7):2645–2653.

28. Vigon I, Florindo C, Fichelson S, et al. Characterization of the murine Mpl proto-oncogene, a member of the hematopoietic cytokine receptor family: molecular cloning, chromosomal location, and evidence for a function in cell growth. Oncogene 1993;8(10):2607–2615.

29. Fishley B, Alexander WS. Thrombopoietin signalling in physiology and disease. Growth Factors 2004;22(3):151–155.

30. Alexander WS, Roberts AW, Nicola NA, et al. Deficiencies in progenitor cells of multiple hematopoietic lineages and defective megakaryocytopoiesis in mice lacking the thrombopoietic receptor c-Mpl. Blood 1996;87(6): 2162–2170.

31. Stoffel R, Wiestner A, Skoda RC. Thrombopoietin in thrombocytopenic mice: evidence against regulation at the mRNA level and for a direct regulatory role of platelets. Blood 1996;87(2):567–573.

32. de Sauvage FJ, Carver-Moore K, Luoh SM, et al. Physiological regulation of early and late stages of megakaryocytopoiesis by thrombopoietin. J Exp Med 1996;183(2):651–656.

33. Ghilardi N, Wiestner A, Skoda RC. Thrombopoietin production is inhibited by a translational mechanism. Blood 1998;92(11):4023–4030.

34. Kuter DJ, Rosenberg RD. The reciprocal relationship of thrombopoietin (c-Mpl ligand) to changes in the platelet mass during busulfan-induced thrombocytopenia in the rabbit. Blood 1995;85(10):2720–2730.

35. Nagata Y, Shozaki Y, Nagahisa H, et al. Serum thrombopoietin level is not regulated by transcription but by the total counts of both megakaryocytes and platelets during thrombocytopenia and thrombocytosis. Thromb Haemost 1997;77(5): 808–814.

36. Shivdasani RA, Fielder P, Keller GA, et al. Regulation of the serum concentration of thrombopoietin in thrombocytopenic NF-E2 knockout mice. Blood 1997;90(5): 1821–1827.

37. Geddis AE, Fox NE, Kaushansky K. The Mpl receptor expressed on endothelial cells does not contribute significantly to the regulation of circulating thrombopoietin levels. Exp Hematol 2006;34(1):82–86.
38. McCarty JM, Sprugel KH, Fox NE, et al. Murine thrombopoietin mRNA levels are modulated by platelet count. Blood 1995;86(10):3668–3675.
39. Hirayama Y, Sakamaki S, Matsunaga T, et al. Concentrations of thrombopoietin in bone marrow in normal subjects and in patients with idiopathic thrombocytopenic purpura, aplastic anemia, and essential thrombocythemia correlate with its mRNA expression of bone marrow stromal cells. Blood 1998;92(1):46–52.
40. Pastos KM, Slayton WB, Rimsza LM, et al. Differential effects of recombinant thrombopoietin and bone marrow stromal-conditioned media on neonatal versus adult megakaryocytes. Blood 2006;108(10):3360–3362.
41. Du X, Williams DA. Interleukin-11: review of molecular, cell biology, and clinical use. Blood 1997;89(11):3897–3908.
42. Tepler I, Elias L, Smith JW, 2nd, et al. A randomized placebo-controlled trial of recombinant human interleukin-11 in cancer patients with severe thrombocytopenia due to chemotherapy. Blood 1996;87(9):3607–3614.
43. Isaacs C, Robert NJ, Bailey FA, et al. Randomized placebo-controlled study of recombinant human interleukin-11 to prevent chemotherapy-induced thrombocytopenia in patients with breast cancer receiving dose-intensive cyclophosphamide and doxorubicin. J Clin Oncol 1997;15(11):3368–3377.
44. Kurzrock R. Thrombopoietic factors in chronic bone marrow failure states: the platelet problem revisited. Clin Cancer Res 2005;11(4):1361–1367.
45. Li J, Yang C, Xia Y, et al. Thrombocytopenia caused by the development of antibodies to thrombopoietin. Blood 2001;98(12):3241–3248.
46. Basser RL, O'Flaherty E, Green M, et al. Development of pancytopenia with neutralizing antibodies to thrombopoietin after multicycle chemotherapy supported by megakaryocyte growth and development factor. Blood 2002;99(7):2599–2602.
47. Bussel JB, Kuter DJ, George JN, et al. AMG 531, a thrombopoiesis-stimulating protein, for chronic ITP. N Engl J Med 2006;355(16):1672–1681.
48. Kuter DJ. New thrombopoietic growth factors. Blood 2007;109(6):4607–4616.
49. Schulze H, Shivdasani RA. Mechanisms of thrombopoiesis. J Thromb Haemost 2005;3(8):1717–1724.
50. Kirito K, Kaushansky K. Transcriptional regulation of megakaryopoiesis: thrombopoietin signaling and nuclear factors. Curr Opin Hematol 2006;13(3):151–156.
51. Szalai G, LaRue AC, Watson DK. Molecular mechanisms of megakaryopoiesis. Cell Mol Life Sci 2006;63(21):2460–2476.
52. Carpinelli MR, Hilton DJ, Metcalf D, et al. Suppressor screen in Mpl-/- mice: c-Myb mutation causes supraphysiological production of platelets in the absence of thrombopoietin signaling. Proc Natl Acad Sci U S A 2004;101(17):6553–6558.
53. Raslova H, Komura E, Le Couedic JP, et al. FLI1 monoallelic expression combined with its hemizygous loss underlies Paris-Trousseau/Jacobsen thrombopenia. J Clin Invest 2004;114(1):77–84.
54. Prchal J, Sokol, L. Benign erythrocytosis and other familial and congenital polycythemias. Eur J Haematol 1996;57:263–268.
55. Forget B, Degar, BA, Arcasoy MO. Familial polycythemia due to truncations of the erythropoietin receptor. Trans Am Clin Climatol Assoc 2000;111:38–44.

56. Perrine G, Prchal JT, Prchal JF. Study of a polycythemic family. Blood 1977;50:134.
57. Prchal J, Crist W, Goldwasser E, et al. Autosomal dominant polycythemia. Blood 1985;66:1208–1214.
58. Juvonen E, Ikkala E, Fyhrquist F, et al. Autosomal dominant erythrocytosis causes by increased sensitivity to erythropoietin. Blood 1991;78:3066–3069.
59. Emanuel P, Eaves C, Broudy V, et al. Familial and congenital polycythemia in three unrelated families. Blood 1992;79:3019–3030.
60. Queisser W, Heim ME, Schmitz JM, et al. Idiopathic familial erythrocytosis. Report on a family with autosomal dominant inheritance. Dtsch Med Wochenschr 1988;113:851–856.
61. Prchal J, Semenza GL, Prchal J, et al. Familial polycythemia. Science 1995;268: 1831–1832.
62. Sokol L, Kralovics R, Hubbell GL, et al. A novel erythropoietin receptor mutation associated with primary familial polycythemia and severe cardiovascular and peripheral vascular disease. Blood 2001;98. Abstract #937.
63. D'Andrea A, Yoshimura A, Youssoufian H, et al. The cytoplasmic region of the erythropoietin receptor contains non-overlapping positive and negative growth-regulatory domains. Mol Cell Biol 1991;11:1980–1987.
64. Winkelmann J, Penny L, Deaven L, et al. The gene for the human erythropoietin receptor: analysis of the coding sequence and assignment to chromosome 19q. Blood 1990;76:24.
65. Gordeuk VR, Stockton DW, Prchal JT. Congenital polycythemias/erythrocytoses. Haematologica 2005;90(1):109–116.
66. Prchal J. Pathogenetic mechanisms of polycythemia vera and congenital polycythemic disorders. Semin Hematol 2001;38:10–20.
67. Kralovics R, Sokol L, Prchal JT. Absence of polycythemia in a child with a unique erythropoietin receptor mutation in a family with autosomal dominant primary polycythemia. J Clin Invest 1998;102(1):124–129.
68. Wajcman H, Galacteros F. Hemoglobins with high oxygen affinity leading to erythrocytosis. New variants and new concepts. Hemoglobin 2005;29:91–106.
69. Labie D, Leroux JP, Najman A, et al. Familial diphosphoglyceratemutase deficiency. Influence on the oxygen affinity curves of hemoglobin. FEBS Lett 1970;9:37–40.
70. Cartier P, Labie D, Leroux JP, et al. Familial diphosphoglycerate mutase deficiency: hematological and biochemical study. French Nouv Rev Fr Hematol 1972;12: 269–287.
71. Gregg X, Prchal JT. Red cell enzymopathies. In: Hoffman RaB E, ed. Hematology: Basic Principles and Practice, 5th ed. 2007. W. B. Saunders Co., Philadelphia, pp 861–876.
72. Liu E, Percy MJ, Amos CI, et al. The worldwide distribution of the VHL 598 C>T mutation indicates a single founding event. Blood 2004;103:1937–1940.
73. Pastore Y, Jelinek J, Ang S, et al. Mutations in the VHL gene in sporadic apparently congenital polycythemia. Blood 2003;101:1591–1595.
74. Pastore Y, Jedlickova K, Guan Y, et al. Mutations of von Hippel-Lindau tumor-suppressor gene and congenital polycythemia. Am J Hum Genet 2003;73: 412–419.
75. Percy M, McMullin MF, Jowitt SN, et al. Chuvash-type congenital polycythemia in four families of Asian and Western European ancestry. Blood 2003;102:1097–1099.

76. Perrotta S, Nobili B, Ferraro M, et al. Von Hippel-Lindau-dependent polycythemia is endemic on the island of Ischia: identification of a novel cluster. Blood 2006;107(2):514–519.
77. Ang S, Chen H, Hirota K, et al. Disruption of oxygen homeostasis underlies congenital Chuvash polycythemia. Nat Genet 2002;32:614–621.
78. Ang S, Chen H, Gordeuk VR, et al. Endemic polycythemia in Russia: mutation in the VHL gene. Blood Cells Mol Dis 2002;28:57–62.
79. Gordeuk VR, Sergueeva AI, Miasnikova GY, et al. Congenital disorder of oxygen sensing: association of the homozygous Chuvash polycythemia VHL mutation with thrombosis and vascular abnormalities but not tumors. Blood 2004;103(10): 3924–3932.
80. Liu E, Percy MJ, Amos CI, et al. The worldwide distribution of the VHL 598 C>T mutation indicates a single founding event. Blood 2004;103(5):1937–1940.
81. Cario H, Schwarz K, Jorch N, et al. Mutations in the von Hippel-Lindau (VHL) tumor suppressor gene and VHL haplotype analysis in patients with presumable congenital erythrocytosis. Haematologica 2005;90:19–24.
82. Friedrich C. Genotype-phenotype correlation in von Hippel-Lindau syndrome. Hum Mol Genet 2001;10:763–767.
83. Maher E, Webster, AR, Richards FM, et al. Phenotypic expression in von Hippel-Lindau disease: correlations with germline VHL gene mutations. J Med Genet 1996;33:328–332.
84. Maher E. Von Hippel-Lindau disease. Curr Mol Med 2004;4:833–842.
85. Clifford S, Cockman ME, Smallwood AC, et al. Contrasting effects on HIF-1alpha regulation by disease-causing pVHL mutations correlate with patterns of tumourigenesis in von Hippel-Lindau disease. Hum Mol Genet 2001;10:1029–1038.
86. Kondo K, Klco J, Nakamura E, et al. Inhibition of HIF is necessary for tumor suppression by the von Hippel-Lindau protein. Cancer Cell 2002;1:237–246.
87. Turner K, Moore JW, Jones A, et al. Expression of hypoxiainducible factors in human renal cancer: relationship to angiogenesis and to the von Hippel-Lindau gene mutation. Cancer Res 2002;62:2957–2961.
88. Bento M, Chang KT, Guan Y, et al. Congenital polycythemia with homozygous and heterozygous mutations of von Hippel-Lindau gene: five new Caucasian patients. Haematologica 2005;90:128–129.
89. Gordeuk V, Stockton DW, Prchal JT. Congenital polycythemias/erythrocytoses. Haematologica 2005;90:109–116.
90. Percy MJ, Zhao Q, Flores A, et al. A family with erythrocytosis establishes a role for prolyl hydroxylase domain protein 2 in oxygen homeostasis. Proc Natl Acad Sci U S A 2006;103(3):654–659.
91. Maran J, Jedlickova K, Stockton D, et al. Finding the novel molecular defect in a family with high erythropoietin autosomal dominant polycythemia. Blood 2003;102:162b.
92. Gregg X, Prchal JT. Recent advances in the molecular biology of congenital polycythemias and polycythemia vera. Curr Hematol Rep 2005;4:238–242.
93. Balduini CL, Iolascon A, Savoia A. Inherited thrombocytopenias: from genes to therapy. Haematologica 2002;87(8):860–880.
94. Kokame K, Miyata T. Genetic defects leading to hereditary thrombotic thrombocytopenic purpura. Semin Hematol 2004;41(1):34–40.

95. Geddis AE. Inherited thrombocytopenia: congenital amegakaryocytic thrombocytopenia and thrombocytopenia with absent radii. Semin Hematol 2006;43(3): 196–203.
96. Wiestner A, Schlemper RJ, van der Maas AP, et al. An activating splice donor mutation in the thrombopoietin gene causes hereditary thrombocythaemia. Nature Genet 1998;18(1):49–52.
97. Kondo T, Okabe M, Sanada M, et al. Familial essential thrombocythemia associated with one-base deletion in the 5'-untranslated region of the thrombopoietin gene. Blood 1998;92(4):1091–1096.
98. Ghilardi N, Wiestner A, Kikuchi M, et al. Hereditary thrombocythemia in a Japanese family is caused by a novel point mutation in the thrombopoietin gene. Br J Haematol 1999;107:310–316.
99. Ghilardi N, Skoda RC. A single-base deletion in the thrombopoietin (TPO) gene causes familial essential thrombocytosis through a mechanism of more efficient translation of TPO mRNA [letter]. Blood 1999;94(4):1480–1482.
100. Jorgensen MJ, Raskind WH, Wolff JF, et al. Familial thrombocytosis associated with overproduction of thrombopoietin due to a novel splice donor site mutation. Blood 1998;92(suppl 1):205a. Abstract.
101. Harrison CN, Gale RE, Wiestner AC, et al. The activating splice mutation in intron 3 of the thrombopoietin gene is not found in patients with non-familial essential thrombocythaemia. Br J Haematol 1998;102(5):1341–1343.
102. Komatsu H, Ding J, Iida M, et al. Familial essentian thrombocythemia associated with a dominant positive acting mutation of the c-MPL gene, which encodes for the receptor for thrombopoietin. Blood 2003;102(11):29.
103. Kitamura T, Onishi M, Yahata T, et al. Activating mutations of the transmembrane domain of MPL in vitro and in vivo: incorrect sequence of MPL-K, an alternative spliced form of MPL [letter]. Blood 1998;92(7):2596–2597.
104. Kunishima S, Mizuno S, Naoe T, et al. Genes for thrombopoietin and c-Mpl are not responsible for familial thrombocythaemia: a case study. Br J Haematol 1998;100(2):383–386.
105. Wiestner A, Padosch SA, Ghilardi N, et al. Hereditary thrombocythaemia is a genetically heterogeneous disorder: exclusion of TPO and MPL in two families with hereditary thrombocythaemia. Br J Haematol 2000;110(1):104–109.
106. Bellanne-Chantelot C, Chaumarel I, Labopin M, et al. Genetic and clinical implications of the Val617Phe JAK2 mutation in 72 families with myeloproliferative disorders. Blood 2006;108(1):346–352.
107. Tecuceanu N, Dardik R, Rabizadeh E, et al. A family with hereditary thrombocythaemia and normal genes for thrombopoietin and c-Mpl. Br J Haematol 2006;135(3):348–351.

5

Management of Polycythemia Vera

Shireen Sirhan

Department of Hematology, McGill University, Montreal, Quebec, Canada

Richard T. Silver

Leukemia and Myeloproliferative Disease Center, Division of Hematology-Oncology, Weill Medical College of Cornell University, New York, New York, U.S.A.

INTRODUCTION

Polycythemia vera (PV) is one of the three Philadelphia chromosome (Ph)-negative myeloproliferative disorders (MPDs) distinguished from the other two, essential thrombocythemia (ET) and primary myelofibrosis (PMF), because of clonal erythrocytosis (1). All three represent stem cell-derived, tri-lineage clonal myeloproliferation, and disease transformation from either PV or ET into a PMF-like phenotype (i.e., post-PV or post-ET MF) may occur (2).

In early 2005, several groups of investigators described a novel Janus kinase 2 (JAK2) mutation (*JAK2V617F*) in association with PV, ET, and PMF (3–6). The majority of subsequent studies that used sensitive detection methods suggest that *JAK2V617F* is found in more than 95% of the patients with PV and approximately 50% of those with either ET or PMF (7,8). Moreover, both JAK2 alleles are mutated in approximately 25% of the PV cases, whereas such homozygous mutation pattern is unusual in either ET or PMF (9). It is now well established that *JAK2V617F* is also present in a substantial minority of the patients with atypical MPDs (10) and the myelodysplastic syndromes (MDS) (8,10,11), including refractory anemia with ringed sideroblasts and thrombocytosis (RARS-T) (12). Therefore, *JAK2V617F* is a sensitive, but not specific, marker for PV. This, however, does not mitigate its diagnostic utility because the mutation is absent in healthy individuals (unless supersensitive assays are used) and in those with lymphoid neoplasms, metastatic cancer, or reactive myeloproliferation, including secondary polycythemia (13).

Most recently, other JAK2 mutations (i.e., JAK2 exon 12 mutations) have been described in *JAK2V617F*-negative PV/idiopathic erythrocytosis but neither in ET nor in PMF (14). A different mutation, MPLW515L/K, was described in PMF and ET but not in PV (15,16). Therefore, in PV, JAK2 mutations appear to be an essential component of the pathogenesis of the disease even though they may not represent the original clonogenic event (17). *JAK2V617F* is an exon 14 G to T somatic mutation (nucleotide position 1849) resulting in the substitution of valine to phenylalanine in codon 617. Finally, *JAK2V617F* is not differently distributed in "familial MPD," as opposed to sporadic PV, suggesting that *JAK2V617F* is acquired in familial MPD as well (18).

CLINICAL MANIFESTATIONS OF POLYCYTHEMIA VERA

Thrombosis, bleeding, leukemic transformation, and development of post-PV MF are considered life-threatening complications of PV, whereas pruritus, constitutional symptoms, abdominal discomfort from splenomegaly, and microvascular disturbances, such as erythromelalgia and headaches, primarily affect quality of life. In addition, various symptoms reported by patients with PV can be attributed to hyperviscosity; these include neurological complaints, such as headaches, dizziness, visual disturbances, and ocular migraine.

Thrombosis in PV involves both small and large and venous or arterial vessels. Most investigators consider cerebrovascular accidents, transient ischemic attacks, myocardial infarction, angina pectoris, peripheral artery occlusions, pulmonary embolism, and deep vein thrombosis as major thrombotic events (19–21). Deep vein thrombosis in PV includes abdominal vein thrombosis (AVT), sometimes with catastrophic consequences. PV-associated AVT might be underreported since a substantial proportion of "idiopathic" AVT might represent latent PV or other MPDs, as has been recently indicated by *JAK2V617F* mutational analysis of such cases (22–24). Superficial thrombophlebitis and microvascular disturbances such as erythromelalgia are considered inflammatory, rather than thrombotic, events since they represent a separate platelet-vessel pathology that often responds to aspirin therapy (25). However, some investigators consider these events as well as recurrent fetal loss and intrauterine growth retardation as consequences of thrombotic complications (26). Bleeding in PV occurs less frequently than thrombosis and has been linked to an acquired von Willebrand syndrome in the presence of extreme thrombocytosis (27).

Tables 1 (at diagnosis) and 2 (during follow-up) present incidence figures of "major" thrombotic, bleeding, and microvascular events in a selected series of large studies in PV. The incidence of major thrombosis at diagnosis ranges from 34% to 38.6% and during follow-up from 8.1% to 19% (Tables 1 and 2). Arterial events are generally twice as prevalent as venous events (31). Also, thrombosis

Table 1 Thrombotic, Hemorrhagic, and Microvascular Events in Polycythemia Vera (PV) Reported at Diagnosis

References	n	Major thrombosis (%)	Major arterial thrombosis[a] (%)	Major venous thrombosis[a] (%)	MVD (%)	Total bleeds (%) [major (%)]
(28)[b]	1213	34	~66[b]	~33[b]	NA	NA
(29)	163	34	64	36	24	3 [NA]
(21)	1638	38.6	~75	~25	5.3	8.1 [4.8]

Source: Modified from Ref. 32.
[a]% of total major thrombotic events.
[b]Estimate per Gruppo Italiano Studio Policitemia (GISP).
Abbreviations: MVD, microvascular disturbances; NA, not available.

Table 2 Thrombotic and Hemorrhagic Events in Polycythemia Vera (PV) Reported at Follow-Up

References	n	Major thrombosis (%)	Major arterial thrombosis (%)[a]	Major venous thrombosis (%)[a]	Total bleeds (%) [major (%)]	% of deaths from hemorrhage	% of deaths from thrombosis
(28)	1213	19	62.5	37.5	NA	2.6	29.6
(29)	163	18.4	80	15	NA [1.8%]	6	19
(21)	1638	13.4	57.1	42.9	2.9% [0.8%]	4.3	41
(30)	396	8.1	59.4	40.6	NA	2	20

Source: Modified from Ref. 32.
[a]Percent of total major thrombotic events.

is more relevant than bleeding as a cause of death in these disorders (Table 2). However, in a smaller series of 55 patients from a single institution, meticulous attention to hematocrit levels, platelet count, and associated medical factors, such as diabetes, hypertension, and avoidance of birth control pills, can significantly reduce this risk to virtually zero (33).

Advanced age, history of thrombosis, and tobacco use have been identified as risk factors for thrombosis in PV (34). Most recently, leukocytosis has been implicated as an additional thrombogenic feature in PV. In a recent report (35) leukocytosis > 15×10^9/L, as opposed to ≤ 10×10^9/L, was identified as an independent predictor of myocardial infarction. [Other studies have also implicated leukocytosis as a significant risk factor for thrombosis in ET as well (19,36)]. This potential thrombogenic relevance of leukocytosis is consistent with the proven antithrombotic activity of hydroxyurea (HU) in both ET and PV (37,38) as well as the fact that granulocytes in PV display increased baseline/induced platelet P-selectin expression, platelet-granulocyte/platelet-monocyte complexes,

Table 3   Risk-Based Treatment Algorithm in Polycythemia Vera

Risk category	Variables	Treatment
Low risk	Age below 60 years *and* no history of thrombosis	Phlebotomy + Aspirin[a] (81 mg/day)
High risk	Age 60 years or older *or* a positive history of thrombosis or high phlebotomy requirements	Phlebotomy + Aspirin[a] + Hydroxyurea[b] *or* interferon-alpha (rIFN-α)

[a]In the absence of aspirin contraindications.
[b]Substitute interferon-alpha for hydroxyurea in women of childbearing potential (see text for more elaboration).

granulocyte activation, and baseline/lipopolysaccharide-induced expression of tissue factor by both monocytes and neutrophils (39).

One of the most troubling and poorly explained symptoms associated with PV is aquagenic pruritus, which occurs in some patients during the course of their disease (40). This particular symptom can sometimes become severe enough to prevent patients from taking daily showers and also interferes with their social activities. Interferon (rIFN-α) is the only medication, which will reliably reduce the intensity of and relieve the symptoms in most cases. Leukemic transformation in PV is a dreaded complication with no effective therapy (41). The incidence is estimated at approximately 5–10% in the first 10 years of the disease and at least twice as much in the second decade of the disease (42). This particular complication is primarily attributed to the intrinsic biology of the disease and is further modified by modern therapeutic agents. The relative contribution is open to debate and will be elaborated in a later section.

RISK STRATIFICATION IN POLYCYTHEMIA VERA

Data emanating from a series of studies performed by the European Collaboration on Low-dose Aspirin in Polycythemia Vera (ECLAP) have confirmed the heterogeneity among PV patients in terms of their risk of thrombosis (21). Accordingly, two distinct categories are identified (Table 3). The two most recognized risk factors for thrombosis in PV are advanced age (> 60–70 years) and a prior vascular event. The presence of either one of these characteristics puts the patient into a high-risk category and their absence in a low-risk category. In the low-risk disease, the presence of either extreme thrombocytosis (defined variably as above 1000×10^9/L or 1500×10^9/L) or cardiovascular risk factors (e.g. smoking, diabetes mellitus, hypertension, hypercholesterolemia, congestive heart failure, and the use of birth control pills) is considered by us to be sufficiently important to upgrade risk to an "intermediate" status, although, the prognostic relevance of either cardiovascular risk factors or extreme thrombocytosis in PV, in terms of thrombosis risk, has not been proved. Regardless, the physician should aggressively manage the risk factors mentioned (43,44). Attention to such details has yielded a median thrombosis-free survival of at least 10 years in one study (33). This includes screening for acquired von Willebrand syndrome before instituting aspirin therapy in the presence of extreme thrombocytosis (27). The platelet count in PV, by itself, has not yet been correlated with thrombosis risk (45,46). On the other hand, recent information suggests that leukocytosis might contribute to the risk of thrombosis and this particular possibility should be explored further in larger studies (35).

MANAGEMENT OF POLYCYTHEMIA VERA

PV is a rare disease, with an incidence of 2 per 100,000 (47). Accordingly, the number of randomized controlled trials assessing various treatment modalities in this disease is limited. Evidence for the management of the patient with PV is based on a combination of a few randomized controlled trials, a larger number of prospective cohort and observational studies, and indirect evidence extrapolated from studies performed on patients with ET (48). Current consensus favors the use of both phlebotomy and daily aspirin (40–100 mg), in the absence of contraindications to aspirin use, in all patients with PV, regardless of risk category (49,50). Such therapy is usually considered adequate for low-risk disease. Early randomized clinical trials have demonstrated the value of cytoreductive therapy in preventing thrombosis at the early stages of the disease, especially in those with high-risk disease (50). However, certain drugs, such as chlorambucil and radiophosphorus (32p), were shown to increase the risk of leukemic transformation and their replacement with less leukemogenic drugs has not been evaluated in a controlled randomized study in PV (51). Regardless, nonrandomized studies have suggested that both HU and interferon alfa (rIFN-α) might confer protection from thrombosis without being leukemogenic (52–54). As such, high-risk PV patients are currently treated with either one of these two agents to minimize their risk of thrombosis (Table 3). The decision to treat low-risk disease associated with either extreme thrombocytosis or with cardiovascular risk factors with cytoreductive therapy is made on an individual basis, taking into consideration such factors as proliferative symptoms, pregnancy plans, and patient preference.

In addition to the above-stated risk-adapted approach to the use of cytoreductive therapy in PV, certain instances might require the institution of cytoreductive therapy for proliferative symptoms in the absence of adverse risk factors for thrombosis. Such instances include the presence of severe iron deficiency, progressive and symptomatic splenomegaly, drenching night sweats, or other hypercatabolic symptoms or frequency of phlebotomy.

SPECIFIC TREATMENT MODALITIES IN POLYCYTHEMIA VERA

Phlebotomy

Phlebotomy has long been the mainstay of treatment for PV and was recommended by Osler as early as the beginning of the twentieth century (55). The Polycythemia

Vera Study Group (PVSG) conducted their first study (PVSG-01) in 1967 (50); this is the only randomized trial comparing phlebotomy alone with phlebotomy combined with myelosuppressive therapy. Patients were randomized to three arms: phlebotomy, phlebotomy and 32p, or phlebotomy and chlorambucil. Although the results revealed an increase in the incidence of thrombosis in the first three years in the phlebotomy-alone arm, a significant overall survival advantage in patients treated with phlebotomy only was also seen: median survivals of 13.9, 11.8, and 8.9 years for each of the aforementioned treatment arms, respectively. This study reinforced the perceived value of phlebotomy as the cornerstone of therapy in PV, since older studies had suggested a median survival of less than 2 years without phlebotomy (43,56).

The optimal hematocrit target in PV has never been addressed in a controlled fashion. Regardless, many investigators, including us, recommend a hematocrit target of < 45% in men and < 42% in women (57), based primarily on data showing a progressive increase in the incidence of vascular occlusive episodes at hematocrit levels higher than 44% (58) and changes in blood viscosity above 45% (59). This particular notion is supported by laboratory studies showing suboptimal cerebral blood flow at a higher hematocrit level (60). The lower hematocrit target in women is derived from the physiological difference between sexes, rather than direct evidence (61). However, a recent ECLAP study of PV patients, most of whom were receiving aspirin as part of their treatment, did not reveal differences in thrombosis incidence across the range of hematocrit between 45% and 50% (21). A recent physician survey indicated that 16% of US hematologists aim for 50% as their preferred target hematocrit (62), whereas the same target is sought after by 20% of Swedish hematologists (63). We believe, nevertheless, as do others (64), that it is prudent to err on the side of caution and target a lower hematocrit of 45% for men and 42% for women (57).

Cytoreductive Therapy

Much controversy remains regarding the cytoreductive drug of choice in PV (65). The main issue has revolved around drug leukemogenicity. Is the propensity to develop acute leukemia in patients with PV inherent to the disease, a consequence of the therapies administered, or a combination of both? The concern regarding leukemogenic risk of therapy in PV was raised long before the publication of the PVSG-01 study (66). The PVSG-01 study confirmed the anecdotal concerns in a randomized fashion (50). While an increase in acute myelogenous leukemia (AML) was noted in the groups treated with either chlorambucil or P32, the incidence of AML in the phlebotomy-only treated patients was 1.5% in the first decade of the disease. This was regarded as the disease-intrinsic rate at which PV is expected to transform into AML. On the other hand, the rate in the 32P- and chlorambucil-treated patients was 5.2% and 13%, respectively. The PVSG subsequently carried out a nonrandomized prospective study using HU as the myelosuppressive agent supplementing phlebotomy and reported an increased incidence of AML (9.8%) compared to that observed in a historical control group of patients treated with phlebotomy only (3.7%) (53); this was not considered to be statistically significant (53). Comparing two noncontemporaneous studies to determine relative risk of leukemia for HU is obviously statistically fallacious. The observation that underlies the current concern regarding the leukemogenicity of the use of HU in both PV and ET, even in more recent studies, are not adequate since the median duration of follow up was 2–4 years, an inadequate duration to determine leukemogenicity or not (30,54).

Hydroxyurea

HU is an antimetabolite that interferes with DNA synthesis by inhibiting the enzyme ribonucleotide reductase. Its effects include dose-related bone marrow suppression leading to macrocytic anemia, neutropenia, and thrombocytopenia. Its use is also associated with ulcerations of the oral mucosa and the skin, particularly the lower extremities, and nail discoloration (67). In the last report by the PVSG in 1997 (53), a group of 51 patients were treated with HU in a prospective nonrandomized fashion and displayed fewer incidences of myelofibrosis and total death as compared to historical controls (7.8% vs. 12.7% and 39.2% vs. 55.2%, respectively). Despite this fallacious statistical comparison previously mentioned, HU became the most commonly used cytoreductive agent in the treatment of PV. However, the concern emanating from the aforementioned PVSG study has led to continued surveillance since then and has resulted in the search for alternative agents.

The Gruppo Italiano Studio Policitemia (GISP) described the natural history of PV in a group of more than 1000 patients, followed for 20 years (56). The particular study did not reveal an association between single-agent HU use and incidence of post-PV AML. However the incidence of AML was significantly higher in patients exposed to HU as well as other alkylating drugs. Most other studies have arrived at similar conclusions (31,54). To date, the largest cohort prospectively assessed for this issue is that of the ECLAP study, which followed 1638 patients for more than 6 years (21). HU-alone treatment in the particular study did not appear to enhance the risk of leukemic transformation, in comparison with patients treated with phlebotomy only [hazard ratio 0.86, 95% confidence interval (CI) 0.26–2.88; $p = 0.8$]. On the other hand, the incidence of AML was significantly higher in patients exposed to HU and alkylating agents or 32p (hazard ratio 7.58, 95% CI 1.85–31; $p = 0.0048$).

Evidence for the efficacy of HU in reducing thrombotic events in PV is mostly translated from randomized controlled trials in ET. In the first of these ET studies, 114 patients were randomized to either HU or no cytoreductive therapy; the HU arm displayed a significant reduction in the rate of thrombosis as compared to the control group (1.6%/patient year vs. 10.7%/patient year; $p = 0.003$) (68). In the second ET study, 809 patients were randomized to either HU or anagrelide, each combined with low-dose aspirin therapy (20). At a median follow-up of 39 months, treatment with HU plus aspirin was associated with decreased rates of arterial thrombosis ($p = 0.004$), serious hemorrhage ($p = 0.008$), and progression to myelofibrosis ($p = 0.01$). However, an increased rate of venous thrombosis was observed in the HU arm (14 vs. 3 cases; $p = 0.006$) and the explanation remains elusive. The composite end point (i.e., risk of arterial thrombosis, venous thrombosis, serious hemorrhage, or death from thrombotic or hemorrhagic causes) was reached in only 36 patients in the HU arm versus 56 patients in the anagrelide arm ($p = 0.03$).

The only randomized study investigating HU in PV was carried out in France, and it randomized patients to treatment with either HU or pipobroman (69). Pipobroman is similar in structure to alkylating agents, but its mechanism of action differs in that it also involves competition with pyrimidine bases. In this study, no significant differences were observed in overall survival or rate of thrombosis, but the incidence of secondary leukemia in both arms of the study was approximately 10% at 13 years.

Taking the results of all the above, it can be concluded that HU is efficacious in controlling the hematocrit level and reducing the thrombotic complications in PV. The majority of the evidence suggestively supports a leukemogenic role if its use is continued for more than 10 years. It is prudent to avoid using this drug in patients previously exposed to alkylating agents and in women who are pregnant or planning a pregnancy in the near future.

Interferon-α

Interferon-α (rIFN-α) is characterized by several properties that make it a potentially efficacious therapeutic agent in the management of PV. It has myelosuppressive effects and in vitro inhibits erythroid progenitors and erythroid burst-forming units (70). The effects of rIFN-α extend to megakaryocytes where the drug inhibits progenitor cell proliferation and reduces thrombopoietin-induced Mpl receptor signaling (71). rIFN-α antagonizes the action of several cytokines, including platelet-derived growth factor (PDGF), transforming growth factor-beta, and basic fibroblast growth factor, which are implicated in the pathogenesis of myelofibrosis (72). In addition, the drug is not known to be leukemogenic or teratogenic.

Evidence for the use of rIFN-α in PV is derived mostly from single-center series (33,52,73–76). A review published in 2000 analyzed the cumulative experience with rIFN-α from 16 studies (77). Based on the 279 patients included, it was found that there was a 50% overall response rate for hematocrit reduction to < 45% without the need for concomitant phlebotomies. The review also showed a 77% reduction in spleen size, and a 75% decrease in pruritus. The most recent and largest series with long-term follow-up was published in 2006 (32). Fifty-five patients with PV, previously treated with either phlebotomy alone or phlebotomy and HU, were followed for a median of 13 years. Within 1–2 years of treatment with rIFN-α, the majority of the patients reached a complete response defined by a hematocrit less than 45% without phlebotomy and a platelet count below 600×10^9/L. The spleen size also decreased in 90% of the patients with splenomegaly. Remarkably, no thrombohemorrhagic events were reported during the follow-up period. Starting and maintenance doses in the particular study were 1 and 3 million units three-times-a-week, respectively (33).

rIFN-α needs to be administered parentally and its use is mostly limited by the frequent occurrence of side effects; the most frequent in this regard are flu-like symptoms. More severe rIFN-α side effects include myalgias, weight loss, and depression and their occurrence might lead to treatment withdrawal rates approaching 40% (77). However, most recent series report adverse drop-out rates of as low as 15% (33). Moreover, the newer semisynthetic pegylated forms might have a more favorable side-effect profile.

There is no doubt that rIFN-α treatment in PV is very promising, and is based on plausible biological effects. Furthermore, recent observations suggest that treatment of PV with rIFN-α decreases *JAK2V617F* allele burden, although not to a significant extent, nor is it comparable to that seen with imatinib mesylate (IM) therapy for CML (78–79). Regardless, the drug needs to be evaluated in larger controlled trials to study long-term clinical outcomes and its advantage over HU therapy. For now, rIFN-α is the treatment of choice for childbearing women with PV and in the presence of intractable pruritus (80) and should be considered for all patients under the age of 65 years who require cytoreductive therapy. We have found it to be particularly effective in patients with progressive splenomegaly and a hypercellular bone marrow with little evidence of fibrosis.

Busulfan

Busulfan is an alkylating agent; its use in PV in recent years has not been widespread. Busulfan was studied in a randomized clinical trial by the European Organization for Research and Treatment of Cancer between 1967 and 1978 (81). In one particular study, 293 PV patients were randomized to treatment with either busulfan or 32P. The 10-year survival was higher in the busulfan arm of the study (70% vs. 55%; $p = 0.02$) because of mainly the lower number of vascular deaths. There was no difference in the rates of progression to AML or myelofibrosis between the two groups. In addition, several single-arms studies have evaluated busulfan in the treatment of PV, including a single-center, retrospective study of 65 patients where overall median survival was reported at 11.1 years; AML incidence was 3% (82). Side effects of busulfan include hyperpigmentation, protracted pancytopenia, and pulmonary fibrosis in occasional cases (83). There is also concern regarding drug leukemogenicity, although this has not been proven in a controlled study in PV. We currently favor the use of busulfan as secondary therapy in elderly patients with a life expectancy not exceeding 10 years, only if they fail treatment with HU.

Radiophosphorous (32p)

The use of 32p for the treatment of PV was introduced in 1932 (84). As mentioned in a previous section, the PVSG-01 trial demonstrated significantly higher rates of transformation to AML in patients treated with 32p as opposed to those treated with phlebotomy alone (50). An incidence of AML up to 15% was noted in some randomized trials (43,85). Our view in regard to the use of 32P in PV is similar to that stated above for busulfan—salvage therapy after failing HU in elderly patients, especially in the presence of a < 10-year life expectancy and/or compliance issues.

Anagrelide

Anagrelide is an imidazoquinazoline derivative; it inhibits cyclic nucleotide phosphodiesterase and the release of arachidonic acid from phospholipase. At concentrations higher than those used clinically, the drug inhibits platelet aggregation. At therapeutic concentrations, it displays a species-specific platelet-lowering effect in humans (86). In a study of 577 patients with MPD anagrelide therapy substantially reduced the platelet count in over 80% of the patients with PV (87). However, meaningful health outcome has not been evaluated in a controlled study. Furthermore, anagrelide is associated with some serious, albeit rare, side effects such as nonischemic cardiomyopathy (88,89). Additional limiting factors include the results of a recent randomized clinical trail in 809 patients with ET where the patients receiving anagrelide therapy experienced significantly higher rates of arterial thrombosis, serious hemorrhage, and fibrotic transformation (20). Since the platelet count in PV has not been shown to be an independent risk factor for thrombosis (45,46), the role of anagrelide in the treatment of PV remains uncertain. On a high risk patient with a significant increase in platelets in whom asprin is contraindicated, anagrelide may be considered.

Imatinib Mesylate

The use of imatinib mesylate for the treatment of PV has been investigated in some pilot studies. It is a selective and potent inhibitor of tyrosine kinase with significant activity against BCR-ABL, PDGFR, and KIT. In one of the very first studies using IM in PV, 7 patients were treated for approximately 6 months (90). Phlebotomy requirements decreased in 6 of the 7 patients and spleen size in 2 patients. However, thrombocytosis was not controlled despite increased drug doses in 3 patients and 1 patient experienced grade 3 drug-induced dermatitis (90). A recent report of 23 cases of PV, where the patients were given IM therapy, complete remission (phlebotomy-free, normal platelet count, no splenomegaly) was observed in only 22% of the study patients (90–92). Furthermore, IM therapy is suboptimal in reducing *JAK2V617F* allele burden in PV, although marked reductions are sometimes witnessed (77,93).

Antiplatelet Therapy

The use of aspirin as a part of the treatment algorithm for PV fell out of favor in the 1980s largely because of a study conducted by the PVSG; high doses of aspirin (900 mg/day) combined with dipyridamole caused excessive bleeding complications (94). In 1997, the GISP designed a pilot study on the safety of low-dose aspirin (40 mg/day): 112 PV patients with no clear indications or contraindications to aspirin were randomized to low-dose aspirin or placebo. The study confirmed the safety of low-dose aspirin in terms of bleeding complications and led to a larger, phase-III study (95). The ECLAP group (49), carried out a randomized double-blind, placebo-controlled study in order to address both the safety and the efficacy of low-dose aspirin (100 mg) in a larger cohort of PV patients. The study enrolled 518 patients without a clear indication or contraindication to aspirin. Median age at recruitment was 61 years and 59% of the patients were males. The cohort was followed for a median of 2.8 years. The aspirin group had a significantly lower risk of the primary combined endpoint of cardiovascular death, nonfatal myocardial infarction, nonfatal stroke, and major venous thromboembolism (relative risk 0.4, 95% CI 0.18–0.91; $p < 0.0277$) (49). The incidence of major bleeding episodes was not significantly increased in the aspirin group (relative risk, 1.62; 95% CI 0.27–9.71). Following the results of this study, low-dose aspirin is now recommended in all the patients with PV who have no contraindication to its use. Aspirin is also an effective treatment for some of the other manifestations of PV, such as erythromelalgia and ocular migraines (96).

Management of Pruritus in Polycythemia Vera

Although not life-threatening, pruritus in PV can severely compromise quality of life. Pathogenesis of PV-associated pruritus is not known, although histamines (97,98), mast cells (99), platelet activation, and platelet release of prostaglandins and serotonin (100) have all been implicated. Antihistamines are often used as first-line treatment, but their effect is minor with variable response rates (40,101). A recent study demonstrated the efficacy of a serotonin reuptake inhibitor, paroxetine, with a response rate of over 80% (102). Similarly favorable results have been reported with rIFN-α treatment (33,40,103). Therefore, in the presence of high-risk disease, rIFN-α might be selected as a treatment of choice for the patient with intractable pruritus whereas paroxetine can be considered for pruritus associated with low-risk disease (43).

Management of Polycythemia Vera During Pregnancy

Information on pregnancy in PV is very limited and comes mostly from small series of case reports. This is partly due to the rarity of the disease in younger age groups; only 15% of the patients with PV are below the age of 40 years at diagnosis (47). The estimated incidence of PV in women between ages 20 years and 34 years is 0.04 per 100,000 (104). Some of the evidence is also extrapolated from ET; where pregnancy is a more common event due to the higher prevalence of the disease amongst young women (105).

In a comprehensive review of the literature on pregnancy in PV (26), a total of 36 pregnancies in 18 patients were reported, with a live birth rate of 58%. It is worth noting that 11 of these pregnancies were prior to 1970, before the results of the PVSG studies were published (26). Most of the fetal complications were due to either early pregnancy loss or intrauterine growth restriction (26). It is assumed

Table 4   Management of Polycythemia Vera During Pregnancy

Have patient followed by an obstetrician experienced in high-risk pregnancies, in addition
    to the hematologist.
Discontinue drugs with potential teratogenic activity. These include hydroxyurea and
    instead, use interferon alpha for high-risk disease.
The hematocrit should be kept at the normal range, by phlebotomy, expected for the stage
    of gestation.
All patients should be started on low dose aspirin prior to pregnancy and treatment should
    continue during the pregnancy and after delivery, in the absence of contraindications.
The use of cytoreductive medications should be avoided in low-risk patients.
The drug of choice for high-risk disease, based on anecdotal evidence of safety, is rIFN-α.
The use of low–molecular-weight heparin (LMWH) in pregnant PV patients is
    controversial. Regardless, it is reasonable to consider LMWH therapy, at a prophylactic
    dose range, in patients with previous history of thrombosis and for the treatment to
    continue until 6 weeks postpartum. Some investigators also recommend LMWH in all
    PV patients, regardless of risk category, in the 6 weeks postpartum.
Fetal monitoring with serial ultrasound scans and frequent Doppler studies to assess
    placental function are advised.

that these complications arise from placental dysfunction similar to that found
in other thrombophilias (26,106,107). Less common complications included late
pregnancy loss, abruptio placentae, and pre-eclampsia (107,108). Maternal morbidity varies between series, depending on the management strategies applied. In
some series, significant maternal morbidity included major thrombotic or hemorrhagic events (26). A review published in 2005 describing 36 pregnancies reported
maternal complications in 22% of the pregnancies: 1 death due to disseminated
intravascular coagulation and a pulmonary embolus, 2 pulmonary emboli, 1 postpartum hemorrhage, and 4 cases of pre-eclampsia (26). However, in another study,
maternal morbidity was not as pronounced with a pulmonary embolus occurring in
1 patient and pre-eclampsia in 3 of 18 pregnancies (109). In the most recently published series of 18 pregnancies in 8 women with PV (109), aggressive management
was credited for improved fetal and maternal outcomes. Current recommendations
for the management of PV during pregnancy are not necessarily evidence-based
they aspire to minimize complication for both the fetus and mother by extrap-
olating information from the literature on the management of ET and inherited
thrombophilias in pregnancy and from the experience from some case series dis-
cussing specific management algorithms (Table 4) (28).

CONCLUDING REMARKS

The discovery of the *JAK2V617F* mutation has revolutionized the field of MPDs
and has identified JAK2 as a legitimate drug target (110–113). Accordingly, specific JAK2-inhibiting small molecules are currently under development and hold
the long anticipated promise of molecularly targeted therapies in PV. Quantitative

JAK2V617F allele burden measurement assays are currently available and should serve a useful function during laboratory correlative studies of anti-JAK2 clinical trials. In the meantime, it is important to emphasize that modern therapy has significantly extended life expectancy in PV with median survival estimates of more than 15 years (31). Similarly, the combination of cytoreductive and antiplatelet therapies have managed to keep the disease-specific risk of thrombosis below 10% in most patients. However, the long-term complications of leukemic or fibrotic transformation remain unaffected by the current therapy and it is this aspect of the disease that requires the most attention at the present time, in our opinion.

REFERENCES

1. Dameshek W. Some speculations on the myeloproliferative syndromes. Blood 1951;6:372–375.
2. Adamson JW, Fialkow PJ, Murphy S, et al. Polycythemia vera: stem-cell and probable clonal origin of the disease. N Engl J Med 1976;295:913–916.
3. Baxter EJ, Scott LM, Campbell PJ, et al. Acquired mutation of the tyrosine kinase JAK2 in human myeloproliferative disorders. Lancet 2005;365:1054–1061.
4. Levine RL, Wadleigh M, Cools J, et al. Activating mutation in the tyrosine kinase JAK2 in polycythemia vera, essential thrombocythemia, and myeloid metaplasia with myelofibrosis. Cancer Cell 2005;7:387–397.
5. Kralovics R, Passamonti F, Buser AS, et al. A gain of function mutation in JAK2 is frequently found in patients with myeloproliferative disorders. N Engl J Med 2005;352:1779–1790.
6. James C, Ugo V, Le Couedic JP, et al. A unique clonal JAK2 mutation leading to constitutive signalling causes polycythaemia vera. Nature 2005;434:1144–1148.
7. Tefferi A, Pardanani A. Mutation screening for JAK2V617F: when to order the test and how to interpret the results. Leuk Res 2006;30:739–744.
8. Vizmanos JL, Ormazabal C, Larrayoz MJ, et al. JAK2 V617F mutation in classic chronic myeloproliferative diseases: a report on a series of 349 patients. Leukemia 2006;20:534–535.
9. Scott LM, Scott MA, Campbell PJ, et al. Progenitors homozygous for the V617F mutation occur in most patients with polycythemia vera, but not essential thrombocythemia. Blood 2006;108:2435–2437.
10. Jones AV, Kreil S, Zoi K, et al. Widespread occurrence of the JAK2 V617F mutation in chronic myeloproliferative disorders. Blood 2005;106:2162–2168.
11. Steensma DP, Dewald GW, Lasho TL, et al. The JAK2 V617F activating tyrosine kinase mutation is an infrequent event in both "atypical" myeloproliferative disorders and myelodysplastic syndromes. Blood 2005;106:1207–1209.
12. Ceesay MM, Lea NC, Ingram W, et al. The JAK2 V617F mutation is rare in RARS but common in RARS-T. Leukemia 2006;20:2060–2061.
13. Tefferi A, Gilliland DG. The JAK2V617F tyrosine kinase mutation in myeloproliferative disorders: status report and immediate implications for disease classification and diagnosis. Mayo Clin Proc 2005;80:947–958.

14. Scott LM, Tong W, Levine R, et al. JAK2 exon 12 mutations in polycythemia vera and idiopathic erythrocytosis. N Engl J Med 2007;356:459–468.

15. Pikman Y, Lee BH, Mercher T, et al. MPLW515L is a novel somatic activating mutation in myelofibrosis with myeloid metaplasia. PLoS Med 2006;3:e270.

16. Pardanani AD, Levine RL, Lasho T, et al. MPL515 mutations in myeloproliferative and other myeloid disorders: a study of 1182 patients. Blood 2006;108: 3472–3476.

17. Kralovics R, Teo SS, Li S, et al. Acquisition of the V617F mutation of JAK2 is a late genetic event in a subset of patients with myeloproliferative disorders. Blood 2006;108:1377–1380.

18. Bellanne-Chantelot C, Chaumarel I, Labopin M, et al. Genetic and clinical implications of the Val617Phe JAK2 mutation in 72 families with myeloproliferative disorders. Blood 2006;108:346–352.

19. Wolanskyj AP, Schwager SM, McClure RF, et al. Essential thrombocythemia beyond the first decade: life expectancy, long-term complication rates, and prognostic factors. Mayo Clin Proc 2006;81:159–166.

20. Harrison CN, Campbell PJ, Buck G, et al. Hydroxyurea compared with anagrelide in high-risk essential thrombocythemia. N Engl J Med 2005;353:33–45.

21. Marchioli R, Finazzi G, Landolfi R, et al. Vascular and neoplastic risk in a large cohort of patients with polycythemia vera. J Clin Oncol 2005;23:2224–2232.

22. Patel RK, Lea NC, Heneghan MA, et al. Prevalence of the activating JAK2 tyrosine kinase mutation V617F in the Budd-Chiari syndrome. Gastroenterology 2006;130:2031–2038.

23. Colaizzo D, Amitrano L, Tiscia GL, et al. The JAK2 V617F mutation frequently occurs in patients with portal and mesenteric venous thrombosis. J Thromb Haemost 2007;5:55–61.

24. Boissinot M, Lippert E, Girodon F, et al. Latent myeloproliferative disorder revealed by the JAK2-V617F mutation and endogenous megakaryocytic colonies in patients with splanchnic vein thrombosis. Blood 2006;108:3223–3224.

25. Michiels JJ, Abels J, Steketee J, et al. Erythromelalgia caused by platelet-mediated arteriolar inflammation and thrombosis in thrombocythemia. Ann Intern Med 1985;102:466–471.

26. Harrison C. Pregnancy and its management in the Philadelphia-negative myeloproliferative diseases. Br J Haematol 2005;129:293–306.

27. Budde U, Schaefer G, Mueller N, et al. Acquired von Willebrand's disease in the myeloproliferative syndrome. Blood 1984;64:981–985.

28. Polycythemia vera: the natural history of 1213 patients followed for 20 years. Gruppo Italiano Studio Policitemia. Ann Intern Med 1995;123:656–664.

29. Passamonti F, Brusamolino E, Lazzarino M, et al. Efficacy of pipobroman in the treatment of polycythemia vera: long-term results in 163 patients. Haematologica 2000;85:1011–1018.

30. Passamonti F, Rumi E, Pungolino E, et al. Life expectancy and prognostic factors for survival in patients with polycythemia vera and essential thrombocythemia. Am J Med 2004;117:755–761.

31. De Stefano V, Za T, Rossi E, et al. Recurrent thrombosis in patients with polycythemia vera or essential thrombocythemia: efficacy of treatment in preventing rethrombosis in different clinical settings. Blood 2006;108:Abstract 119.

32. Tefferi A, Elliot M. Thrombosis in myeloproliferative disorders: prevalence, prognostic factors, and the role of leukocytosis and JAK2V617F. Semin Thromb Hemost 2007;33:313–320.

33. Silver RT. Long-term effects of the treatment of polycythemia vera with recombinant interferon-alpha. Cancer 2006;107:451–458.

34. Finazzi G. A prospective analysis of thrombotic events in the European collaboration study on low-dose aspirin in polycythemia (ECLAP). Pathol Biol (Paris) 2004;52:285–288.

35. Landolfi R, Di Gennaro L, Barbui T, et al. Leukocytosis as a major thrombotic risk factor in patients with polycythemia vera. Blood 2007;109:2446–2452.

36. Carobbio A, Finazzi G, Guerini V, et al. Leukocytosis is a risk factor for thrombosis in essential thrombocythemia: interaction with treatment, standard risk factors, and JAK2 mutation status. Blood 2007;109:2310–2313.

37. Cortelazzo S, Finazzi G, Ruggeri M, et al. Hydroxyurea for patients with essential thrombocythemia and a high risk of thrombosis. N Engl J Med 1995;332:1132–1136.

38. Berk PD, Wasserman LR, Fruchtman SM, et al. Treatment of polycythemia vera: a summary of clinical trials conducted by the polycythemia vera study group. In: Wasserman LR, Berk PD, Berlin NI, eds. Polycythemia Vera and the Myeloproliferative Disorders. Philadelphia, PA: W.B. Saunders, 1995, pp. 166–194.

39. Falanga A, Marchetti M, Barbui T, et al. Pathogenesis of thrombosis in essential thrombocythemia and polycythemia vera: the role of neutrophils. Semin Hematol 2005;42:239–247.

40. Diehn F, Tefferi A. Pruritus in polycythaemia vera: prevalence, laboratory correlates, and management. Br J Haematol 2001;115:619–621.

41. Passamonti F, Rumi E, Arcaini L, et al. Leukemic transformation of polycythemia vera: a single center study of 23 patients. Cancer 2005;104:1032–1036.

42. Najean Y, Rain JD, Dresch C, et al. Risk of leukaemia, carcinoma, and myelofibrosis in P-32- or chemotherapy-treated patients with polycythaemia vera—a prospective analysis of 682 cases. Leuk Lymphoma 1996;22:111–119.

43. Tefferi A. Polycythemia vera: a comprehensive review and clinical recommendations. Mayo Clin Proc 2003;78:174–194.

44. McMullin MF, Bareford D, Campbell P, et al. Guidelines for the diagnosis, investigation, and management of polycythaemia/erythrocytosis. Br J Haematol 2005;130:174–195.

45. Elliott MA, Tefferi A. Thrombosis and haemorrhage in polycythaemia vera and essential thrombocythaemia. Br J Haematol 2005;128:275–290.

46. Di Nisio M, Barbui T, Di Gennaro L, et al. The haematocrit and platelet target in polycythemia vera. Br J Haematol 2007;136:249–259.

47. Ania BJ, Suman VJ, Sobell JL, et al. Trends in the incidence of polycythemia vera among Olmsted County, Minnesota residents, 1935–1989. Am J Hematol 1994;47:89–93.

48. Barbui T, Finazzi G. Evidence-based management of polycythemia vera. Best Pract Res Clin Haematol 2006;19:483–493.

49. Landolfi R, Marchioli R, Kutti J, et al. Efficacy and safety of low-dose aspirin in polycythemia vera. N Engl J Med 2004;350:114–124.

50. Berk PD, Goldberg JD, Donovan PB, et al. Therapeutic recommendations in poly-cythemia vera based on Polycythemia Vera Study Group protocols. Semin Hematol 1986;23:132–143.

51. Berk PD, Goldberg JD, Silverstein MN, et al. Increased incidence of acute leukemia in polycythemia vera associated with chlorambucil therapy. N Engl J Med 1981;304:441–447.

52. Silver RT. Interferon alfa: effects of long-term treatment for polycythemia vera. Semin Hematol 1997;34:40–50.

53. Fruchtman SM, Mack K, Kaplan ME, et al. From efficacy to safety—a Polycythemia Vera Study Group Report on Hydroxyurea in Patients with Polycythemia Vera. Semin Hematol 1997;34:17–23.

54. Finazzi G, Caruso V, Marchioli R, et al. Acute leukemia in polycythemia vera. An analysis of 1638 patients enrolled in a prospective observational study. Blood 2005;105:2664–2670.

55. Osler W. Erythremia (polycythemia with cyanosis, Maladie de Vaquez). Lancet 1908;1:143–146.

56. Anonymous. Polycythemia vera: the natural history of 1213 patients followed for 20 years. Gruppo Italiano Studio Policitemia. Ann Intern Med 1995;123:656–664.

57. Tefferi A, Spivak JL. Polycythemia vera: scientific advances and current practice. Semin Hematol 2005;42:206–220.

58. Pearson TC, Wetherley-Mein G. Vascular occlusive episodes and venous haematocrit in primary proliferative polycythaemia. Lancet 1978;2:1219–1222.

59. Pearson TC. Rheology of the absolute polycythaemias. Builliere's Clin Haemat 1987;1:637.

60. Thomas DJ et al. Cerebral blood flow in polycythemia. Lancet 1977;2:161–163.

61. Natvig H, Vellar OD. Studies on hemoglobin values in Norway. 8. Hemoglobin, hematocrit and MCHC values in adult men and women. Acta Med Scand 1967;182:193–205.

62. Streiff MB, Smith B, Spivak JL. The diagnosis and management of polycythemia vera in the era since the Polycythemia Vera Study Group: a survey of American Society of Hematology members' practice patterns. Blood 2002;99:1144–1149.

63. Andreasson B, Lofvenberg E, Westin J. Management of patients with poly-cythaemia vera: results of a survey among Swedish haematologists. Eur J Haematol 2005;74:489–495.

64. Finazzi G, Barbui T. How we treat patients with polycythemia vera. Blood 2007;109:5104–5111.

65. Barbui T. The leukemia controversy in myeloproliferative disorders: Is it a natural progression of disease, a secondary sequela of therapy, or a combination of both? Semin Hematol 2004;41:15–17.

66. Osgood EE. Leukaemogenic effect of ionising-irradiation treatment in poly-cythaemia. Lancet 1964;67:967.

67. Guillot B, Bessis D, Dereure O. Mucocutaneous side effects of antineoplastic chemotherapy. Expert Opin Drug Saf 2004;3:579–587.

68. Cortelazzo S, Finazzi G, Ruggeri M, et al. Hydroxyurea for patients with essential thrombocythemia and a high risk of thrombosis. N Engl J Med 1995;332:1132–1136.

69. Najean Y, Rain JD. Treatment of polycythemia vera—the use of hydroxyurea and pipobroman in 292 patients under the age of 65 years. Blood 1997;90:3370–3377.

70. Means RT, Jr., Krantz SB. Inhibition of human erythroid colony-forming units by gamma interferon can be corrected by recombinant human erythropoietin. Blood 1991;78:2564–2567.
71. Wang Q, Miyakawa Y, Fox N, et al. Interferon-alpha directly represses megakaryopoiesis by inhibiting thrombopoietin-induced signaling through induction of SOCS-1. Blood 2000;96:2093–2099.
72. Martyre MC. Critical review of pathogenetic mechanisms in myelofibrosis with myeloid metaplasia. Curr Hematol Rep 2003;2:257–263.
73. Silver RT. Recombinant interferon-alpha for treatment of polycythaemia vera [letter]. Lancet 1988;2:403.
74. Silver RT. A new treatment for polycythemia vera: recombinant interferon alfa [see comments]. Blood 1990;76:664–665.
75. Silver RT. Interferon-alpha 2b: a new treatment for polycythemia vera. Ann Intern Med 1993;119:1091–1092.
76. Silver RT. Treatment of polycythemia vera with recombinant interferon. Int J Hematol 2002;76(Suppl 2):294–295.
77. Lengfelder E, Berger U, Hehlmann R. Interferon alpha in the treatment of polycythemia vera. Ann Hematol 2000;79:103–109.
78. Jones AV, Silver RT, Waghorn K, et al. Minimal molecular response in polycythemia vera patients treated with imatinib or interferon alpha. Blood 2006;107:3339–3341.
79. Kiladjian JJ, Cassinat B, Turlure P, et al. High molecular response rate of polycythemia vera patients treated with pegylated interferon alpha-2a. Blood 2006;108:2037–2040.
80. Elliott MA, Tefferi A. Interferon-alpha therapy in polycythemia vera and essential thrombocythemia. Semin Thromb Hemost 1997;23:463–472.
81. Anonymous. Treatment by radiophosphorus versus busulfan in polycythemia vera: a randomized trial (E.O.R.T.C.'s) "leukemias and hematosarcomas" group. Recent Results Cancer Res 1977;62:104–109.
82. Messinezy M, Pearson TC, Prochazka A, et al. Treatment of primary proliferative polycythaemia by venesection and low-dose busulphan: retrospective study from one centre. Br J Haematol 1985;61:657–666.
83. Littler WA, Kay JM, Hasleton PS, et al. Busulphan lung. Thorax 1969;24:639–655.
84. Lawrence JH. Nuclear physics and therapy: preliminary report on a new method for the treatment of leukemia and polycythemia vera. Radiology 1940;35:51–60.
85. Najean Y, Rain JD. Treatment of polycythemia vera—use of P-32 alone or in combination with maintenance therapy using hydroxyurea in 461 patients greater than 65 years of age. Blood 1997;89:2319–2327.
86. Tefferi A, Silverstein MN, Petitt RM, et al. Anagrelide as a new platelet-lowering agent in essential thrombocythemia: mechanism of action, efficacy, toxicity, current indications. Semin Thromb Hemost 1997;23:379.
87. Anonymous. Anagrelide, a therapy for thrombocythemic states: experience in 577 patients. Anagrelide Study Group. Am J Med 1992;92:69–76.
88. Dingli D, Tefferi A. A critical review of anagrelide therapy in essential thrombocythemia and related disorders. Leuk Lymphoma 2005;46:641–650.
89. Engel PJ, Johnson H, Baughman RP, et al. High-output heart failure associated with anagrelide therapy for essential thrombocytosis. Ann Intern Med 2005;143:311–313.

90. Silver RT. Imatinib mesylate (Gleevec(TM)) reduces phlebotomy requirements in polycythemia vera. Leukemia 2003;17:1186–1187.
91. Silver RT, Fruchtman S, Feldman EJ, et al. Imatinib mesylate is effective in the treatment of polycythemia vera: a multi-institutional clinical trial (Abstract). Blood 2004;104:189a.
92. Silver RT. Treatment of polycythemia vera with recombinant interferon alpha (rIF-Nalpha) or imatinib mesylate. Curr Hematol Rep 2005;4:235–237.
93. Kiladjian JJ, Cassinat B, Turlure P, et al. High molecular response rate of polycythemia vera patients treated with pegylated interferon alpha-2a. Blood 2006;108:2037–2040.
94. Tartaglia AP, Goldberg JD, Berk PD, et al. Adverse effects of antiaggregating platelet therapy in the treatment of polycythemia vera. Semin Hematol 1986;23:172–176.
95. Low-dose aspirin in polycythaemia vera: a pilot study. Gruppo Italiano Studio Policitemia (GISP). Br J Haematol 1997;97:453–456.
96. van Genderen PJ, Michiels JJ. Erythromelalgia: a pathognomonic microvascular thrombotic complication in essential thrombocythemia and polycythemia vera. [Review] [23 refs]. Semin Thromb Hemost 1997;23:357–363.
97. Gilbert HS, Warner RR, Wasserman LR. A study of histamine in myeloproliferative disease. Blood 1966;28:795–806.
98. Steinman HK, Kobza-Black A, Lotti TM, et al. Polycythaemia rubra vera and water-induced pruritus: blood histamine levels and cutaneous fibrinolytic activity before and after water challenge. Br J Dermatol 1987;116:329–333.
99. Jackson N, Burt D, Crocker J, et al. Skin mast cells in polycythaemia vera: relationship to the pathogenesis and treatment of pruritus. Br J Dermatol 1987;116:21–29.
100. Fjellner B, Hagermark O. Pruritus in polycythemia vera: treatment with aspirin and possibility of platelet involvement. Acta Derm Venereol 1979;59:505–512.
101. Weick JK, Donovan PB, Najean Y, et al. The use of cimetidine for the treatment of pruritus in polycythemia vera. Arch Intern Med 1982;142:241–242.
102. Tefferi A, Fonseca R. Selective serotonin reuptake inhibitors are effective in the treatment of polycythemia vera-associated pruritus. Blood 2002;99:2627.
103. Foa P, Massaro P, Caldiera S, et al. Long-term therapeutic efficacy and toxicity of recombinant interferon-alpha 2a in polycythaemia vera. Eur J Haematol 1998;60:273–277.
104. McNally RJ, Roman E, Cartwright RA. Leukemias and lymphomas: time trends in the UK, 1984–93. Cancer Causes Control 1999;10:35–42.
105. Wright CA, Tefferi A. A single institutional experience with 43 pregnancies in essential thrombocythemia. Eur J Haematol 2001;66:152–159.
106. Griesshammer M, Struve S, Harrison CM. Essential thrombocythemia/polycythemia vera and pregnancy: the need for an observational study in Europe. Semin Thromb Hemost 2006;32:422–429.
107. Barbui T, Finazzi G. Myeloproliferative disease in pregnancy and other management issues. Hematology Am Soc Hematol Educ Program Book 2006:246–252.
108. Barbui T, Barosi G, Grossi A, et al. Practice guidelines for the therapy of essential thrombocythemia. A statement from the Italian Society of Hematology, the Italian Society of Experimental Hematology and the Italian Group for Bone Marrow Transplantation. Haematologica 2004;89:215–232.

109. Robinson S, Bewley S, Hunt BJ, et al. The management and outcome of 18 pregnancies in women with polycythemia vera. Haematologica 2005;90:1477–1483.
110. Pardanani A, Hood J, Lasho T, et al. TG101209, a selective JAK2 kinase inhibitor, suppresses endogenous and cytokine-supported colony formation from hematopoietic progenitors carrying JAK2V617F or MPLW515K/L mutations (Abstract). Blood 2006;108:758a.
111. Gaikwad AS, Prchal JT. Efficacy of tyrosine kinase inhibitors in polycythemia vera (Abstract). Blood 2006;108:762a.
112. Hood J, Cao J, Hanna E, et al. JAK2 inhibitors for the treatment of myeloprolifertive disorder (Abstract). Blood 2006;118:1038a.
113. Thiele J, Kvasnicka HM, Vardiman J. Bone marrow histopathology in the diagnosis of chronic myeloproliferative disorders: a forgotten pearl. Best Pract Res Clin Haematol 2006;19:413–437.

6

Management of Essential Thrombocythemia

Guido Finazzi

Departments of Transfusion Medicine and Hematology, Ospedali Riuniti, Bergamo, Italy

Tiziano Barbui

Department of Hematology, Ospedali Riuniti, Bergamo, Italy

Among the chronic myeloproliferative disorders (MPD), essential thrombo-cythemia (ET) is characterized by longer median survival as well as lower trans-formation rates into acute leukemia or post-ET myelofibrosis (MF) (1,2). The clinical course is marked by thrombotic and hemorrhagic episodes that occur more frequently in older patients and those with previous vascular events. There is an ongoing debate as to whether the evolution to acute leukemia is part of the natural history of the disease or is related to the use of cytoreductive agents given to control the myeloproliferation and avoid vascular complications. Hence, the best strategy is to limit the cytotoxic therapy to patients stratified on the basis of their risk for developing vascular events.

This chapter reviews recent progress in the management of ET with partic-ular emphasis upon four key areas: clinical course, risk stratification, risk-adapted therapy, and management of pregnancy.

CLINICAL COURSE

Frequency

According to population-based epidemiological studies (3,4), the incidence rates of ET range from 15 to 25 cases per million inhabitants annually. These figures are in agreement with a systematic screening for erythrocytosis and thrombocy-tosis in 10,000 consecutive persons living in the city of Vicenza, Italy (5). This cross-sectional study of healthy people led to the identification of four cases of ET (platelet count $\geq 600 \times 10^9$/L) with an estimated prevalence of 400 cases per million inhabitants [95% confidence interval (CI) 109–1.020/million]. Interestingly, no thrombotic or hemorrhagic complications occurred over 5 years of follow-up in these incidentally discovered ET patients.

The disorder appears to affect primarily middle-aged people, with an average age at diagnosis of about 55 years (6). There is a higher prevalence of females (3,6), mainly due to a second peak frequency at around 30 years of age for women. This predisposition of young women to develop ET is relevant for the issue of pregnancy discussed below.

Incidence and Type of Thrombotic and Bleeding Complications

Thrombosis and hemorrhage are the most frequent clinical complications observed in ET patients (7). In uncontrolled studies, reported cumulative rates for thrombosis and hemorrhage during follow-up ranged from 7% to 17% and 8% to 14%, respectively (8). In one study that also evaluated a control population (9), the incidence of thrombotic episodes was 6.6% per patient-year in ET versus 1.2% per patient-year in control subjects and the rate of major hemorrhagic complications was 0.33% per patient-year in ET versus 0% per patient-year in controls.

The most frequent types of major thrombosis include stroke, transient ischemic attack, myocardial infarction, peripheral arterial thrombosis, and deep venous thrombosis often occurring in unusual sites, such as hepatic (Budd-Chiari syndrome), portal, and mesenteric veins. In addition to large vessel occlusions, ET patients may suffer from microcirculatory symptoms, including vascular headaches, dizziness, visual disturbances, distal paresthesia, and acrocyanosis. The most characteristic of these disturbances is erythromelalgia, consisting of congestion, redness, and burning pain to ischemia, as well as gangrene of distal portions of toes and fingers (10). The most frequent bleeding events are hemorrhages from the gastrointestinal tract followed by hematuria and other mucocutaneous hemorrhages. Hemarthrosis and large-muscle hematomas are uncommon.

Progression of Disease and Survival

ET may transform to MF or acute leukemia as part of the natural history. In a series of 195 patients followed for a median of 7.2 years (range, 1.9–24), conversion to post-ET MF was observed in 13 cases, with an actuarial probability of 2.7% at 5 years, 8.3% at 10 years, and 15.3% at 15 years (11). In a long-term cohort study of 322 consecutive patients followed for a median of 13.6 years, survival was similar to that of the control population in the first decade of disease (risk ratio 0.72, 95% CI 0.50–0.99) but became significantly worse thereafter (risk ratio 2.21, 95% CI 1.74–2.76). The risk of leukemic or any myeloid disease transformation was low in the first 10 years (1.4% and 9.1%, respectively) but increased substantially in the second (8.1% and 28.3%, respectively) and third (24.0% and 58.5%, respectively) decades of the disease (6). A more recent analysis of 605 patients followed in the same institution for a median of 84 months allowed to construct prognostic models for survival and leukemic transformation (12). Adverse factors for survival included age $\geq$ 60 years, hemoglobin level below normal (females $<$ 120 g/L; males $<$ 135 g/L), and leukocyte count $>$ 15 $\times$ 10^9/L. Low-risk (no adverse factors), intermediate-risk (at least one adverse factor), and high-risk ($\geq$ 2 adverse factors) groups showed respective median survivals of 278, 200, and 111 months ($p < 0.0001$). Leukemic conversion was predicted by two risk factors, including below-normal hemoglobin level and platelet count $\geq$ 1000 $\times$ 10^9/L. Low-risk (no risk factors), intermediate-risk (one), and high-risk (both risk factors) groups showed transformation rates of 0.4, 4.8, and 6.5% months, respectively ($p < 0.0001$).

RISK STRATIFICATION BASED ON THROMBOHEMORRHAGIC RISK

Age over 60 years and a previous thrombotic event were identified as major risk factors for thrombosis in most studies (summarized in Table 1). Additional risk factors have been recognized in some series of patients, including clonal disease, impaired expression of c-Mpl in bone marrow megakaryocytes, presence of factor V Leiden, and antiphospholipid antibodies (reviewed in Ref. 8). The risk is increased by the concomitant presence of hypertension, hypercholesterolemia, and smoking, but it should be recognized that these associations are not consistently found in all studies.

Recently, a prognostic role for leukocytosis in MPD has been advocated. Three large-cohort studies have demonstrated that an increased leukocyte count is a novel, independent risk factor for both thrombosis and inferior survival (6,12,17). In one study, a correlation between leukocytosis and the JAK2V617F mutation was reported (17). In ET, in vivo leukocyte activation has been shown to occur and to be associated with signs of activation of both platelets and endothelial cells (19). Platelet activation is particularly increased in patients carrying the JAK2V617F mutation (20). Thus, leukocyte and platelet activation may play a role in the generation of the prethrombotic state that characterizes this disease.

The presence of the JAK2V617F mutation in about 50% of the patients with ET raises the question whether mutated and nonmutated patients differ in terms of thrombotic risk. The largest relevant study on 806 patients suggested that JAK2 mutation was associated with venous, but not arterial, events (21). An increased risk of thrombosis in JAK2-mutated patients with essential thrombocythemia was also reported by other investigators (22,23). However, the rate of vascular complications was not affected by the presence of the mutation in two other relatively large studies, including 150 and 130 patients, respectively (24,25). It is possible that the higher age distribution, hematocrit and leukocyte levels consistently found in mutation-positive patients (21–25) contributed to the apparent association between JAK2V617F and thrombosis reported in some studies.

Paradoxically, a very high platelet count ($>$ 1500 $\times$ 10^9/L) was found to be a major predictor of bleeding rather than of thrombosis (26) (Table 1). The

Table 1 Cohort Studies of Risk Factors for Thrombosis and Bleeding in Essential Thrombocythemia Including at least 100 Patients

		Risk factors for thrombosis (RR or P)				
Study (Ref)	No. of Patients	Age > 60	Previous thrombosis	Platelet count	Leukocytosis	Cardiovascular risk factors[a]
Cortelazzo et al. (9)	100	10.3 (2.05–51.5)	13 (4.1–41.5)	NS	–	NS
Besses et al. (13)	148	3.3 (1.5–7.4)	3.0 (1.5–6.0)	NS	–	4.7 (1.8–11.8)
Colombi et al. (14)	103	NS	$p < 0.001$	NS	–	–
Jantunen et al. (15)	132	NS	–	NS	–	$p = 0.01$
Bazzan et al. (16)	187	NS (age > 55)	–	NS	NS	
Wolanskyi et al. (6)	322	1.51 (1.05–2.18)	2.3 (1.25–4.24) (arterial only)	–	1.74 (1.15–2.66) (WBC $\geq 15 \times 10^9$/L)	NS
Carobbio et al. (17)	439	2.3 (1.3–3.9) (age > 60 and previous thrombosis evaluated together)		NS	2.3 (1.4–3.9) (WBC $\geq 8.7 \times 10^9$/L)	–

Study (Ref)	Patients, no.	Risk factor for bleeding Platelet count
van Genderen et al. (10)	200 (review of published cases)	$p < 0.001$ (platelets > 1.000×10^9/L)
Fenaux et al. (18)	147	"higher risk" (platelets > 2.000×10^9/L)
Wolanskyi et al. (6)	322	NS

[a] At least one of the following: smoking, hypertension, hypercholesterolemia, or diabetes. NS, not significant; –, not evaluated.

explanation of this comes from the impairment of von Willebrand factor multimers found both in patients with ET and those with reactive thrombocytosis (7,26). Large von Willebrand factor multimers have been found to be decreased in parallel with the degree of thrombocythemia, and normalization of the platelet count was accompanied by restoration of a normal plasma von Willebrand factor multimeric distribution and correction of bleeding tendency. However, in a retrospective study of 99 consecutive young patients (aged < 60 years) who presented with extreme thrombocytosis (platelet count $\geq 1000 \times 10^9$/L) and without a previous history of thrombohemorrhagic complications, the incidences of major thrombosis and hemorrhage during the follow-up were similar between those who were treated with prophylactic cytoreductive therapy and those who did not receive such therapy (27). This clinical observation challenges the role of extreme thrombocytosis as a major risk factor for vascular events in otherwise low-risk patients with ET.

RISK-ADAPTED THERAPY

Before deciding whether to start platelet-lowering treatment, ET patients should be evaluated for a history of thrombotic or hemorrhagic events and the presence of cardiovascular risk factors (i.e., smoking, hypertension, hypercholesterolemia, and diabetes). Then, they should be stratified according to their probability of developing major bleeding or thrombosis (Table 2) (1,28).

Low Risk

Avoiding cytoreduction is recommended in low-risk ET patients. The natural history of such patients left untreated was prospectively evaluated in a controlled study that compared 65 low-risk patients with 65 age- and sex-matched normal controls (29). After a median follow-up of 4.1 years, the incidence of thrombosis was not significantly higher in patients than in controls (1.91% vs. 1.5% per patient-year; age- and sex-adjusted risk ratio 1.43, 95% CI 0.37–5.4). No major bleeding was observed. Thrombotic deaths seem very rare in low-risk ET subjects, and there are no data indicating that fatalities can be prevented by starting cytoreductive drugs early. Therefore, withholding chemotherapy is justifiable in young, asymptomatic ET patients with a platelet count below 1500×10^9/L. This policy is based on the low risk of complications and the potential leukemogenicity of cytotoxic drugs. However, the strength of these recommendations is based on studies having a small number of patients, and further data from large clinical trials are needed.

Aspirin at different doses (30–500 mg/day) has been found to control microvascular symptoms, such as erythromelalgia, and transient neurological and ocular disturbances, including dysarthria, hemiparesis, scintillating scotomas, amaurosis fugax, migraine, and seizures (7). The efficacy and safety of aspirin, 100 mg daily, in preventing major thrombotic events has been formally assessed in a randomized clinical trial in polycythemia vera (PV) (30). Aspirin significantly

Table 2   Classification of Essential Thrombocythemia Based on
Thrombotic and Hemorrhagic Risk

Low risk	Age < 60 years, no history of thrombosis or major bleeding, and platelet count < 1500×10^9/L
Intermediate risk	Neither low risk nor high risk
High risk	Age > 60 years, or a previous history of thrombosis or major bleeding

Correction of cardiovascular risk factors (i.e., smoking, hypertension, hypercoles-
terolemia, and diabetes) is recommended in all patients.

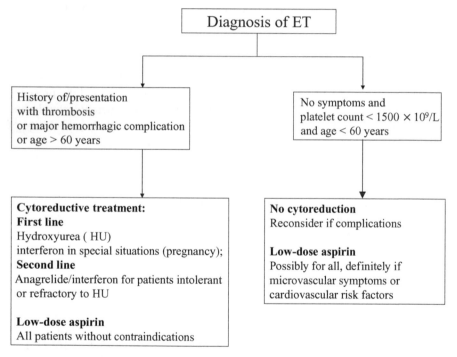

Figure 1   An algorithm of risk-adapted treatment recommendations in patients with ET.

lowered the risk of a primary combined end point, including cardiovascular death,
nonfatal myocardial infarction, nonfatal stroke, and major venous thromboembolism (relative risk 0.4 [95% CI 0.18–0.91]; $p = 0.0277$) without increasing
major bleeding (relative risk 1.6, 95% CI 0.27–9.71). Based on these findings, an
antithrombotic preventive strategy with low-dose aspirin is recommended in all
PV patients. Translating evidence from this study to ET can be considered, but
formal clinical trials have not hitherto been produced (Fig. 1).

Intermediate Risk

Whether some patients may be classified as at "intermediate risk" of thrombosis is more contentious. The rationale for assigning this risk category is the increase in incidence of thrombotic events in the age range 40–60 years compared to less than 40 years (9) and the uncertainty over the weighting that might be ascribed to weaker or more controversial risk factors. The Italian Consensus Criteria define "intermediate risk" as age 40–60 years, platelets less than $1000 \times 10^9/L$, and either vascular risk factors or familial thrombophilia with no consensus on treatment (8).

In a recent review, Elliott and Tefferi suggested that those aged less than 60 years and with no thrombosis and a either platelet count greater than $1500 \times 10^9/L$ or cardiovascular risk factor (e.g., smoking, diabetes, etc.) are of intermediate risk and should be treated with aspirin, but concluded there was no consensus on cytoreductive therapy (7).

Finally, in the United Kingdom, intermediate-risk patients, aged 40–60 years with all of the following: platelets less than $1500 \times 10^9/L$, no prior thrombosis or hemorrhage, and no hypertension or diabetes, are entering into an ongoing randomized study comparing hydroxyurea (HU) plus aspirin or aspirin alone (31).

High Risk

Hydroxyurea

HU has emerged as the treatment of choice in high-risk patients with ET because of its efficacy in preventing thrombosis (see "Clinical Trials") and rare acute toxicity (Fig. 1). Hematopoietic impairment, leading to neutropenia and macrocytic anemia, is the main short-term toxic effect of HU. Other less frequent side effects include oral and leg ulcers and skin lesions.

The leukemogenicity of this agent is still debated. Some long-term studies found that a proportion of ET patients treated with HU developed acute leukemia (32,33). In other studies, however, this drug was rarely associated with secondary malignancies when used alone (34–37). In an analysis of 25 ET patients younger than 50 years and treated with HU for a high risk of thrombosis, no leukemic or neoplastic transformation occurred after a median follow-up of 8 years (range, 5–14) (34). In 1638 patients with PV enrolled in a prospective study, HU alone did not enhance the risk of leukemia in comparison with patients treated with phlebotomy only (hazard ratio 0.86, 95% CI 0.26–2.88; $p - 0.8$), whereas this risk was significantly increased by any other cytoreductive drug, namely radiophosphorus, busulfan, or pipobroman, either used alone or in combination (hazard ratio 5.46, 95% CI 1.84–16.25; $p = 0.002$) (35). The incidence of acute leukemic transformation is higher in patients with ET treated with HU if they have cytogenetic abnormalities (32,33) or have received other cytotoxic drugs with different mechanisms of action (32,35–37).

Anagrelide

Anagrelide, an imidazo quinazinoline derivative, has been shown to reduce the platelet count in a species-specific manner (38,39). The mechanism by which anagrelide induces thrombocytopenia is unclear, but current attention is focused upon the inhibition of megakaryocytes differentiation and maturation (39). Major side effects of the drug include palpitations, headaches, noncardiac edema, and congestive cardiac failure (39). In one report, patients treated with anagrelide developed cardiomyopathy (40).

There is an extensive experience of the use of this drug, which is licensed in the United States, as a first-line agent for the control of thrombocytosis associated with any MPDs. In Europe, the drug has been granted a license only for ET patients refractory or intolerant of first-line therapy. The criteria for defining resistance or intolerance to HU have been recently established by an International Working Group (41). They include platelet count greater than 600×10^9/L after 3 months of at least 2 g/day of HU (2.5 g/day in patients with a body weight over 80 kg); platelet count greater than 400×10^9/L and WBC less than 2.5×10^9/L or hemoglobin less than 10 g/dL at any dose of HU; presence of leg ulcers or other unacceptable mucocutaneous manifestations at any dose of HU; and HU-related fever.

Until recently, studies of anagrelide in ET were nonrandomized, lacked a control arm, and had relatively limited follow-up. The largest study to date evaluated 934 ET patients for efficacy and 2251 ET patients for safety and had a maximum follow-up of 7 years; there was no evidence that anagrelide increased conversion to acute leukemia and no mention was made of MF (42). A study of 35 consecutive young ET patients treated with anagrelide, with a median follow-up of 10.7 years, demonstrated that 20% had thrombotic complications and a similar proportion had major hemorrhagic complications, raising a question about the efficacy of this drug (43). These events occurred when the platelet count was above 400×10^9/L, suggesting that control of the platelet count to below 400 $\times 10^9$/L might reduce this risk. A second major finding from this study was the development of a significant anemia of more than 3 g/dL in one-quarter of patients.

Interferon-alpha (IFN-α)

IFN-α has been evaluated in several cohorts of ET patients (reviewed in Ref. 44). Platelet count was reduced to below 600×10^9/L in about 90% of cases after about 3 months, with an average dose of 3 million international units (IU) daily. The time and degree of platelet reduction during the induction phase were dose-dependent. The IFN-α dose can be tapered during maintenance, but after its discontinuation, the platelet count rebounds in the majority of patients. IFN-α is not known to be teratogenic and does not cross the placenta. Thus, it has been used successfully throughout pregnancy in some ET patients with no adverse fetal or maternal effects.

Side effects are a major problem with this drug. Besides flu-like symptoms observed in the early treatment phase, signs of chronic toxicity include weakness, myalgia, weight and hair loss, gastrointestinal toxicity, and depression. In a series of 273 ET patients (44), IFN-α therapy was terminated in 25% (67 cases) before completion of the treatment. The rate of withdrawal ranged between 0% and 66% in the different studies. This wide range may be partly explained by the difference in observation times that ranged from 1 month to 4 years. So far, no leukemogenic effects have been reported.

Recently, semisynthetic pegylated forms of interferon-α (peg-IFNα) have been used to treat MPD, which in a limited number of studies (reviewed in 45), have been shown to be superior to unmodified IFN as related to its adverse event profile and efficacy. Interestingly, the use of peg-IFNα-2 a in 27 patients with PV was able to decrease the percentage of mutated JAK2 allele in 24 cases (89%) from a mean of 49% to a mean of 27% (46). However, a more limited effect on JAK2 mutational status of another form of peg-IFNα (peg-IFNα-2b) in patients with PV and ET has been reported (47). Despite its high cost and toxicity, IFN remains a useful agent in the cytoreductive treatment of ET, especially in very young patients and pregnant women.

Clinical Trials

Two randomized clinical trials assessing benefits and risks of myelosuppressive therapy in ET patients at high risk of thrombosis have been carried out so far.

The first was performed about 10 years ago in Italy and evaluated HU versus untreated controls (48): 114 ET patients were randomized to HU or no cytoreductive treatment. During a median follow-up of 27 months, 2 thromboses were recorded in the HU-treated group (1.6%/patient-year) compared with 14 in the control group (10.7%/patient-year; $p = 0.003$). This study provided the basis for considering HU as the standard therapy for high-risk ET patients and the reference arm for other randomized trials.

The second trial was carried out in the United Kingdom and compared HU plus aspirin with anagrelide plus aspirin in 809 high-risk ET patients analyzed with a median follow-up of 39 months (49). Overall, patients randomized to anagrelide and aspirin were more likely to reach the composite primary end point of major thrombosis (arterial or venous), major hemorrhage, or death from a vascular cause ($p = 0.03$). When individual end points were assessed, arterial thrombosis, major hemorrhage, and MF were all significantly more frequent for patients treated with anagrelide ($p = 0.004$, 0.008, and 0.01, respectively). However, anagrelide and aspirin seem to offer at least partial protection from thrombosis, as the prevalence of thrombotic events was significantly lower than the control arm of the Italian study (48) (actuarial rate of first thrombosis 8% versus 26% at 2 years, respectively), while the HU arms were approximately equivalent (actuarial rate of first thrombosis 4% at 2 years in both trials). The success of HU is likely to reflect the importance of additional factors, such as the hematocrit, leukocyte count, or leukocyte activity (50) in the pathogenesis of thrombosis. Intriguingly, venous thrombosis was less frequent in patients treated with anagrelide ($p = 0.006$).

Major hemorrhage was increased for anagrelide plus aspirin treatment ($p = 0.008$). The most frequent of these end points were gastrointestinal hemorrhages. Hemorrhagic events may result from some subtle effect upon platelet function possibly accentuated by aspirin or in relation to combined gastric toxicity.

Myelofibrotic transformation was seen in 16 patients treated with anagrelide in comparison with 5 treated with HU. It seems logical that anagrelide might be less effective than HU at suppressing the natural evolution of ET to MF, as the number of megakaryocytes remains elevated in ET patients treated with anagrelide compared to those given HU. The incidence of MF in the anagrelide arm (3.95%) at the median follow-up of 39 months is approximately in accordance with what has been previously reported (0.9% per annum) (11), supporting the view that HU may be more effectively suppressing MF.

MANAGEMENT OF PREGNANCY

Normal pregnant women are at an increased risk of thrombosis, calculated to be approximately six times higher than in nonpregnant women, and the risk is compounded if they also have MPD. Women with MPD may present a high incidence not only of pregnancy-related venous thromboembolism, but also of other vascular complications of pregnancy involving occlusion of the placental circulation (51,52). However, the paucity of published data, summarized in Table 3, makes it difficult to obtain a clear view of the overall risk of these events.

Clinical epidemiology and risk factors

In the Italian guidelines for the therapy of ET (8), the outcomes of 461 pregnancies reported in retrospective and prospective cohort studies were pooled. Most reports dealt with single cases or small numbers and there is some suspicion of reporting bias, since there seems to be a tendency to describe patients with complications rather than those with an uncomplicated pregnancy. Elliott and Tefferi (60) restricted their review to series comprising at least 6 patients but, interestingly, the results were no different from those in the systematically retrieved literature that formed the basis of the ET Italian guidelines.

The mean age at pregnancy was 29 years, with a mean platelet count at the beginning of pregnancy being 1000×10^9/L. During the second trimester, a spontaneous decline was registered to a nadir of 599×10^9/L. This decrease seems larger than the reduction seen in normal pregnancies, which is attributed to an increase in plasma volume. The mechanism is not known, but could involve placental or fetal production of a factor that down-regulates platelet production. In the postpartum period, the platelet counts rise back up to their earlier levels and rebound thrombocytosis may occur in some patients. This increases the probability of vascular complications at this time, which is a period of high thrombotic risk, as in other conditions of thrombophilia as well as in normal women.

Overall, 50–70% of ET women had successful live births; first-trimester loss occurred in about 25–40% and late pregnancy loss in 10% of the cases. Abruptio placentae was reported in 3.6% of the cases, higher than in the general population (1%) (8). Pre-eclampsia rates were similar to the normal population (1.7%) and intrauterine growth retardation was reported in 4–5% (8).

Maternal thrombosis or hemorrhage may occur. In the pooled analysis cited above (8), postpartum thrombotic episodes were reported in 13 patients, occurring in 5.2% of pregnancies, and minor or major, pre- or postpartum bleeding events in other 13 cases. The maternal vascular risk may be higher in women with previous venous or arterial events or hemorrhages attributed to MPD, independent of whether they occurred in a previous pregnancy or not. Similarly, severe complications in a previous pregnancy, such as three or more first-trimester losses or one or more second- or third-trimester losses, birth weight less than fifth centile of gestation, preeclampsia, intrauterine death, or stillbirth, are considered to raise the risk of subsequent events for the mother and the fetus. Other vascular risk factors in pregnant women are age, obesity, immobilization, and other causes of genetic and acquired thrombophilia, including antiphospholipid antibodies.

Treatment

A detailed personal and family history should be taken and a woman with ET who plans a pregnancy should be put under the joint care of a hematologist and an obstetrician experienced in the care of patients with high-risk pregnancies in order to assess the risks and agree on the most appropriate therapy. It is recommended that the patient stop any possibly teratogenic drugs at least 3 months before conception. Depending on the risk of maternal vascular events and pregnancy morbidity, the various treatment options range from no therapy, aspirin alone, low-molecular-weight heparin (LMWH) to cytoreductive therapy (Table 4).

Aspirin

The rationale for the use of low-dose aspirin in MPD is supported by the results of a randomized clinical trial carried out in patients with PV (30). However, the largest series of pregnant ET patients published to date failed to find any benefit of aspirin even in women with previous fetal losses (58). In a systematic literature review up to October 2003 (8), pregnancy was successful in 74% of the ET patients treated with aspirin (79 of 106), compared to only 55% of the women not receiving aspirin (80 of 145). The Italian guidelines concluded that although there was no direct evidence of the efficacy of aspirin in pregnant ET women, the drug is recommended for these women if they have a history of microvascular symptoms or at least one previous adverse pregnancy event (8). According to Harrison (51) and Griesshammer (52), in the absence of clear contraindications, all patients with ET should be given aspirin (75 or 100 mg daily) throughout pregnancy and for at

Table 3 Case Series of Pregnancies in Essential Thrombocythemia Including at Least 5 Patients

Study (Ref)	No. of patients	No. of pregnancies	Treatment during pregnancy (no. of pts.)	Outcomes	Maternal thrombohemorrhagic complications	No. of live births (%)
Beard et al. (53)	6	9	None (3) Aspirin alone (4) Aspirin + heparin (2) + antepartum platelet apheresis (1)		1 hemorrhage postpartum 1 hemorrhage after abortion 1 superficial thrombophlebitis	8 (89%)
Beressi et al. (54)[a]	18	34	None (10) Aspirin alone (18) Other antiplatelet drugs (2) Cytoreductive drugs (4) + antepartum platelet apheresis (3)		5 vaginal bleeding (mild to moderate)	17 (50%) (2 elective abortions; 1 ectopic pregnancy)
Pagliaro et al. (55)	9	15	None (5) Aspirin alone (3) Aspirin + heparin (7)		1 abdominal vein thrombosis	9 (60%) (1 elective abortion)
Randi et al. (56)	13	16	None (9) Aspirin alone (7)		1 cerebral thrombosis 2 abdominal vein thrombosis	13 (81%)
Bangerter et al. (57)	9	17	None (11) Aspirin alone (1) Aspirin + heparin (5)		3 major vaginal bleeding 2 minor bleeding (epistaxis) 1 transient visual loss	11 (65%)

Wright et al. (58)[a]	20	43	None (16) Aspirin alone (24) Heparin (1) Cytoreductive drugs (2) + antepartum platelet apheresis (3)	3 vaginal bleeding (mild to moderate)	22 (51%) (2 elective abortions; 1 ectopic pregnancy)
Niittyvuopio et al. (59)	16	40	None (27) Aspirin alone (5) Aspirin + interferon-alpha (5) Cytoreductive drugs (3)	2 cerebral and visual disturbances	25 (62%)

[a]Case series coming from the same institution.

Table 4   Risk-Adapted Management of Pregnancy in ET

1. Risk stratification
   At least one of the following defines high-risk pregnancy:
   - previous major thrombotic or bleeding complication
   - previous severe pregnancy complications[a]
   - platelet count $> 1500 \times 10^9$/L
2. Therapy
   a) Low-risk pregnancy
      - Aspirin 100 mg/day
      - LMWH 4000 U/day after delivery until 6 weeks postpartum

   High-risk pregnancy
   As above, plus
   - If previous major thrombosis or severe pregnancy complications: LMWH
     throughout pregnancy (stop aspirin if bleeding complications)
   - If platelet count $> 1500 \times 10^9$/L: consider IFN-α
   - If previous major bleeding: avoid aspirin and consider IFN-α to reduce
     thrombocytosis

[a]Severe pregnancy complications: ≥ 3 first-trimester or ≥ 1 second- or third-trimester losses, birth weight < 5th centile of gestation, pre-eclampsia, intrauterine death, or stillbirth.

least 6 weeks after delivery. Low-dose aspirin is considered safe in pregnancy and should preferably be started before conception to facilitate placental and fetal development. Bleeding complications are rare, but particular attention should be paid to patients with a platelet count above $1000–1500 \times 10^9$/L, since the risk of bleeding may increase significantly.

Low-Molecular Weight Heparin (LMWH)

LMWH in pregnancy is indicated for prophylaxis and treatment of deep venous thrombosis in selected high-risk ET women, and to reduce fetal morbidity. The suggested dose of enoxaparin is 4000 U (40 mg) once-daily increasing to 4000 U twice-daily from 16 weeks, dropping to 4000 U daily for 6 weeks postpartum. To increase the antithrombotic efficacy in very high-risk situations LMWH was used in combination with low-dose aspirin. Randomized clinical trials in antiphospholipid syndrome patients indicated that the combination of heparin plus low-dose aspirin significantly improved the live birth rate, to 71–80%, and was superior to aspirin alone (live birth rate about 40%) (reviewed in (61)).

These results cannot be translated directly to MPD patients in whom the pathogenesis of vascular occlusion may be different, with an apparently prominent role of leukocyte activation and interaction between platelets, leukocytes and endothelium (19). Nonetheless, LMWH may be considered in addition to low-dose aspirin in high-risk ET women with a history of late fetal loss, preterm delivery, and intrauterine growth retardation (51,52).

Cytoreductive Therapy

During pregnancy, platelet count may undergo a natural fall and this could reduce the need of cytoreductive drugs in patients with ET. Platelet-lowering therapy in pregnancy is controversial, since the available data does not indicate a relation between the platelet count and the adverse pregnancy outcome. According to the Italian guidelines (8) and expert judgment (51,52), candidates for platelet-lowering drugs are women with a previous history of major thrombosis or major bleeding, or when platelet count is greater than $1000-1500 \times 10^9/L$, or when familial thrombophilia or cardiovascular risk factors are documented. If cytoreduction has to be given, IFN-α is probably the safest option. Other cytotoxic drugs, such as HU, busulfan, and anagrelide, should be avoided, particularly during organogenesis in the first trimester.

In conclusion, evidence-based recommendations for the most appropriate treatment of pregnancy in women with ET cannot be given to date, since only anedoctal data or, at best, retrospective studies have been published. Within the European LeukemiaNet, a prospective observational registry of pregnancies in MPDs was established with the aim to address the numerous questions still unanswered (52).

REFERENCES

1. Tefferi A, Barbui T. *BCR/ABL* negative, classic myeloproliferative disorders: diagnosis and treatment. Mayo Clin Proc 2005;80:1220–1232.
2. Finazzi G, Harrison C. Essential thrombocythemia. Semin Hematol 2005;42: 230–238.
3. Mesa RA, Silverstein MN, Jacobsen SJ, et al. Population-based incidence and survival figures in essential thrombocythemia and agnogenic myeloid metaplasia: an Olmsted County study, 1976–1995. Am J Hematol 1999;61:10–15.
4. Johansson P, Kutti J, Andreasson B, et al. Trends in the incidence of chronic Philadelphia chromosome – negative (Ph-) myeloproliferative disorders in the city of Goteborg, Sweden, during 1983–1999. J Intern Med 2004;256:161–165.
5. Ruggeri M, Tosetto A, Frezzato M, et al. The rate of progression to polycythemia vera or essential thrombocythemia in patients with erythrocytosis or thrombocytosis. Ann Intern Med 2003;139:470–475.
6. Wolanskyj AP, Schwager SM, McClure RF, et al. Essential thrombocythemia beyond the first decade: Life expectancy, long-term complication rates, and prognostic factors. Mayo Clin Proc 2006;81:159–166.
7. Elliott MA, Tefferi A. Thrombosis and haemorrhage in polycythemia vera and essential thrombocythaemia. Br J Haematol 2005;128:275–290.
8. Barbui T, Barosi G, Grossi A, et al. Evidence- and consensus-based practice guidelines for the therapy of essential thrombocythemia. A statement from the Italian Society of Hematology. Haematologica 2004;89:215–232.
9. Cortelazzo S, Viero P, Finazzi G, et al. Incidence and risk factors for thrombotic complications in a historical cohort of 100 patients with essential thrombocythemia. J Clin Oncol 1990;8:556–562.

10. van Genderen PJ, Michiels JJ. Erythromelalgic, thrombotic, and hemorrhagic manifestations of thrombocythemia. Presse Med 1994;23:73–77.

11. Cervantes F, Alvarez-Larran A, Talarn, et al. Myelofibrosis with myeloid metaplasia following essential thrombocythemia: actuarial probability, presenting characteristics, and evolution in a series of 195 patients. Br J Haematol 2002;118: 786–790.

12. Gangat N, Wolanskyj AP, McClure RF, et al. Risk stratification for survival and leukemic transformation in essential thrombocythemia: a single institutional study in 605 patients. Leukemia 2007;21:270–276.

13. Besses C, Cervantes F, Pereira A, et al. Major vascular complications in essential thrombocythemia: a study of the predictive factors in a series of 148 patients. Leukemia 1999;13:150–154.

14. Colombi M, Radaelli F, Zocchi L, et al. Thrombotic and hemorrhagic complications in essential thrombocythemia. A retrospective study of 103 patients. Cancer 1991;67:2926–2930.

15. Jantunen R, Juvonen E, Ikkala E, et al. The predictive value of vascular risk factors and gender for the development of thrombotic complications in essential thrombocythemia. Ann Hematol 2001;80:74–78.

16. Bazzan M, Tamponi G, Schinco P, et al. Thrombosis-free survival and life expectancy in 187 consecutive patients with essential thrombocythemia. Ann Hematol 1999;78:539–543.

17. Carobbio A, Finazzi G, Guerini V, et al. Leukocytosis is a risk factor for thrombosis in essential thrombocythemia: interaction with treatment, standard risk factors, and JAK2 mutation status. Blood 2007;109:2310–2313.

18. Fenaux P, Simon M, Caulier MT, et al. Clinical course of essential thrombocythemia in 147 cases. Cancer 1990;66:549–556.

19. Falanga A, Marchetti M, Barbui T, et al. Pathogenesis of thrombosis in essential thrombocythemia and polycythemia vera: the role of neutrophils. Semin Hematol 2005;42:239–247.

20. Arellano-Rodrigo E, Alvarez-Larran A, Reverter JC, et al. Increased platelet and leukocyte activation as contributing mechanisms for thrombosis in essential thrombocythemia and correlation with the JAK2 mutation status. Haematologica 2006;91:169–175.

21. Campbell PJ, Scott LM, Buck G, et al. Definition of subtypes of essential thrombocythaemia and relation to polycythaemia vera based on JAK2 V617F mutation status: a prospective study. Lancet 2005;366:1945–1953.

22. Cheung B, Radia D, Pantedelis P, et al. The presence of the JAK2 V617F mutation is associated with higher haemoglobin and increased risk of thrombosis in essential thrombocythaemia. Br J Haematol 2005;132:244–250.

23. Finazzi G, Rambaldi A, Guerini V, et al. Risk of thrombosis in patients with essential thrombocythemia and polycythemia vera according to JAK2 V617 F status. Haematologica 2007;92:135–136.

24. Antonioli E, Guglielmelli P, Pancrazzi A, et al. Clinical implications of the JAK2 V617 F mutation in essential thrombocythemia. Leukemia 2005;19:1847–1849.

25. Wolanskyj AP, Lasho TL, Schwager SM, et al. JAK2 V617 F mutation in essential thrombocythaemia: clinical associations and long-term prognostic relevance. Br J Haematol 2005;131:208–213.

26. van Genderen PJ, Budde U, Michiels JJ, et al. The reduction of large von Willebrand multimers in plasma in essential thrombocythemia is related to the platelet count. Br J Haematol 1996;93:962–965.
27. Tefferi A, Gangat N, Wolanskyj AP. Management of extreme thrombocytosis in otherwise low-risk essential thrombocythemia: does number matter? Blood 2006;108:2493–2494.
28. Barbui T, Finazzi G. When and how to treat essential thrombocythemia. N Engl J Med 2005; 85–86.
29. Ruggeri M, Finazzi G, Tosetto A, et al. No treatment for low-risk essential thrombocythemia: results from a prospective study. Br J Haematol 1998;103:772–777.
30. Landolfi R, Marchioli R, Kutti J, et al. Efficacy and safety of low-dose aspirin in polycythemia vera. N Engl J Med 2004;350:114–124.
31. Harrison CN, Green AR. Essential thrombocythemia. Hematol Oncol Clin North Am 2003;17:1175–1190.
32. Sterkers Y, Preudhomme C, Lai J-L, et al. Acute myeloid leukemia and myelodyslastic syndromes following essential thrombocythemia treated with hydroxyurea: high proportion of cases with 17p deletion. Blood 1998;91:616–622.
33. Lofvenberg E, Nordenson I, Walhlin A. Cytogenetic abnormalities and leukemic transformation in hydroxyurea-treated patients with Philadelphia chromosome – negative, chronic myeloproliferative disease. Cancer Genet Cytogenet 1990;49: 57–67.
34. Finazzi G, Ruggeri M, Rodeghiero F, et al. Efficacy and safety of long-term use of hydroxyurea in young patients with essential thrombocythemia and a high risk of thrombosis. Blood 2003;101:3749.
35. Finazzi G, Caruso V, Marchioli R, et al. Acute leukemia in polycythemia vera. An analysis of 1638 patients enrolled in a prospective observational study. Blood 2005;105:2664–2670.
36. Finazzi G, Ruggeri M, Rodeghiero F, et al. Second malignancies in patients with essential thrombocythemia treated with busulphan and hydroxyurea: long-term follow-up of a randomized clinical trial. Br J Haematol 2000;110:577–583.
37. Murphy S, Peterson P, Iland H, et al. Experience of the Polycythemia Vera Study Group with essential thrombocythemia: a final report on diagnostic criteria, survival, and leukemic transition by treatment. Semin Hematol 1997;34:29–39.
38. Anagrelide study group. Anagrelide, a therapy for thrombocythemic states: experience in 577 patients. Anagrelide Study Group. Am J Med 1992;92:69–76.
39. Wagstaff AJ, Keating GM. Anagrelide. A review of its use in the management of essential thrombocythaemia. Drugs 2006;66:111–131.
40. Jurgens DJ, Moreno-Aspitia A, Tefferi A. Anagrelide-associated cardiomyopathy in polycythemia vera and essential thrombocythemia. Haematologica 2004;89: 1394–1395.
41. Barosi G, Besses C, Birgegard G, et al. A unified definition of clinical resistance/intolerance to hydroxyurea in essential thrombocythemia: results of a consensus process by an international working group. Leukemia 2007;21:277–280.
42. Fruchtman SM, Petitt RM, Gilbert HS, et al. Anagrelide: analysis of long-term safety and leukemogenic potential in myeloproliferative disorders. Leuk Res 2005;29: 481–491.
43. Storen EC, Tefferi A. Long-term use of anagrelide in young patients with essential thrombocythemia. Blood 2001;97:863–866.

44. Lengfelder E, Griesshammer M, Hehlmann R. Interferon-alpha in the treatment of essential thrombocythemia. Leuk Lymphoma 1996;22(suppl 1):135–142.
45. Quintas-Cardama A, Kantarjian HM, Giles F, et al. Pegylated interferon therapy for patients with Philadelphia chromosome–negative myeloproliferative disorders. Semin Thromb Hemost 2006;32:409–416.
46. Kiladjian JJ, Cassinat B, Turlure P, et al. High molecular response rate of polycythemia vera patients treated with pegylated interferon α-2a. Blood 2006;108:2037–2040.
47. Samuelsson J, Mutschler M, Birgegard G, et al. Limited effects on JAK2 mutational status after pegylated interferon α-2b therapy in polycythemia vera and essential thrombocythemia. Haematologica 2006;91:1281–1282.
48. Cortelazzo S, Finazzi G, Ruggeri M, et al. Hydroxyurea in the treatment of patients with essential thrombocythemia at high risk of thrombosis: a prospective randomized trial. N Engl J Med 1995;332:1132–1136.
49. Harrison CN, Campbell P, Buck G, et al. Hydroxyurea compared with anagrelide in high-risk essential thrombocythemia. N Engl J Med 2005;353:33–45.
50. Maugeri N, Giordano G, Petrilli MP, et al. Inhibition of tissue factor expression by hydroxyurea in polymorphonuclear leukocytes from patients with myeloproliferative disorders: a new effect for an old drug? J Thromb Haemost 2006;4:2593–2598.
51. Harrison C. Pregnancy and its management in the Philadelphia-negative myeloproliferative diseases. Br J Haematol 2005;129:293–306.
52. Griesshammer M, Struve S, Harrison C. Essential thrombocythemia/polycythemia vera and pregnancy: the need for an observational study in Europe. Semin Thromb Haemost 2006;32:422–429.
53. Beard J, Hillmen P, Anderson CC, et al. Primary thrombocythemia in pregnancy. Br J Haematol 1991;77:371–374.
54. Beressi AH, Tefferi A, Silverstein MN, et al. Outcome analysis of 34 pregnancies in women with essential thrombocythemia. Arch Intern Med 1995;155:1217–1222.
55. Pagliaro P, Arrigoni L, Muggiasca ML, et al. Primary thrombocythemia in pregnancy: treatment and outcome in fifteen cases. Am J Hematol 1996;53:6–10.
56. Randi ML, Rossi C, Fabris F, et al. Essential thrombocythemia in young adults: treatment and outcome of 16 pregnancies. J Intern Med 1999;246:517–518.
57. Bangerter M, Guthner C, Beneke H, et al. Pregnancy in essential thrombocythemia: treatment and outcome of 17 patients. Eur J Haematol 2000;65:165–169.
58. Wright CA, Tefferi A. A single institutional experience with 43 pregnancies in essential thrombocythemia. Eur J Haematol 2001;66:152–159.
59. Niittyvuopio R, Juvonen E, Kaaja R, et al. Pregnancy in essential thrombocythemia: experience with 40 pregnancies. Eur J Haematol 2004;73:431–436.
60. Elliott MA, Tefferi A. Thrombocythaemia and pregnancy. Best Pract Res Clin Hematol 2003;16:227–242.
61. Robertson L, Wu O, Langhorne P, et al. Thrombophilia in pregnancy: a systematic review. Br J Haematol 2005;132:171–196.

7

Management of Myelofibrosis

Francisco Cervantes

Hematology Department, Hospital Clinic, IDIBAPS,
University of Barcelona, Spain

Giovanni Barosi

Unit of Clinical Epidemiology and Center for the Study of Myelofibrosis, IRCCS
Policlinico San Matteo, Pavia, Italy

INTRODUCTION

Myelofibrosis, also known as myelofibrosis with myeloid metaplasia or agnogenic myeloid metaplasia, is a chronic myeloproliferative disorder characterized by bone marrow fibrosis, extramedullary hemopoiesis with splenomegaly, anemia with dacryocytes, and a leukoerythroblastic blood picture (1). The disease can present as a de novo disorder (primary myelofibrosis or PMF) or appear as an evolutive form of a previously known polycythemia vera or essential thrombocythemia (post-PV MF or post-ET MF) (2). Although the marrow fibrosis is the distinctive feature of myelofibrosis, it actually represents a reactive phenomenon to the clonal proliferation of a pluripotent hemopoietic stem cell that, due to a somatic mutation, acquires a proliferative advantage over the benign progenitors (3,4). The resulting abnormal cell population releases several cytokines and growth factors in the bone marrow, leading to the secondary appearance of the fibrosis, and through the blood stream colonizes extramedullary organs, such as the spleen and the liver (1). The recent demonstration of the JAK2 mutation V617F in approximately one-half of PMF patients (5) and the MPL mutation in a proportion of those without the JAK2 mutation (6,7) has allowed a better understanding of the pathogenesis of the

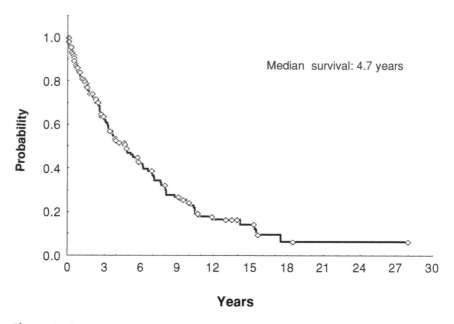

Figure 1 Survival curve of 167 patients diagnosed with primary myelofibrosis at the Hospital Clinic of Barcelona, Spain.

disease. However, despite the latter progresses, there is no specific marker for the disease and its diagnosis remains of exclusion.

PMF is an infrequent disease, with an estimated incidence in the Western countries of 0.4–0.7 new cases per 100,000 person/year (8). It affects mainly elderly people, since median age at presentation is about 65 years, but 22% of patients are 55 years old or younger at diagnosis (9). In modern series (10,11), median survival of PMF patients ranges from 3.5 to 5 years (Fig. 1). However, there is a wide variability, with some patients dying within 1 or 2 years from diagnosis while others surviving for even decades. This fact has lead to the identification of prognostic factors at disease diagnosis and the elaboration of several prognostic scoring systems (9,10,12) (Table 1). The presentation and evolution of PMF is also heterogeneous and, thus, the clinical spectrum of the disease ranges from patients who are asymptomatic at diagnosis and may not require treatment for years to others who present with symptoms derived from anemia and splenomegaly and constitutional symptoms. In turn, the hematologic profile of PMF is also variable, ranging from leukopenia to leukocytosis and from thrombocytopenia to thrombocytosis. Such heterogeneity makes it necessary to adjust the treatment of the disease to its characteristics in every individual.

Except for the minority of patients who can receive an allogeneic stem cell transplantation, PMF remains an incurable disease, with its therapy being merely palliative and primarily aimed at alleviation of the symptoms and improvement in patients' quality of life, but without having a real impact on survival. This, and the

Table 1 Prognostic Scoring Systems for Patients with Primary Myelofibrosis Overall (Dupriez), for Patients 55 Years Old or Younger (Cervantes) and for Patients 60 Years Old or Younger (Elliot)

	Dupriez score	Cervantes score	Elliott score
Adverse factors	H Hb < 100 g/L WBC < 4 × 10⁹/L or > 30 × 10⁹/L	Hb < 100 g/L Blood blasts ≥ 1% Constitutional symptoms	H Hb < 100 g/L WBC < 4 × 10⁹/L or > 30 × 10⁹/L Platelets < 100 × 10⁹/L Monocytes > 1 × 10⁹/L
Prognostic groups	Low risk: 0 factors Intermed. risk: 1 factor High risk: 2 factors	Low risk: 0–1 factor High risk: 2–3 factors	Low risk: 0 factors Intermed. risk: 1 factor High risk: ≥ 2 factors

fact that many patients do not respond to the available therapies and all eventually die from complications of the disease, has stimulated the interest for the search of new modalities for the treatment of myelofibrosis.

The present review summarizes the current status of the treatment of myelofibrosis, with special emphasis being made on conventional treatment and stem cell transplantation options. While the drugs of more recent introduction will also be considered, they will be reviewed in more detail in another chapter of this book.

CONVENTIONAL TREATMENT

Since most currently available therapies do not have a clear impact on patient survival, at the time of making a therapeutic decision in a patient with PMF, it is important to consider the possible benefit that could derive from treatment institution. In this sense, to date, it is generally agreed that if the patient has no symptoms or do not show risk factors for developing complications (e.g., marked thrombocytosis), a wait-and-see approach is a reasonable option, with treatment being delayed until significant changes are observed in the patient's clinical or hematological situation upon periodic and watchful observation (13). It is likely, however, that such a conservative approach will progressively change as more effective therapies for PMF become available.

Cytoreductive Therapy

In the "hyperproliferative" forms of myelofibrosis, with constitutional symptoms or bone pain, marked and often symptomatic splenomegaly, leukocytosis, and/or thrombocytosis, there is an indication for the institution of cytolytic treatment, with hydroxyurea being the drug of choice. Hydroxyurea can reduce the spleen and liver size, relief the constitutional symptoms, and control the leukocytosis and the thrombocytosis in a substantial proportion of patients (14,15). The drug dose varies from patient to patient and must be adjusted to the individual hematologic tolerability, since accentuation of the anemia is sometimes observed following treatment institution. Because of this, it is recommended to start with a low dose (e.g., 500 mg daily), in order to identify those patients who are more sensitive to the drug and minimize toxicity, and to progressively increase the dose according to the patient's hematologic tolerability and the evolution of the clinical status.

Busulfan can also be used in the proliferative forms of PMF (16) but, due to its prolonged effect in the bone marrow, with the risk of provoking long-lasting cytopenia, it requires a close control, which makes it inconvenient for the treatment in clinical practice.

In one study, low-dose melphalan (2.5 mg for 3 days a week, with progressive increase up to a maximum dose of 2.5 mg a day), administered after 2 months or more of low-dose danazol (200 mg/day) or prednisone (0.25 mg/kg per day) yielded favorable responses in 66 of 99 patients with hyperproliferative myelofibrosis (17). Splenic size, leukocytosis, and thrombocytosis normalized in 23%, 86%, and 93% of patients, respectively. Anemia improved in 12 of 20 patients not requiring transfusion and 6 of 16 became transfusion independent. However, although acute transformation is considered as part of the natural history of PMF, the leukemogenic potential of melphalan probably explains its scarce use in clinical practice.

2-chlorodeoxyadenosine, a purine nucleoside analog of intravenous administration, has been reported to have a role for the treatment of progressive hepatomegaly and symptomatic thrombocytosis that develop after splenectomy (18).

Androgens

Once treatable causes of the anemia of myelofibrosis are excluded, such as iron or vitamin B12 deficiency or autoimmune hemolysis, androgens are a therapeutic option. The efficacy of testosterone in the anemia of myelofibrosis was first shown in the early 1960s (19,20) and its main mechanism of action seems to be the stimulation of the bone marrow function (21). According to the published studies, nandrolone, fluoxymesterolone, methandrostenolone, and oxymetholone improve the anemia in 30–60% of patients (22–24), with an abnormal karyotype and severely compromised hemopoiesis being the factors associated with a low chance of achieving a favorable response to treatment (23). Side effects include fluid retention, hirsutism, virilization, abnormal liver function tests, and, more rarely, liver and prostate tumors. Similar results, but with less toxicity, can be obtained using danazol, a semisynthetic attenuated androgen that can also correct the thrombocytopenia. A sufficient dose of the drug (from 600 to 800 mg daily, depending on patient's weight) must be administered and should be maintained for a minimum of 6 months, unless toxicity develops, since a substantial proportion of responses are seen between 3 and 6 months of treatment institution (25). Once a response has been obtained, the dose must be progressively reduced to the minimum necessary dose to maintain the response, usually 200 mg/day. Liver function must be monitored and periodic ultrasound imaging surveillance performed in order to detect the possible appearance of liver tumors, whereas systematic screening for prostate cancer must be carried out in men.

Erythropoietin and Darbepoetin-α

Recombinant human erythropoietin (rHuEPO) is currently used to treat the anemia of myelofibrosis (26–29). In an analysis of 20 patients treated with rHuEPO, the response rate was 45%, with 20% of patients maintaining the response in the long term (29). When the above 20 patients plus 31 from the literature were pooled together, the overall response rate was 55%, including 31% complete responses, and the median duration of the responses was 12 months. At the multivariate study, inappropriate serum erythropoietin (Epo) levels ($<$ 125 mU/mL) was the only pre-treatment variable associated with a favorable response to rHuEPO, whereas lack of transfusion support at treatment start had borderline significance. Therefore, Epo should be restricted to patients with anemia and inappropriate Epo levels. Since the responses are usually seen at few weeks of treatment start, erythropoietin would be the choice therapy for such a subgroup of patients. Similar results can be obtained using darbepoetin-α, an erythropoietin-stimulating protein that can be administered at longer time intervals, being more convenient to the patient (30). Again, the favorable responses are restricted to patients with inappropriate Epo levels.

Other Drugs

There have been many reports on the use of interferon-α in PMF, although most of them refer to small series of patients (31–36). In some studies, interferon had no effect in the anemia and the splenomegaly and, although it often decreased the leukocytes and the platelets, this was sometimes rather an undesirable effect than a therapeutic response (31,32). This, and the frequent side effects, led to treatment discontinuation in most patients. Better results were reported in other studies that included patients with the hyperproliferative form of PMF, in which interferon reduced the leukocytosis and the thrombocytosis, although it did not improve the anemia (33–35). In a more recent study of patients with hyperproliferative myelofibrosis, no beneficial effect of interferon was noted in spleen size, marrow fibrosis, or microvessel density, whereas side effects led to treatment withdrawal in 7 of 11 patients (36). Thus, interferon would have a minor role in myelofibrosis, given its limited efficacy and frequent toxicity. However, it could be occasionally considered in patients with hyperproliferative disease refractory to cytolytic treatment (33–35).

Besides autoimmune hemolytic anemia, corticosteroids have been reported to improve nonhemolytic anemia in some patients with PMF (37). Cyclosporin A has been employed in patients with severe anemia and autoimmune features, including positive Coombs' test, antinuclear and antimitochondrial antibodies, and circulating immune complexes, who are refractory to prednisone. In a series of 10 such patients, 3 of the 6 who could complete 6 months of treatment responded favorably, with a high CD4/CD8 ratio being the best predictor of the response (38). Finally, anagrelide can be useful to treat the thrombocytosis that is uncontrollable by hydroxyurea (39).

Antifibrosing agents such as d-penicillamin, 1,25-dihydroxy-vitamin D_3 (40), and pirfenidone (41) have shown minimal therapeutic activity in myelofibrosis patients and are no longer used in this disease.

Splenectomy

Splenectomy is considered occasionally as a palliative measure for PMF patients, especially those with massive and painful splenomegaly or refractory cytopenias. However, the decision of removing the spleen should be carefully taken, given the substantial risk associated with the procedure in PMF patients. Thus, in a retrospective analysis of 15 series of the literature, including a total of 321 patients submitted to splenectomy, operative mortality was 13.4%, early morbidity 45.3%, and late morbidity 16.3% (42). In two single institution series (43,44), operative morbidity was 39.3% and 31%, and mortality 8.4% and 9%, respectively, with the latter increasing up to 26% when the 3-month postsplenectomy period was considered (44). Main complications of splenectomy are bleeding (especially hemoperitoneum), infections, and thrombosis. In addition, massive hepatomegaly due to compensatory myeloid metaplasia of the liver develops in 16–24% of patients, some of which die from liver failure (44). Postsplenectomy thrombocytosis that increases the risk of thrombosis, especially in the splenoportal vein tract (45), is observed in 20–22% of patients, mainly in those with presurgical platelet values higher than 50×10^9/L (46). Moreover, following splenectomy, a higher rate of blast transformation has been registered in one study (47). Since the procedure is not associated with a higher risk of developing acute leukemia in healthy individuals, it has been speculated with a possible effect of the splenectomy in accelerating a preexisting myeloid proliferation.

Splenectomy has been considered for symptomatic splenomegaly refractory to treatment, transfusion-dependent anemia unresponsive to therapy, severe constitutional symptoms, uncontrollable hemolysis, portal hypertension secondary to increased portal flow, and marked thrombocytopenia (44). The benefits vary, depending on the indication. Thus, in the series of the Mayo Clinic, durable responses in constitutional symptoms, transfusion-dependent anemia, portal hypertension, and severe thrombocytopenia were obtained in 67%, 23%, 50%, and 0% of cases, respectively (44). Since no survival prolongation from splenectomy has been demonstrated, the risks of splenectomy should be balanced against the possible advantages in every patient, in order to restrict the procedure to those most likely to benefit. In this sense, thrombocytosis would be a formal contraindication for splenectomy, given the high probability of provoking uncontrollable thrombocytosis and subsequent thrombosis, whereas severe thrombocytopenia should no longer be considered an indication for the procedure.

Radiation Therapy

Splenic irradiation can reduce spleen size and procure rapid symptom relief to PMF patients. The doses used have been variable, with the total doses ranging from 0.15 to 65 Gy per course, administered in fractioned doses. In the largest published series, which included 22 patients, the median dose administered per course was 2.8 Gy (48). Splenic irradiation can be considered in patients who are poor candidates to surgery and, especially, for palliation of severe pain from spleen infarction (49,50). However, its effect is not durable, whereas the risk of provoking severe and long-lasting cytopenias, probably due to an effect on the circulating progenitors (51), is high. The latter complication is registered in up to one-third of patients and can be life-threatening, due to the risk of severe infection or bleeding (48). Therefore, routine use of splenic irradiation in patients with myelofibrosis should not be recommended. Finally, an increased risk of postoperative bleeding has been observed in patients who were submitted to splenic irradiation to reduce the spleen size before splenectomy (48).

Low-dose radiation therapy is the choice therapy for symptomatic extramedullary hemopoiesis, in places such as the spinal cord, the peritoneum or the pleura, granulocytic sarcomas of the bone causing local pain, and pulmonary hypertension secondary to diffuse myeloid metaplasia of the lung (52–55). It has also been given for symptomatic hepatomegaly, but its effect is always transient whereas myelosuppression often develops.

ANTIANGIOGENIC AND IMMUNOMODULATORY DRUGS

Patients with PMF have prominent neovascularization in the bone marrow, due to the release in the marrow microenvironment of several cytokines, such as the vascular endothelial growth factor (VEGF), the basic fibroblast growth factor (bFGF), the transforming growth factor-beta, and others (56,57). Based on this, antiangiogenic drugs are increasingly being administered in this disease.

Thalidomide inhibits VEGF- and bFGF-dependent angiogenesis and the tumor necrosis factor alpha. In a pooled analysis of 62 patients with myelofibrosis treated with thalidomide in five phase II trials (58), in which the starting daily dose ranged from 100 to 200 mg, treatment withdrawal was 21% within the first 4 weeks, 49% before 3 months, and 66% before 6 months due to toxicity. In addition to the general side effects of thalidomide, such as constipation, fatigue, paresthesiae, and sedation, in a proportion of patients the disease worsened coincidently with treatment. Thus, 8% of them had a decrease in Hb, 10% developed thrombocytopenia, and 10% neutropenia. Moreover, in almost 20% of cases, myeloproliferative acceleration of myelofibrosis was seen in temporal association with treatment, although disease progression, per se, may have occurred. Among patients assessable for response, the anemia improved in 29% of cases, the thrombocytopenia in 38%, and the splenomegaly in 41%. The results were better in the early phases of the disease as well as in untreated patients.

In an attempt to minimize toxicity, lower doses of thalidomide have been given. Thus, 21 patients from the Mayo Clinic received a dose of 50 mg/day plus oral prednisone, 30 mg daily for 3 months, and then tapered (59). Treatment withdrawal was only 5%. Anemia improved in 70% of patients, with 40% becoming transfusion independent, and thrombocytopenia in 75%, whereas spleen size reduction was noted in 19% of cases. Responses were mostly durable after prednisone discontinuation. In a second study including 63 patients from several European institutions, thalidomide dose was also 50 mg, but prednisone was not given (60). Treatment withdrawal was 49%, thrombocytopenia improved in 38% of cases, and splenomegaly in 36%, whereas amelioration of anemia was registered in only 11% of patients. Therefore, the combination of low-dose thalidomide and prednisone seems to be a well-tolerated treatment for myelofibrosis, which would be especially effective in patients with anemia or thrombocytopenia.

The efficacy of thalidomide in PMF has been questioned by the results of two recent studies, one from the Swedish group (61) and, especially, the prospective study of the French group (62). The latter investigators randomized 52 patients with myelofibrosis and anemia to receive standard-dose thalidomide or placebo and found that patients receiving thalidomide showed a high rate of side effects and discontinuation, whereas they did not show a significant improvement in the anemia, as compared with the patients in the placebo arm. Taking into account these observations, it could be speculated that the efficacy of low-dose thalidomide plus prednisone might be ascribed rather to the prednisone than to the thalidomide itself, although a drug synergy would be a second possibility.

Lenalidomide, a thalidomide derivative, resulted in 22% responses for the anemia, with normalization of the Hb in 9 cases, 33% for the splenomegaly, and 50% for the thrombocytopenia in 69 myelofibrosis patients from two institutions. Due to side effects, treatment discontinuation rate was high (39–48%) (63).

TYROSINE KINASE INHIBITORS

The rationale for the use of imatinib mesylate in PMF was its inhibition of the receptor of the platelet-derived growth factor (PDGF-R) and the c-kit. In five studies including a total of 73 patients, side effects were frequent and led to treatment withdrawal in many cases (13,64,65). Thus, neutropenia developed in 15–60% of patients, usually in those with low leukocyte counts at treatment start, whereas 48–82% of them developed leukocytosis and/or thrombocytosis. Extrahematologic toxicity was also frequent. On the other hand, no or only a minor effect on the anemia, the thrombocytopenia, or the splenomegaly was noted. Therefore, the role of imatinib in myelofibrosis would be a minor one, if any.

R115777, a farnesyl transferase inhibitor, has in vitro antiproliferative activity in the hemopoietic progenitors from PMF. In a trial including 8 patients, this drug provided 25% favorable responses in the anemia and the splenomegaly, with the responses being significantly associated with higher VEGF plasma levels at treatment start (66). In another study of 13 patients, an effect was seen on the splenomegaly, but not in the anemia (67). In turn, the preliminary results of SU5416, a VEGF tyrosine kinase inhibitor, indicate minimal therapeutic activity in PMF (68).

The next candidates for the treatment of myelofibrosis are newer and hopefully better tolerated immunomodulatory drugs, the proteasome inhibitors, the VEGF neutralising antibodies, and the JAK2 inhibitors. In this sense, with the prospect of the availability of newer drugs for the treatment of PMF, a panel of international experts, the so-called International Working Group for Myelofibrosis Research and Treatment (IWG-MRT), recently reached a consensus for the use of uniform criteria for the evaluation of the therapeutic response in this disease (69) (Table 2).

STEM CELL TRANSPLANTATION

Allogeneic hemopoietic stem cell transplantation (allo-SCT) remains the only curative therapy of myelofibrosis. Despite initial concern on the possible adverse effect of severe marrow fibrosis on hematologic recovery after allo-SCT (70), some case reports and small series of patients published in the late 1980s and early 1990s showed the feasibility of the procedure (71,72). Since then, several series of conventional conditioning allo-SCT in myelofibrosis patients have been published (73–77) but, for the purpose of the present review, we will focus on the two larger published studies (73,77), which actually included patients from several of the previously reported series.

Guardiola et al. (73) analyzed the results of allo-SCT in 55 patients (median age at transplantation 42 years, range: 4–53) from several institutions. Graft failure occurred in 9% of cases and 1-year transplant-related mortality was 27%. At 5 years of transplant, the probability of survival and disease-free survival was 47% and 39%, respectively. The variables with a negative influence on engraftment were osteosclerosis and lack of splenectomy. Hb < 10 g/dL, a high-risk Dupriez score (10), osteosclerosis, and the presence of karyotypic abnormalities had an adverse effect on survival, whereas increased age, karyotypic abnormalities, and the absence of or mild graft-versus-host disease were associated with posttransplant relapse. In an update of the series extended to 66 patients, the outcome of patients transplanted over the age of 45 years was poor, since only 14% of them survived at 5 years, versus 62% of younger patients (74).

In a single-institution study of 56 patients from the Seattle group (77), engraftment was achieved in all but 3 patients and transplant related mortality was 36%. At 3 years, the probability of survival and disease-free survival was 58% and 64%, respectively. Dupriez score, cytogenetic abnormalities, and the degree of fibrosis were the most important prognostic factors for transplant-related mortality. Disappearance of the splenomegaly was observed in 27 patients not previously submitted to splenectomy. In patients older than 45 years, the survival probability was 50% at 3 years. Except for the higher frequency of graft failure, the results

Table 2 International Working Group (IWG) Consensus Criteria for Treatment
Response in Myelofibrosis

1. *Complete remission* (CR). Requires all of the following in the absence of both
   transfusion and growth factor support
     (i) Complete resolution of disease-related symptoms and signs, including palpable
         hepatosplenomegaly
     (ii) Peripheral blood count remission defined as Hb > 11 g/dL, platelet count $\geq$ 100 $\times$
          10^9/L, and absolute neutrophil count $\geq$ 1.0 $\times$ 10^9/L
     (iii) Normal leukocyte differential, including disappearance of nucleated red blood
           cells and immature myeloid cells in blood, in the absence of splenectomy
     (iv) Bone marrow histological remission, defined as the presence of age-adjusted
          normocellularity, < 5% myeloblasts, and an osteomyelofibrosis grade of $\leq$ 1
2. *Partial remission* (PR). Requires all of the above criteria for CR except for bone
   marrow histological remission. However, a repeat bone marrow biopsy is required in
   the assessment of PR and may or may not show favorable changes that do not, however,
   fulfill criteria for CR
3. *Clinical improvement* (CI). Requires one of the following in the absence of both disease
   progression (as outlined below) and CR/PR assignment (CI response is validated only if
   it lasts for $\geq$ 8 wk)
     (i) A $\geq$ 2 g/dL increase in Hb level or becoming transfusion independent (applicable
         only for patients with baseline Hb < 10 g/dL)
     (ii) Either a $\geq$ 50% reduction in palpable splenomegaly of a spleen that is $\geq$ 10 cm at
          baseline or a spleen that is palpable at > 5 cm at baseline becomes not palpable
     (iii) A $\geq$ 100% increase in platelet count and an absolute platelet count of $\geq$ 50 $\times$
           10^9/L (applicable only for patients with baseline platelet count of < 50 $\times$ 10^9/L)
     (iv) A $\geq$ 100% increase in ANC and an ANC of $\geq$ 0.5 $\times$ 10^9/L (applicable only for
          patients with baseline absolute neutrophil count of < 1 $\times$ 10^9/L)
4. *Progressive disease*. Requires one of the following
     (i) Progressive splenomegaly that is defined by the appearance of a previously
         absent splenomegaly that is palpable at > 5 cm below the left costal margin or a
         $\geq$ 100% increase in palpable distance for baseline splenomegaly of 5–10 cm or a
         $\geq$ 50% increase in palpable distance for baseline splenomegaly of > 10 cm
     (ii) Leukemic transformation confirmed by a bone marrow blast count of 20%
     (iii) An increase in blood blast percentage of $\geq$ 20% that lasts for $\geq$ 8 weeks
5. *Stable disease*. None of the above
6. *Relapse*. Loss CR, PR, and CI: a patient with CR or PR is considered to have undergone
   relapse when no longer fulfills the criteria for even CI

in the 20 patients transplanted from unrelated donors were comparable to those
transplanted from family donors.

The procedure-related mortality around 30% and the morbidity associated
with allogeneic SCT must be balanced versus the expected survival of younger
patients with PMF. Median survival of patients 55 years old or younger is
10.7 years (9) and, based on the presence of three bad prognostic factors (namely,
Hb < 10 g/dL, constitutional symptoms, and blasts $\geq$ 1% in peripheral blood),

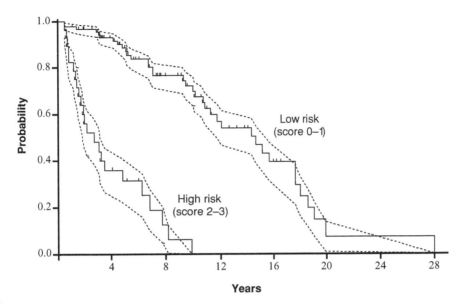

Figure 2 Prognostic groups in patients ≤ 55 years at diagnosis of primary myelofibrosis (*n* = 121; see Table 1 for prognostic factors).

two subgroups of patients can be clearly identified: a low-risk group (with none or only one poor prognostic factor) and a high-risk group (with two or the three bad prognostic features) (Fig. 2). The low-risk group encompasses three-quarters of the patients and its median survival approaches 15 years, versus 33 months for patients in the high-risk group. These data may be of help at the time of making the decision of performing a transplant in a patient with myelofibrosis (78). Thus, whereas the indication for performing an allo-SCT upfront in young individuals with high-risk PMF is clear, for low-risk patients a wait-and-see approach or conventional treatment first seems reasonable, delaying transplantation until the appearance of poor-risk features or resistance to conventional therapy.

There is not sufficient evidence to recommend routine splenectomy before transplantation in myelofibrosis. The faster hematologic recovery, as well as the debulky effect in patients with massive splenomegaly, would favor spleen removal. In turn, the substantial morbidity and mortality associated with the procedure and the observation that even marked splenomegalies can resolve following transplantation (77) would argue against splenectomy as a preparation maneuver for transplantation. Therefore, the decision must be taken on an individual basis. In this sense, until more solid evidence is available, it seems reasonable to restrict the procedure to those patients with osteosclerosis or massive splenomegaly, taking into account the higher risk of graft failure in such cases (73).

With regard to the conditioning regimen, it has been suggested that busulfan, with doses adjusted to achieve adequate plasma levels of the drug, would result

Table 3   Results of Reduced-Intensity Conditioning Allogeneic Stem Cell
Transplantation for Myelofibrosis

Author	No. of patients	Conditioning regimen	Full chimerism	Remission rate	Survival rate
Devine	4	Flu/Mel	4	100%	100%
Kröger	21	Flu/Bu/ATG	20	75%[a]	84%[b]
Rondelli	21	Several	20	81%[c]	86%[a]
Merup	10	Flu/Bu-Mel	10	90%[d]	90%[c]

[a] Median follow-up: 31 months.
[b] Median follow-up: 22 months.
[c] Median follow-up: ± 30 months.
Abbreviations: Flu, fludarabine; Mel, melphalan; Bu, busulfan; ATG, antithymocyte globulin.

in lower transplant-related mortality and higher survival than TBI-based regimens
(77).

   Based on the demonstration of a graft-versus-myelofibrosis effect (79,80),
reduced-intensity conditioning (RIC) allo-SCT is currently being performed in
myelofibrosis (Table 3). Devine et al. (81) reported for the first time the results
of RIC allo-SCT using fludarabine (30 mg/m^2/day for 5 days) plus melphalan
(70 mg/m^2/day for 2 days) as conditioning regimen in 4 patients aged 48– to
58 years with intermediate- or high-risk disease. In all cases, engraftment was
observed and full-donor chimerism was demonstrated by day 30, persisting at
14-month follow-up, when all patients remained alive and without signs of the
disease, including a normal marrow biopsy.

   Kröger et al. (82) analyzed RIC allo-SCT in 21 patients, most of them conditioned with fludarabine, busulfan, and antithymocyte globulin. Full chimerism
was observed in 20 cases and, after a median follow-up of 22 months, complete
histopathological remission rate was 75%, with an estimated 3-year overall and
disease-free survival of 84%. In another multicentric study including 21 patients
with intermediate- or high-risk myelofibrosis (83), all but 1 patient achieved full
engraftment and posttransplant donor cell chimerism was > 95% in 19 cases, while
the other 2 achieved complete donor chimerism following donor lymphocyte infusion. Three patients died from acute GVHD, infection, and relapse, respectively,
and 18 remained alive at a median posttransplant follow-up of 31 months (range,
12–122). More recently, Merup et al. (84) have compared retrospectively the
results of conventional and RIC regimens for allo-SCT in myelofibrosis, showing
that transplant-related mortality was 30% in the 17 patients receiving conventional
transplants versus 10% in the 10 patients submitted to a RIC procedure.

   In a recent study, Kröger et al. (85) reported the results of monitoring
residual disease by quantitative PCR in 22 RIC allo-SCT procedures performed
in 21 patients with JAK2-positive myelofibrosis. Of the 21 patients, 17 (78%)
became PCR negative and 15 remained JAK-2 negative after a median follow-up of
20 months. JAK2 negativity was achieved after a median of 89 days after allograft

and a significant inverse correlation was observed between JAK2 positivity and donor-cell chimerism. Of note, 4 of the 5 patients who never achieved JAK2 negativity fulfilled the criteria for complete remission of the IWG-MRT (69), suggesting that quantification of JAK2 positive cells after allogeneic SCT would be a more precise tool to define complete remission.

In summary, the short-term results of RIC allo-SCT in myelofibrosis are encouraging, since the procedure has a substantially lower treatment-related mortality than conventional allo-SCT while apparently maintaining the capacity to eradicate the disease. There are some aspects of RIC allo-SCT that need to be clarified; among them is the optimal conditioning regimen or the role of splenectomy. Risk stratification is important in order to select those patients most likely to benefit from this treatment. For the time being, until the long-term results of RIC allo-SCT are available, this transplant modality should be restricted to patients 45–70 years old with intermediate- or high-risk PMF or who are resistant to conventional treatment.

Autologous SCT (auto-SCT) has been performed in myelofibrosis, based on the high number of hemopoietic progenitors circulating in the peripheral blood of these patients. In a retrospective multicentric study of 21 patients, a sufficient number of $CD34^+$ cells could be obtained in all cases (86). However, use of G-CSF was recommended, taking into account that in PMF most circulating $CD34^+$ cells are committed progenitors lacking the capacity to sustain the hemopoiesis. Graft failure was registered in 3 patients and 5 required backup stem cell infusion. At 2 years, the actuarial survival rate was 61%, with 6 patients having died, 3 from graft failure or infection and 3 from disease progression. Symptomatic splenomegaly improved in 7 of 10 patients, transfusion independence was achieved in 10 of 17, and thrombocytopenia resolved in 4 of 8, whereas significant reduction in the marrow fibrosis was seen in 6 cases. Therefore, auto-SCT can be considered as a palliative treatment for myelofibrosis patients younger than 70 years who are resistant to treatment and lack a suitable donor for allogeneic transplantation.

REFERENCES

1. Barosi G. Myelofibrosis with myeloid metaplasia: diagnostic definition and prognostic classification for clinical studies and treatment guidelines. J Clin Oncol 1999;17:2954–2970.
2. Mesa RA, Verstovsek S, Cervantes F, et al. Primary myelofibrosis (PMF), post–polycythemia vera myelofibrosis (post-PV MF), post essential thrombocythemia myelofibrosis (post-ET MF), blast phase PMF (PMF-BP): consensus on terminology by the International Working Group for Myelofibrosis Research and Treatment (IWG-MRT). Leuk Res pub ahead of print 2007;31:737–740.
3. Jacobson RJ, Salo A, Fialkow PJ. Agnogenic myeloid metaplasia: a clonal proliferation of hematopoietic stem cells with secondary myelofibrosis. Blood 1978;51: 189–194.

4. Buschle M, Janssen JW, Drexler H, et al. Evidence of pluripotent stem cell origin of idiopathic myelofibrosis: clonal analysis of a case characterized by a N-ras gene mutation. Leukemia 1988;2:658–660.

5. Kralowics R, Passamonti F, Buser AS, et al. A gain-of-function mutation of JAK2 in myeloproliferative disorders. N Engl J Med 2005;352:1779–1790.

6. Pikman Y, Lee BH, Mercher T, et al. MPLW515L is a novel somatic activating mutation in myelofibrosis with myeloid metaplasia. PloS Med 2006;3:1140–1151.

7. Pardanani AD, Levine RL, Lasho T, et al. MPL515 mutations in myeloproliferative and other myeloid disorders: a study of 1182 patients. Blood 2006;108:3472–3476.

8. Mesa RA, Silverstein MN, Jacobsen SJ, et al. Population-based incidence and survival figures in essential thrombocythemia and agnogenic myeloid metaplasia: an Olmsted County study, 1975–1995. Am J Hematol 1999;61:10–15.

9. Cervantes F, Barosi G, Demory JL, et al. Myelofibrosis with myeloid metaplasia in young individuals: disease characteristics, prognostic factors, and identification of risk groups. Br J Haematol 1998;102:684–690.

10. Dupriez B, Morel P, Demory JL, et al. Prognostic factors in agnogenic myeloid metaplasia: a report on 195 cases with a new scoring system. Blood 1996;88: 1013–1018.

11. Cervantes F, Pereira A, Esteve J, et al. Identification of "long-lived" and "short-lived" patients at presentation of primary myelofibrosis. Br J Haematol 1997;97:635–640.

12. Elliott MA, Verstovsek S, Dingli D, et al. Monocytosis is an adverse prognostic factor for survival in younger patients with primary myelofibrosis. Leuk Res epub ahead of print 2007.

13. Cervantes F. Modern management of myelofibrosis. Br J Haematol 2005;128: 583–592.

14. Lofvenberg E, Wahlin A, Roos G, et al. Reversal of myelofibrosis by hydroxyurea. Eur J Haematol 1990;44:33–38.

15. Manoharan A. Management of myelofibrosis with intermittent hydroxyurea. Br J Haematol 1991;77:252–254.

16. Oishi N, Swisher SN, Troup SB. Busulfan therapy in myeloid metaplasia. Blood 1960;15:863–872.

17. Petti MC, Latagliata R, Spadea T, et al. Melphalan treatment in patients with myelofibrosis with myeloid metaplasia. Br J Haematol 2002;116:576–581.

18. Tefferi A, Silverstein MN, Li C-Y. 2-chlorodeoxyadenosine treatment after splenectomy in patients who have myelofibrosis with myeloid metaplasia. Br J Haematol 1997;99:352–357.

19. Kennedy BJ. Effect of androgenic hormone in myelofibrosis. JAMA 1962;182: 114–119.

20. Silver RT, Jenkins DE, Jr., Engle RL. Use of testosterone and busulfan in the treatment of myelofibrosis with myeloid metaplasia. Blood 1964;23:341–353.

21. Reilly JT. Idiopathic myelofibrosis: pathogenesis, natural history, and management. Blood Rev 1997;11:233–242.

22. Hast R, Engstedt L, Jameson S, et al. Oxymetholone treatment in myelofibrosis. Blut 1978;37:19–26.

23. Besa EC, Nowell PC, Geller NL, et al. Analysis of the androgen response of 23 patients with agnogenic myeloid metaplasia: the value of chromosomal studies in predicting response and survival. Cancer 1982;49:308–313.

24. Brubaker LH, Briere J, Laszlo J, et al. Treatment of anemia in myeloproliferative disorders: a randomized study of fluoxymesterone v transfusions only. Arch Intern Med 1982;142:1533–1537.
25. Cervantes F, Alvarez-Larrán A, Domingo A, et al. Efficacy and tolerability of danazol as a treatment for the anemia of myelofibrosis with myeloid metaplasia: long-term results in 30 patients. Br J Haematol 2005;129:771–775.
26. Bourantas KL, Tsiara S, Christou L, et al. Combination therapy with recombinant human erythropoietin, interferon-α-2b and granulocyte-macrophage colony-stimulating factor in idiopathic myelofibrosis. Acta Haematol 1996;96:79–82.
27. Rodríguez JN, Martino ML, Diéguez JC, et al. RHuEpo for the treatment of anemia in myelofibrosis with myeloid metaplasia. Experience in 6 patients and meta-analytical approach. Haematologica 1998;83:616–621.
28. Hasselbalch HC, Clausen NT, Jensen BA. Successful treatment of anemia in idiopathic myelofibrosis with recombinant human erythropoietin. Am J Hematol 2002;70:92–99.
29. Cervantes F, Alvarez-Larrán A, Hernández-Boluda JC, et al. Erythropoietin treatment of the anaemia of myelofibrosis with myeloid metaplasia: results in 20 patients and review of the literature. Br J Haematol 2004;127: 399–403.
30. Cervantes F, Alvarez-Larrán A, Hernández-Boluda JC, et al. Efficacy and safety of darbepoetin-alpha in the anaemia of myelofibrosis with myeloid metaplasia. Br J Haematol 2006;134:184–186.
31. Hasselbalch H. Interferon in myelofibrosis. Lancet 1988;i:355.
32. List AF, Doll DC. Alpha-interferon in the treatment of idiopathic myelofibrosis. Br J Haematol 1992;80:566–567.
33. Barosi G, Liberato LN, Costa A, et al. Cytoreductive effect of recombinant alpha interferon in patients with myelofibrosis with myeloid metaplasia. Blut 1988;58: 271–274.
34. Gilbert HS. Long-term treatment of myeloproliferative disease with interferon alpha-2b: feasibility and efficacy. Cancer 1998;83:1205–1213.
35. Bachleitner-Hofmann T, Gisslinger H. The role of interferon-α in the treatment of idiopathic myelofibrosis. Ann Hematol 1999;78:533–538.
36. Radin AI, Kim HT, Grant BW, et al. Phase II study of alpha interferon in the treatment of the chronic myeloproliferative disorders (E5487): a trial of the Eastern Cooperative Oncology Group. Cancer 2003;98:100–109.
37. Jack FR, Smith SR, Saunders PWG. Idiopathic myelofibrosis: anaemia can respond to low-dose dexamethasone. Br J Haematol 1994;87:876–884.
38. Centenara E, Guarnone R, Ippoliti G, et al. Cyclosporin-A in severe refractory anemia of myelofibrosis with myeloid metaplasia: a preliminary report. Haematologica 1998;83:622–626.
39. Yoon SY, Li CY, Mesa RA, et al. Bone marrow effects of anagrelide therapy in patients with myelofibrosis with myeloid metaplasia. Br J Haematol 1999;106: 682–688.
40. McCarthy DM, Hibbin JA, Goldman JM. A role for 1,25-hydroxyvitamin D_3 in control of BM collagen deposition. Lancet 1984;i:78–80.
41. Mesa RA, Tefferi A, Elliott MA, et al. A phase II trial of pirfenidone (5-methyl-1-phenyl-2-[1H]-pyridone), a novel anti-fibrosing agent, in myelofibrosis with myeloid metaplasia. Br J Haematol 2001;114:111–113.

42. Benbassat J, Penchas S, Ligumski M. Splenectomy in patients with agnogenic myeloid metaplasia: an analysis of 321 published cases. Br J Haematol 1979;42: 207–214.

43. Barosi G, Ambrosetti A, Buratti A, et al. Splenectomy for patients with myelofibrosis with myeloid metaplasia: pretreatment variables and outcome prediction. Leukemia 1993;7:200–206.

44. Tefferi A, Mesa RA, Nagomey DN, et al. Splenectomy in myelofibrosis with myeloid metaplasia: a single-institution experience with 223 patients. Blood 2000;95: 2226–2233.

45. Chaffanjon PC, Brichon PY, Ranchoup Y. Portal vein thrombosis following splenectomy for hematologic disease: retrospective study with Doppler color flow imaging. World J Surg 1998;22:1082–1086.

46. Barosi G, Ambrosetti A, Buratti A, et al. Splenectomy for patients with myelofibrosis with myeloid metaplasia: pretreatment variables and outcome prediction. Leukemia 1993;7:200–206.

47. Barosi G, Ambrosetti A, Centra A, et al. Splenectomy and risk of blast transformation in myelofibrosis with myeloid metaplasia. Blood 1998;91:3630–3636.

48. Elliott MA, Chen MG, Silverstein MN, et al. Splenic irradiation for symptomatic splenomegaly associated with myelofibrosis with myeloid metaplasia. Br J Haematol 1998;103:505–511.

49. Wagner H, Jr., McKeough PG, Desforges J, et al. Splenic irradiation in the treatment of patients with chronic myelogenous leukemia or myelofibrosis with myeloid metaplasia. Results of daily and intermittent fractionation with and without concomitant hydroxyurea. Cancer 1986;58:1204–1207.

50. Bouabdallah R, Coso D, Gonzague-Casabianca L, et al. Safety and efficacy of splenic irradiation in the treatment of patients with idiopathic myelofibrosis: a report on 15 patients. Leuk Res 2000;24:491–495.

51. Koeffler HP, Cline MJ, Golde DW. Splenic irradiation in myelofibrosis: effect on circulating myeloid progenitor cells. Br J Haematol 1979;43:69–77.

52. Price F, Bell H. Spinal cord compression due to extramedullary hematopoiesis. Successful treatment in a patient with longstanding myelofibrosis. JAMA 1985;253: 2876–2877.

53. Leinweber C, Order SE, Calkins AR. Whole-abdominal irradiation for the management of gastroinstestinal and abdominal manifestations of agnogenic myeloid metaplasia. Cancer 1991;68:1251–1254.

54. Barlett RP, Greipp PR, Tefferi A, et al. Extramedullary hematopoiesis manifesting as a symptomatic pleural effusion. Mayo Clin Proc 1995;70:1161–1164.

55. Steensma DP, Hook CC, Stafford SL, et al. Low-dose, single-fraction, whole-lung radiotherapy for pulmonary hypertension associated with myelofibrosis with myeloid metaplasia. Br J Haematol 2002;118:813–816.

56. Thiele J, Rompeik V, Wagner S, et al. Vascular architecture and collagen type IV in primary myelofibrosis and polycythaemia vera: an immunomorphometric study on trephine biopsies of the marrow. Br J Haematol 1992;80: 227–234.

57. Mesa RA, Hanson CA, Rajkumar VS, et al. Evaluation and clinical correlations of bone marrow angiogenesis in myelofibrosis with myeloid metaplasia. Blood 2000;96:3374–3380.

58. Barosi G, Elliott M, Canepa M, et al. Thalidomide in myelofibrosis with myeloid metaplasia: a pooled-analysis of individual patient data from 5 studies. Leuk Lymphoma 2002;43:2301–2307.

59. Mesa RA, Steensma DP, Pardanani A, et al. A phase II trial of combination low-dose thalidomide and prednisone for the treatment of myelofibrosis with myeloid metaplasia. Blood 2003;101:2534–2541.

60. Marchetti M, Barosi G, Balestri F, et al. Low-dose thalidomide ameliorates cytopenias and splenomegaly in myelofibrosis with myeloid metaplasia: a phase II trial. J Clin Oncol 2004;22:424–431.

61. Merup M, Kutti J, Birgergard G, et al. Negligible effects of thalidomide in patients with myelofibrosis with myeloid metaplasia. Med Oncol 2002;19:79–86.

62. Abgrall JF, Guibaud I, Bastie JN, et al. Thalidomide versus placebo in myeloid metaplasia with myelofibrosis: a prospective, randomized, double-blind, multicenter study. Haematologica 2006;91:1027–1032.

63. Tefferi A, Cortes J, Verstovsek S, et al. Lenalidomide therapy in myelofibrosis with myeloid metaplasia. Blood 2006;108:1158–1164.

64. Tefferi A, Mesa RA, Gray LA, et al. Phase II trial of imatinib mesylate in myelofibrosis with myeloid metaplasia. Blood 2002;99:3854–3856.

65. Hasselbalch HC, Bjerrum OW, Jensen BA, et al. Imatinib mesylate in idiopathic and postpolycythemic myelofibrosis. Am J Hematol 2003;74:238–242.

66. Cortes J, Albitar M, Thomas D, et al. Efficacy of the farnesyl transferase inhibitor R115777 in chronic myeloid leukemia and other hematologic malignancies. Blood 2003;101:1692–1697.

67. Mesa RA, Tefferi A, Gray LA, et al. In vitro antiproliferative activity of the farnesyltransferase inhibitor R115777 in hematopoietic progenitors from patients with myelofibrosis with myeloid metaplasia. Leukemia 2003;17:849–855.

68. Giles FJ, Cooper MA, Silverman L, et al. Phase II study of SU5416—a small-molecule, vascular endothelial growth factor tyrosine-kinase receptor inhibitor—in patients with refractory myeloproliferative diseases. Cancer 2003;97:1920–1928.

69. Tefferi A, Barosi G, Mesa R, et al. International Working Group (IWG) consensus criteria for treatment response in myelofibrosis with myeloid metaplasia, from the IWG for Myelofibrosis Research and Treatment (IWG-MRT). Blood 2006;108: 1497–1503.

70. Rajantie J, Sale GE, Deeg HJ, et al. Adverse effect of severe marrow fibrosis on hematologic recovery after chemoradiotherapy and allogeneic bone marrow transplantation. Blood 1986;67:1693–1697.

71. Dokal I, Jones L, Deenmamode M, et al. Allogeneic bone marrow transplantation for primary myelofibrosis. Br J Haematol 1989;71:158–160.

72. Singhal S, Powles R, Treleaven J, et al. Allogeneic bone marrow transplantation for primary myelofibrosis. Bone Marrow Transplant 1995;16:743–746.

73. Guardiola P, Anderson JE, Bandini G, et al. Allogeneic stem cell transplantation for agnogenic myeloid metaplasia: a European Group for Blood and Marrow Transplantation, Societé Française de Greffe de Moelle, Gruppo Italiano per il Trapianto del Midollo Osseo, and Fred Hutchinson Cancer Research Center Collaborative Study. Blood 1999;93:2831–2838.

74. Guardiola P, Anderson JE, Gluckman E. Myelofibrosis with myeloid metaplasia (letter). N Engl J Med 2000;343:659.

75. Daly A, Song K, Nevill T, et al. Stem cell transplantation for myelofibrosis: a report from two Canadian centers. Bone Marrow Transplant 2003;32:35–40.
76. Ditschkowski M, Beelen DW, Trenschel R, et al. Outcome of allogeneic stem cell transplantation in patients with myelofibrosis. Bone Marrow Transplant 2003;34: 807–813.
77. Deeg HJ, Gooley TA, Flowers ME, et al. Allogeneic hematopoietic stem cell transplantation for myelofibrosis. Blood 2003;102:3912–3918.
78. Maziarz RT, Mesa RA, Tefferi A. Allogeneic stem cell transplantation for chronic myeloproliferative disorders and myeloproliferative disorders and myelodysplastic syndromes: the question is "when." Mayo Clin Proc 2003;78:941–943.
79. Byrne JL, Beshti H, Clark D, et al. Induction of remission after donor leukocyte infusion for the treatment of relapsed chronic idiopathic myelofibrosis following allogeneic transplantation: evidence for a "graft vs. myelofibrosis" effect. Br J Haematol 2000;108:430–433.
80. Cervantes F, Rovira M, Urbano-Ispizua A, et al. Remission of idiopathic myelofibrosis following donor lymphocyte infusion after failure of allogeneic stem cell transplantation. Bone Marrow Transplant 2000;26:697–699.
81. Devine SM, Hoffman R, Verma A, et al. Allogeneic blood cell transplantation following reduced-intensity conditioning is effective therapy for older patients with myelofibrosis with myeloid metaplasia. Blood 2002;99:2255–2258.
82. Kröger N, Zabelina T, Schieder H, et al. Pilot study of reduced-intensity conditioning followed by allogeneic stem cell transplantation from related and unrelated donors in patients with myelofibrosis. Br J Haematol 2005;128:690–697.
83. Rondelli D, Barosi G, Bacigalupo A, et al. Allogeneic stem cell transplantation with reduced intensity conditioning in intermediate- and high-risk patients with myelofibrosis with myeloid metaplasia. Blood 2005;105:4115–4119.
84. Merup M, Lazarevic V, Nahi H, et al. Different outcome of allogeneic transplantation in myelofibrosis using conventional or reduced-intensity conditioning regimens. Br J Haematol 2006;135:367–373.
85. Kröger N, Badbaran A, Holler E, et al. Monitoring of the JAK2-V617F mutation by highly sensitive quatitative real-time PCR after allogeneic stem cell transplantation in patients with myelofibrosis. Blood 2007;109:1316–1321.
86. Anderson JE, Tefferi A, Craig F, et al. Myeloablation and autologous peripheral blood stem cell rescue results in hematologic and clinical responses in patients with myelofibrosis. Blood 2001;98:586–593.

8

New Drugs in Myeloproliferative Disorders

Srdan Verstovsek

Department of Leukemia, MD Anderson Cancer Center, Houston, Texas, U.S.A.

Ruben A. Mesa

Division of Hematology, Mayo Clinic, College of Medicine, Rochester, Minnesota, U.S.A.

TREATING THE MYELOPROLIFERATIVE DISEASES: WHY THE NEED FOR "NEW DRUGS?"

Which Groups of Patients?

The classic BCR-ABL–negative myeloproliferative disorders (MPDs) include polycythemia vera (PV), essential thrombocythemia (ET), and agnogenic myeloid metaplasia. Included in this latter group are also postthrombocythemic and post-polycythemic myeloid metaplasia (1). This last group has been the subject of focus and nomenclature changes by the International Working Group for Myelofibrosis Research and Treatment (IWG-MRT). Primary myelofibrosis (PMF) is designated for de novo presentations, and the myelofibrosis (MF) that develops in the setting of either ET or PV is referred to as post-ET MF or post-PV MF, respectively.

Why the need for therapy?

Phenotypically, the MPDs have a wide range of manifestations, including a variable age of diagnosis [typically around the age of 60 (2), although patients in the third, fourth, and fifth decades of life are common]. Clinically, these disorders

143

share a variable spectrum of symptoms arising from myeloproliferation (erythrocytosis, leukocytosis, or thrombocytosis) as well as target organ damage from the intramedullary proliferative state [organomegaly (3), vascular complications (4), skin manifestations (5), liver dysfunction (6), pulmonary hypertension (7), etc.]. Individuals with advancing disease, PMF or post-ET/PV MF, have worsening cytopenias, constitutional symptoms, risk of leukemic transformation, and risk of premature death.

SETTING THE INITIAL THERAPEUTIC PLAN: TRANSPLANT VERSUS THERAPY

A variable prognostic outlook for the MPDs (PMF, post ET/PV MF) complicates the design of a therapeutic plan for a particular patient. It is generally agreed, however, that PMF is associated with the worst prognosis, with its median survival rivaling that of many lethal solid malignancies. Various prognostic features can help stratify the suspected outcomes in MF patients (8), including anemia (9), karyotypic abnormalities (10), age, the presence of circulating blasts (9), and markedly increased angiogenesis in the marrow (11). Patients with ET and PV can potentially have life expectancies as long as their age matched the controls (12,13). However, such longevity among these patients is not universal as short- and long-term risks of both morbidity and mortality exist.

Currently, in MPD patients, no therapy has been shown to either cure or prolong survival, except for allogeneic stem cell transplantation. The idea of using stem cell transplantation for the therapy of PMF is the most attractive, since this disease has the worst prognosis among the MPD disorders. Initial reports have shown that this therapy does indeed have curative potential in PMF patients (14,15). A 58% 3-year survival was reported in a group of 56 PMF (and post-ET/PV MF) patients (age 10–66 years), with a 32% nonrelapse mortality rate (16). The significant toxicity of full allogeneic transplant in PMF led to nonmyeloablative trials (17–19). These trials have been encouraging in terms of decreased nonrelapse mortality, and because of increasing age of the patients successfully transplanted. However, allogeneic transplant still carries a significant risk of graft-versus-host disease (at least 33%) and the exact role and benefit depends on the long-term prognosis of the patient. Currently, there are no data on the use of stem cell transplantation in ET or PV patients. Indeed, the significant risks of any of the stem cell transplantation procedures make it difficult to justify this therapy for ET and PV given the overall good prognosis of these patients.

LIMITATIONS OF CURRENT THERAPY

ET and PV both share a risk of thrombosis and hemorrhagic events. The exact mechanisms for the development of thrombohemorrhagic complications in MPD patients are several and clearly include uncorrected erythrocytosis, thrombocytosis, and, as recently described, perhaps leukocytosis as well (20). Current data on

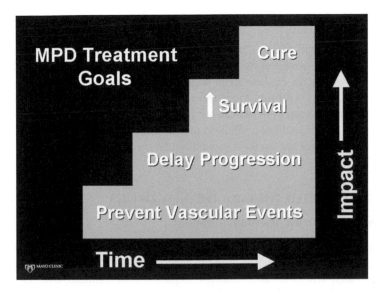

Figure 1 Myeloproliferative disorder therapeutic goals.

the prevention of these events has been limited. Patients with PV benefit from the control of erythrocytosis (by phlebotomy), and the use of low-dose aspirin (21). Hydroxyurea (HU) was shown in a randomized fashion to aid in the prevention of thrombotic events in patients with high-risk ET (22). The PT-1 (primary thrombocythemia 1) trial compared in a randomized fashion HU and anagrelide (both along with low-dose aspirin) for ET patients and found HU plus aspirin to be superior in regard to preventing arterial events, hemorrhage, and transformation to post-ET MF (23). There remains a lack of uniform agreement as to the outcomes of this latter trial (in terms of the nature of the arterial events, and the pathologic interpretations employed to determine transformation to post-ET MF); additionally, there are other trials ongoing. Nevertheless, given the current randomized data, we recommend HU as the standard therapy for those patients who require a platelet-lowering therapy (high risk because of prior vascular events, age, or cardiovascular risk factors). However, concerns linger whether HU accelerates an MPD toward leukemic transformation. This has never been proven when HU has been used as a single agent (24). Moreover, not all patients are able to tolerate or achieve adequate control with single agent HU.

In the MPDs, no medical therapy (specifically HU, anagrelide, or interferon) has definitively helped to decrease the long-term risks of transformation to myelofibrosis or acute leukemia, accentuating the need for developing newer therapies. Indeed, looking at the stepwise approach to the impact of our therapies for ET and PV (Fig. 1), they remain strictly "first level," (i.e., preventing thrombohemorrhagic events only). Historically, the medical therapy for PMF and post-ET/PV MF can best be described as being empirically derived, resulting in palliative outcomes at best (25). Cytopenias have improved in subsets of patients with erythropoietin supplementation (26), androgens (27), and/or corticosteroids. Similarly, nonspecific myelosuppressive regimens, such as HU (28), busulfan (29), melphalan (30), and cladribine (31), have all been reported to provide palliative reduction of painful splenomegaly. However, all of these prior therapies have shared the following disappointing features: (1) inability to improve intramedullary manifestations of the disease, (2) no improvement in the disease course, and (3) no prolongation of survival. Therapy of PMF (including MF associated with post-ET and PV) remains palliative. This accentuates the need for more effective and targeted treatments.

PATHWAYS TO TARGETED THERAPY: THE NEW DRUGS

Targeting the Bone Marrow Microenvironment

In addition to ineffective erythropoiesis, PMF is characterized by a prominent bone marrow stromal reaction occurring in the early stages of the disease, which has been associated with increased marrow expression of profibrogenic and pro-angiogenic cytokines such as transforming growth factor beta (TGF-β), platelet-derived growth factor (PDGF), tumor necrosis factor alpha (TNF-α), basic fibroblast growth factor, and vascular endothelial growth factor (VEGF) (32). Therapies aimed at the molecular targets involved in the aforementioned pathogenetic pathways represent the cornerstone of current clinical trials in PMF.

Immunomodulatory Inhibitory Drugs (IMIDs): Thalidomide, Lenalidomide, and Pomalidomide

The group of inhibitory cytokine and antiangiogenic agents collectively known as IMIDs have shown great promise in the MPDs, and most specifically in PMF and post-ET/PV MF. Initial dose-escalating pilot studies with thalidomide in PMF started with doses of 100 mg/day (33). These studies revealed improvement of anemia and splenomegaly in approximately 20% of the patients and of thrombocytopenia in a higher percentage. However, the dropout rate because of adverse drug side effects was unacceptably high at those doses. Subsequent trials demonstrated that lower doses of thalidomide (50 mg/day), compared to the higher doses, were better tolerated and retained an equivalent degree of therapeutic activity (34). A pooled analysis of the earlier trials found reasonable initial response rates to single-agent thalidomide, without improvement in marrow fibrosis or cytogenetic abnormalities (35) (Table 1). Recently, a single-agent, randomized trial of thalidomide versus placebo in PMF was reported as a negative study (41). However, this latter trial had a severe design flaw. All patients were begun on a dose of thalidomide (400 mg/day) known to be intolerable in PMF patients. Because less than 20% of the patients received the desired duration of treatment, there was a significant dropout rate because of predictable toxicity, obscuring the ability of the trial to detect any activity.

Table 1 Summary of Clinical Experience with IMIDs in Phase II Clinical Trials

Agent	N	Anemia (%)	Thrombocytopenia (%)	Responses reported			Ref
				Splenomegaly (%)	Marrow Fibrosis (%)	Cytogenetics (%)	
Thal	68	29	38	41	0	0	(35)
Thal + Pred	32	62	75	19	0	0	(36)
Thal + Pred + ETAN	15	55	71	33	0	0	(37)
Thal + Pred + EPO	5	100	100	20	0	0	(38)
Thal + Pred + CTX	13	11	10	0	0	0	(39)
LEN	68	22	50	33	3	1.5	(40)
LEN + Pred	*Two Recently Completed Clinical Trials—no data available*						
POM ± Pred	*International Randomized, Placebo-Controlled Trial Ongoing*						

Abbreviations: THAL, thalidomide; ETAN: etanercept; CTX, oral cyclophosphamide; LEN: lenalidomide; POM: pomalidomide.

Based on the promising initial results of low-dose (50 mg/day) thalidomide, combination trials were investigated. The initial trial compared a 3-month trial of prednisone (beginning at 40 mg/day) subsequently "tapered" to long-term, low-dose thalidomide (36). Steroids were added due to the synergy observed in other hematologic malignancies, such as myeloma, and the single-agent activity of prednisone in PMF. Responses observed for anemia, thrombocytopenia, and splenomegaly remain the most impressive seen to date for PMF trials (Table 1). However, no definitive improvement in marrow morphology or cytogenetic abnormalities occurred. Subsequently, attempts were made to improve TNF-α blockade with the addition of the inhibitor etanercept (42) (which had single-agent activity in decreasing constitutional symptoms in PMF). This trial showed similar, but not enhanced, activity over the thalidomide-prednisone (thal-pred) regimen (37) (Table 1). Other attempts at augmenting response with the use of erythropoietin in patients with inadequate baseline erythropoietin levels have been successful in small numbers (38) (Table 1). Efforts to increase the ability of the thal-pred regimen to cytoreduce splenomegaly with the use of low-dose oral cyclophosphamide led to poorer results (39).

Clearly, increasing the activity of the IMIDs requires a new generation of IMIDs rather than alternative combination strategies with thalidomide. Lenalidomide is a second-generation IMID with pleiotropic, cytokine-modulating activity, which is significantly more potent than thalidomide in modulating the cytokines, previously mentioned as important in the pathogenesis of the disease. Based upon the benefits observed with thalidomide, the clinical activity of lenalidomide has been evaluated in two phase II trials involving 68 patients with symptomatic PMF, both primary and secondary to other MPDs (40). In doses of 10 mg/day, lenalidomide therapy resulted in the overall response rates of 22% for anemia, 33% for splenomegaly, and 50% for thrombocytopenia (40). Remarkably, normalization of hemoglobin levels was observed in 8 (17%) of 46 patients who were either transfusion dependent or had a baseline hemoglobin less than 10 g/dL. In addition, 4 of these patients also displayed resolution of leukoerythroblastosis. Of special note, there were 2 patients who had resolution of intramedullary features of fibrosis and angiogenesis, and 1 [with a del5(q)] with a cytogenetic remission (Table 1). Although these latter responses were in a very small subset, they represent the first time such responses have been observed in a PMF trial not involving stem cell transplantation. In aggregate, although the initial response rates to lenalidomide do not appear to differ from the prior experience with thalidomide, the nature of the responses seem more profound. Currently, two large-scale trials are ongoing to evaluate whether combining this agent with corticosteroids will further improve upon the responses observed with single-agent lenalidomide.

Another promising IMID, pomalidomide, is 20,000-fold more potent than thalidomide in inhibiting TNF-α, although cross-resistance with the latter does not appear to occur (43). Due to its excellent oral absorption and adequate pharmacokinetics, pomalidomide is suitable for once-daily administration. In phase I trials in patients with multiple myeloma, the main side effects associated with pomalidomide therapy were related to myelosuppression and deep vein thrombosis (44). Given the promising results obtained with lenalidomide, a randomized, placebo-controlled, international clinical study to determine the activity of pomalidomide (with or without a prednisone taper) in PMF and post-ET/PV MF is currently underway.

Antiangiogenic Agents (Table 2) (Angiogenesis Inhibitors)

Vatalanib (PTK787/ZK 222584), an oral inhibitor of the VEGF receptor-1 (VEGFR-1) and VEGFR-2 tyrosine kinases has been used in clinical trials in patients with MPDs because of its antiangiogenic activity (45). PTK/ZK also inhibits a broad array of additional tyrosine kinases including PDGF receptor, c-KIT, and c-FMS (45). Although, in theory, PTK/ZK should have been quite active in the study patients, the responses observed were quite modest with mainly clinical improvement [CI by IWG-MRT criteria (46) seen (45)]. Twenty-nine patients with MF received a continuous dosing schedule of PTK/ZK of 500 or 750 mg twice-daily. One patient (3%) achieved complete remission and five patients (17%) achieved clinical improvement. Significant decrease in intramedullary angiogenesis was not observed, with only modest reductions in marrow hypercellularity described. Intriguingly, 1 patient did experience a complete remission [by IWG-MRT criteria (46)], suggesting a particularly sensitive target (not identified) in this individual.

It is interesting that the results of the PTK/ZK trial parallel the modest results reported with the other VEGFR inhibitor SU5416 in MF (47). SU5416 is a synthetic inhibitor of VEGFR-2, KIT, and FLT-3. In a multicenter phase II study, intravenous SU5416 145 mg/m^2 was given twice-weekly for a median of three 4-week cycles to 32 adult MPD patients, including 3 with MF. One of the patients with MF attained a partial response. However, the overall clinical activity was marginal and the tolerability was poor (47). Sunitinib (SU11248) is an orally bioavailable, multitargeted kinase inhibitor with selectivity for PDGF receptors, VEGF receptors, KIT, and FLT-3 (48). Sunitinib has been recently reported active in a phase I/II study of patients with acute myeloid leukemia (49), and a phase II study of this agent in MF is underway.

The ability of the nonspecific "angiogenesis inhibitors" such as thalidomide and lenalidomide to provide more profound responses (in the absence of true improvements in angiogenesis), suggests that the clinical activity of these latter agents is independent of the inhibition of angiogenesis.

Fibrogenesis Inhibitors

TGF-β_1 plays a central role in the prominent bone marrow stromal reaction observed in the patients with PMF. Several compounds, originally designed for the treatment of other profibrotic conditions, inhibit TGF-β_1–mediated signaling. GC-1008 is one such agent, as is a pan-specific human anti-TGF-β_1 antibody. GC-1008 is currently undergoing clinical evaluation for several indications, including pulmonary fibrosis, renal cancer, melanoma of the skin, and also for PMF (50).

Table 2 Investigational Medical Therapy for PMF (Including Post-ET/PV MF):
Selected Ongoing Clinical Trials

Agent	Class/type of drug	Route	Major toxicities
Sunitinib	Angiogenesis inhibitor	Oral	Edema, fatigue, mucositis, hypertension
Bortezomib	Proteasome inhibitor	IV	Peripheral neuropathy, hypotension, gastrointestinal disturbances
Dasatinib	Kinase inhibitor	Oral	Myelosuppression, fluid retention, fatigue
GC-1008	Pan-specific human anti-TGF-β antibody	IV	Unknown
CEP-701	JAK2 inhibitor	Oral	Gastrointestinal disturbances
GX15–170	Pan-BCL-2-inhibitor	IV	Somnolence, euphoria
Azacitidine	Hypomethylating agent	SC	Myelosuppression

Abbreviations: IV, intravenous; SC, subcutaneous.

Alternatively, metelimumab (CAT-192) is a human TGF-β_1 monoclonal antibody that is currently undergoing phase I/II trials for patients with scleroderma. A different approach is the employment of TGF-β_1–specific antisense oligonucleotides. AP-11014 is such an example and is currently being developed for human non–small-cell lung, colorectal, and prostate cancers (51). However, delivery and tissue-penetration issues for these antisense therapies might limit their application (50). Several studies have shown the efficacy of using small molecules such as LY580276 (IC_{50} 175 nM) (52), pyrazole 2 (IC_{50} 18 nM) (53), SB-505124 (IC_{50} 47 nM) (54), and SD-208 (55) to inhibit the TGF-β type-I receptor kinase ALK5. Although promising, all these compounds are in preclinical phases of development and their in vivo activity and tolerability are yet to be determined.

Pirfenidone (5-methyl-1-phenyl-2-[1 H]-pyridone) is an oral agent with inhibitory activity against PDGF, TNF-α, and TGF-β that inhibits fibroblast proliferation and deposition of extracellular matrix proteins (56). Unfortunately, in a prospective study, pirfenidone failed to show any significant clinical activity in PMF, in which 16 of the 28 (57%) patients were withdrawn because of disease progression or drug intolerance and only 1 patient had an improvement in anemia and splenomegaly (56). Current evidence suggests that spontaneous nuclear factor kappa beta (NF-κB) pathway activation associated with secretion of the fibrogenic cytokine TGF-β_1 takes place in megakaryocytes, monocytes, and CD34$^+$ cells from patients with PMF (57). Rameshwar et al. reported that monocytes from patients with PMF presented a spontaneous activation of the NF-κB transduction pathway and that NF-κB inhibition by antisense oligonucleotides decreased TGF-β_1 secretion (58). In addition, preliminary data in a murine model of MF suggest that the proteasome inhibitor, bortezomib, inhibits activation of the NF-κB pathway and decreases plasma concentration of TGF-β_1, thus inhibiting the development of MF (59). Based on these latter findings, and the intriguing activity seen in myelodysplastic syndrome (MDS) (60), clinical trials of bortezomib in patients with MF have been initiated.

Targeting the Signal Transduction Pathways

Tyrosine Kinase Inhibitors

Imatinib mesylate is an inhibitor of the tyrosine kinase activity of ABL, PDGFR, KIT, and ARG (61). The employment of imatinib for the therapy of patients with PMF was based on its inhibitory activity against PDGF-mediated signaling and the reduction of bone marrow fibrosis and microvessel density observed in patients with chronic myeloid leukemia , for which imatinib is a standard therapy (62). Results from all the phase II trials of imatinib in patients with PMF reported to date are modest (63,64). Only one study showed significant improvement in splenomegaly, including 4 (29%) patients who had normalization of spleen span (65). Imatinib was administered at doses ranging from 200 to 800 mg daily, but dropout rates were in excess of 50% across all trials due to adverse events (63,64). Recently, imatinib has been shown to increase the number of clonogenic megakaryocytic progenitors in bone marrow, indicating that imatinib may restore megakaryocyte differentiation and be effective for the treatment of thrombocytopenia in PMF (66). Dasatinib (BMS-354825) is a dual SRC- and ABL-kinase inhibitor, 300-fold more potent ABL kinase inhibitor than imatinib (67). In addition, dasatinib effectively inhibits PDGFR-β (IC$_{50}$ 28 nM) (67). Based on these preclinical data and on the results obtained with imatinib, results from an ongoing clinical trial of dasatinib in patients with PMF are eagerly awaited.

Farnesyl Transferase Inhibitors

RAS gene mutations are commonly encountered in hematologic malignancies and are present in 6% of patients with PMF (68). Attachment of RAS to the membrane is critical for its activation and this is accomplished through a posttranslational reaction termed prenylation by an enzyme called farnesyltransferase (Ftase), and to a lesser extent, by geranylgeranyl-protein transferases (69). Inhibition of these enzymes has been sought as a means of interfering with RAS signaling, which led to the development of Ftase inhibitors. Their activity, however, appears to extend beyond RAS inhibition and may be mediated through inhibition of other prenylation-dependent proteins, such as RhoB, CENP-E, and CENP-F (70). Tipifarnib (R115777), a nonpeptidomimetic Ftase inhibitor, was administered at 600 mg orally, twice-daily for 4 weeks out of every 6-week cycle to 8 patients with PMF (71). Two of them had a significant decrease in splenomegaly, 1 had normalization of white blood cell count and differential, and 1 became transfusion independent. Of note, responders had markedly higher pretreatment plasma VEGF concentrations than nonresponders during therapy (71).

In parallel efforts, in vitro testing of tipifarnib demonstrated that aberrant myeloid colony formation was reduced by 50% at concentrations of 34 and 2.7 nM for myeloid and megakaryocytic colonies from PMF patients, respectively. Since these concentrations seemed quite achievable at tolerable dose levels (i.e., 300 mg twice-daily) a phase II trial was undertaken (72). Eligible patients had histologically confirmed PMF and were symptomatic, defined by anemia (hemoglobin < 10 g/dL or transfusion dependent) or palpable hepatosplenomegaly. Patients received 300 mg of tipifarnib orally, twice-daily for the first 21 days of a 28-day cycle (similar to the trial by Kurzrock in MDS (73). The primary end point was the response, as defined by improvement in either anemia or organomegaly. Amongst 34 patients enrolled in the trial, tipifarnib resulted in little improvement in anemia. However, the myelosuppressive aspects of the agent may have masked improvements in cytopenias. In contrast, tipifarnib did cause clinically relevant decreases in organomegaly in 11 patients (33%) (splenomegaly in 3, hepatomegaly in 5, and both in an additional 3), many of whom had previously failed HU. Responses observed did not significantly correlate with reductions in bone marrow fibrosis, osteosclerosis, neoangiogenesis, or resolution of baseline karyotypic abnormalities. Whether this latter benefit is independent of tipifarnib-induced myelosuppression is unclear. Additional MPD patients were treated on a broad phase II trial (15 unclassified MPD patients) (74), and similar to the PMF trial, responses were a nonspecific decrease in leukocytosis.

Other Novel Investigational Agents

Alternative approaches with potential clinical activity in patients with PMF are being investigated. GX15–070 is a synthetic small molecule that inhibits the binding of the antiapoptotic proteins BCL-2, BCL-XL, BCL-W, and MCL-1 to the proapoptotic proteins BAX and BAK, thus reinstituting programmed cell death in transformed cells. In a phase I study of GX15–070 in patients with chronic lymphocytic leukemia, 2 of the 4 patients who were anemic at baseline (1 of them was transfusion dependent) showed significant sustained elevations in their hemoglobin levels (75). Based on this preliminary data, GX15–070 is being investigated in other hematologic malignancies, including PMF, where this compound might improve cytopenias.

Aberrant CpG island hypermethylation in regulatory areas of tumor suppressor genes leading to inactivation is commonly encountered in human cancer (76). Methylation of p15^{INK4B}, p16^{INK4A}, and the retinoic acid receptor β has been observed in advanced-stage PMF (77). Azacitidine and decitabine are DNA methyltransferase inhibitors that induce reactivation of methylated genes (78). Both agents are approved by the Food and Drug Administration in the U.S.A. for the treatment of patients with MDS, and are currently being investigated in phase II studies in PMF.

Targeting the JAK2V617F Mutation and Associated Signal Transduction Pathways

The next generation of targeted therapy for PMF will move beyond agents targeting the stromal reaction, or cytokines, to agents aimed at the aberrant clone and constitutively active proliferative stimuli. The discovery of the activating point mutation in the autoinhibitory pseudokinase domain of JAK2 (the JAK2V617F) was a watershed moment in the understanding of the pathogenesis of the BCR-ABL–negative MPDs (79–82). JAK2V617F is present in only about half of the PMF and post-ET MF patients, but in the vast majority of post-PV MF patients (83). Recent additional discoveries, such as the c-MPLW515 L/K (84,85), and the role of additional mutations in exon 12 of *JAK2* gene in JAK2V617F–negative PV patients (86) have provided further insight into intrinsic myeloproliferative drive in these patients. Although the currently identified molecular defects do not fully explain many issues of MPD pathogenesis, they provide an exciting and hopefully more fruitful therapeutic target. There have already been multiple reports of agents in development that have demonstrated the ability to inhibit the aberrant JAK2V617F, along with the wild-type JAK2, such as TG101209 (87), Go6976 (88), erlotinib (89), MK0457(90), CEP-701 (91) (now in a clinical study), and Z3 (92). Intriguingly, in primary cells from wild-type JAK2 patients, who have the c-MPLW515 L/K, growth inhibition can similarly be accomplished by JAK2 inhibitors, such as TG101209 (87). These latter observations suggest the possibility that even in JAK2 wild-type MPD patients, a growth dependence on the JAK-STAT pathway may exist and agents targeting this pathway may be active regardless of the JAK2 mutation status. This hypothesis is further supported by the continual discovery of aberrations in this pathway, as in exon 12 of *JAK2* gene in JAK2V617F–negative PV patients (86).

There are several challenges as we enter the era of JAK2 inhibitors for PMF and MPD patients. First, who are the most appropriate candidates for agents with uncertain safety profiles, given that there are many patients with JAK2V617F–positive ET and PV, with a good natural history (12), who will be seeking these agents? Second, although there are many agents that may have the ability to inhibit the wild-type JAK2, we must proceed with caution as few have desired specificity for the JAK2 itself, let alone the JAK2V617F. This opens up the possibility of many undesired toxicities related to the inhibition of additional tyrosine kinases. Additional challenges are inherent in the process of clinical research: how to effectively choose which candidate agents from preclinical testing truly merit clinical testing, and how to properly design trials to truly test optimum dose and schedule of these agents. Indeed, concern that significant potential for type II error exists for agents in which we are uncertain as to how to assess their response, that we could prematurely discard beneficial agents by having incorrect assumptions regarding the chronology or rapidity of response.

What effects can we expect to observe from the inhibition of *JAK2* (no medication is likely to strictly inhibit the JAK2V617F)? As we look at MPD therapeutic goals (Fig. 1), will inhibition of the JAK-STAT pathway decrease myeloproliferation? The current published in vitro and murine data would suggest a positive answer. Will JAK-STAT inhibition decrease the development of thrombohemorrhagic events, given the multifactorial nature of their origin? What about the major therapeutic endpoints desired by clinicians and patients, namely delaying or preventing disease progression, or increasing survival? These latter goals are highly desired, but uncertainty exists as to whether the inhibition of JAK2 will accomplish these goals, since the exact role of the JAK2V617F mutation in disease progression or development of PMF-BP remains unclear (93). The observation that *JAK2*-mutant MPD patients have the potential to develop acute leukemia from a JAK2 wild-type clone (94) questions the role of this mutation in disease progression. Therefore, what impact JAK2 inhibition will have on disease progression (i.e., none, decrease, or increase) is quite uncertain and will require close long-term monitoring of patients taking JAK2 inhibitors, to be certain no adverse impact arises from the use of these agents. Finally, if beneficial, will the JAK2 inhibitors lead to the cure? Unlikely at this juncture, but an outcome that parallels the efficacy of imatinib for chronic myeloid leukemia (95) in terms of short- and long-term control of the disease would be greatly welcomed by physician and patient alike.

CONCLUSION

The development of novel therapies for MPD patients has been historically hampered by limited progress regarding the molecular pathogenesis of this disease. However, great strides have been made in this regard over the last decade, culminated by the recent discovery of the gain-of-function JAK2V617F mutation. A challenge for the near future will be the development of targeted agents with acceptable toxicity profiles able to interfere with the JAK-STAT–signaling pathway. The first such agent, CEP-701, is in clinical testing already. In recent years, a number of agents have been tested in clinical studies for MPD patients, with disappointing results, including pirfenidone, imatinib, tipifarnib, vatalanib, and SU5416. However, promising results have been obtained with thalidomide, which has encouraged clinicians and researchers to pursue the development of novel, more potent IMIDs, such as lenalidomide and pomalidomide. Participation in clinical trials involving investigational agents, such as IMIDs, novel antiangiogenic agents, proteosome inhibitors, and novel signal-transduction inhibitors, alone or in combination, is warranted to keep the current pace of discoveries that will eventually lead to more efficacious therapies for the MPDs.

REFERENCES

1. Tefferi A. The Philadelphia chromosome – negative chronic myeloproliferative disorders: a practical overview. Mayo Clin Proc 1998;73:1177–1184.
2. Mesa RA, Silverstein MN, Jacobsen SJ, et al. Population-based incidence and survival figures in essential thrombocythemia and agnogenic myeloid metaplasia: an Olmsted County Study, 1976–1995. Am J Hematol 1999;61:10–15.
3. Tefferi A, Mesa RA, Nagorney DM, et al. Splenectomy in myelofibrosis with myeloid metaplasia: a single-institution experience with 223 patients. Blood 2000;95: 2226–2233.
4. Landolfi R. Bleeding and thrombosis in myeloproliferative disorders. Curr Opin Hematol 1998;5:327–331.

5. van Genderen PJ, Michiels JJ. Erythromelalgia: a pathognomonic microvascular thrombotic complication in essential thrombocythemia and polycythemia vera. Semin Thromb Hemost 1997;23:357–363.
6. Tefferi A, Jimenez T, Gray LA, et al. Radiation therapy for symptomatic hepatomegaly in myelofibrosis with myeloid metaplasia. Eur J Haematol 2001;66:37–42.
7. Dingli D, Utz JP, Krowka MJ, et al. Unexplained pulmonary hypertension in chronic myeloproliferative disorders. Chest 2001;120:801–808.
8. Cervantes F. Prognostic factors and current practice in treatment of myelofibrosis with myeloid metaplasia: an update anno 2000. Pathol Biol (Paris) 2001;49:148–152.
9. Dupriez B, Morel P, Demory JL, et al. Prognostic factors in agnogenic myeloid metaplasia: a report on 195 cases with a new scoring system [see comments]. Blood 1996;88:1013–1018.
10. Tefferi A, Mesa RA, Schroeder G, et al. Cytogenetic findings and their clinical relevance in myelofibrosis with myeloid metaplasia. Br J Haematol 2001;113: 763–771.
11. Mesa RA, Hanson CA, Rajkumar SV, et al. Evaluation and clinical correlations of bone marrow angiogenesis in myelofibrosis with myeloid metaplasia. Blood 2000;96:3374–3380.
12. Passamonti F, Rumi E, Pungolino E, et al. Life expectancy and prognostic factors for survival in patients with polycythemia vera and essential thrombocythemia. Am J Med 2004;117:755–761.
13. Wolanskyj AP, Schwager SM, McClure RF, et al. Essential thrombocythemia beyond the first decade: life expectancy, long-term complication rates, and prognostic factors. Mayo Clin Proc 2006;81:159–166.
14. Guardiola P, Esperou H, Cazalshatem D, et al. Allogeneic bone marrow transplantation for agnogenic myeloid metaplasia. Br J Haematol 1997;98:1004–1009.
15. Guardiola P, Anderson JE, Bandini G, et al. Allogeneic stem cell transplantation for agnogenic myeloid metaplasia: a European Group for Blood and Marrow Transplantation, Societe Francaise de Greffe de Moelle, Gruppo Italiano per il Trapianto del Midollo Osseo, and Fred Hutchinson Cancer Research Center Collaborative Study. Blood 1999;93:2831–2838.
16. Deeg HJ, Gooley TA, Flowers ME, et al. Allogeneic hematopoietic stem cell transplantation for myelofibrosis. Blood 2003;102:3912–3918.
17. Rondelli D, Barosi G, Bacigalupo A, et al. Allogeneic hematopoietic stem cell transplantation with reduced intensity conditioning in intermediate or high-risk patients with myelofibrosis with myeloid metaplasia. Blood 2005;105:4115–4119.
18. Kröger N, Zabelina T, Schieder H, et al. Pilot study of reduced-intensity conditioning followed by allogeneic stem cell transplantation from related and unrelated donors in patients with myelofibrosis. Br J Haematol 2005;128:690–697.
19. Devine SM, Hoffman R, Verma A, et al. Allogeneic blood cell transplantation following reduced-intensity conditioning is effective therapy for older patients with myelofibrosis with myeloid metaplasia. Blood 2002;99:2255–2258.
20. Falanga A, Marchetti M, Vignoli A, et al. Leukocyte-platelet interaction in patients with essential thrombocythemia and polycythemia vera. Exp Hematol 2005;33: 523–530.
21. Landolfi R, Marchioli R, Kutti J, et al. Efficacy and safety of low-dose aspirin in polycythemia vera. N Engl J Med 2004;350:114–124.

22. Cortelazzo S, Finazzi G, Ruggeri M, et al. Hydroxyurea for patients with essential thrombocythemia and a high risk of thrombosis. N Engl J Med 1995;332: 1132–1136.

23. Harrison CN, Campbell PJ, Buck G, et al. Hydroxyurea compared with anagrelide in high-risk essential thrombocythemia. N Engl J Med 2005;353:33–45.

24. Finazzi G, Caruso V, Marchioli R, et al. Acute leukemia in polycythemia vera: an analysis of 1638 patients enrolled in a prospective observational study. Blood 2005;105:2664–2670.

25. Mesa RA. Myelofibrosis with myeloid metaplasia: therapeutic options in 2003. Curr Hematol Rep 2003;2:264–270.

26. Cervantes F, Alvarez-Larran A, Hernandez-Boluda JC, et al. Erythropoietin treatment of the anaemia of myelofibrosis with myeloid metaplasia: results in 20 patients and review of the literature. Br J Haematol 2004;127:399–403.

27. Cervantes F, Hernandez-Boluda JC, Alvarez A, et al. Danazol treatment of idiopathic myelofibrosis with severe anemia. Haematologica 2000;85:595–599.

28. Lofvenberg E, Wahlin A, Roos G, et al. Reversal of myelofibrosis by hydroxyurea. Eur J Haematol 1990;44:33–38.

29. Chang JC, Gross HM. Remission of chronic idiopathic myelofibrosis to busulfan treatment. Am J Med Sci 1988;295:472–476.

30. Petti MC, Latagliata R, Spadea T, et al. Melphalan treatment in patients with myelofibrosis with myeloid metaplasia. Br J Haematol 2002;116:576–581.

31. Faoro LN, Tefferi A, Mesa RA. Long-term analysis of the palliative benefit of 2-chlorodeoxyadenosine for myelofibrosis with myeloid metaplasia. Eur J Haematol 2005;74:117–120.

32. Xu M, Bruno E, Chao J, et al. The constitutive mobilization of bone marrow–repopulating cells into the peripheral blood in idiopathic myelofibrosis. Blood 2005;105:1699–1705.

33. Barosi G, Grossi A, Comotti B, et al. Safety and efficacy of thalidomide in patients with myelofibrosis with myeloid metaplasia. Br J Haematol 2001;114:78–83.

34. Marchetti M, Barosi G, Balestri F, et al. Low-dose thalidomide ameliorates cytopenias and splenomegaly in myelofibrosis with myeloid metaplasia: a phase II trial. J Clin Oncol 2004;22:424–431.

35. Barosi G, Elliot MA, Canepa L, et al. Thalidomide in myelofibrosis with myeloid metaplasia: a pooled-analysis of individual patient data from five studies. Leuk Lymphoma 2002;43:2301–2307.

36. Mesa RA, Steensma DP, Pardanani A, et al. A phase II trial of combination low-dose thalidomide and prednisone for the treatment of myelofibrosis with myeloid metaplasia. Blood 2003;101:2534–2541.

37. Mesa RA, Stensma DP, Li CY, et al. Phase II study of the combination of low-dose thalidomide, prednisone, and etanercept (PET regimen) in the treatment of anemia, splenomegaly, and constitutional symptoms associated with myelofibrosis with myeloid metaplasia (MMM). Blood 2005;106:a2576.

38. Benetatos L, Chaidos A, Alymara V, et al. Combined treatment with thalidomide, corticosteroids, and erythropoietin in patients with idiopathic myelofibrosis. Eur J Haematol 2005;74:273–274.

39. Mesa RA, Pardanani A, Steensma DP, et al. Phase II Study of the Combination of Low-Dose Thalidomide, Prednisone, and Oral Cyclophosphamide (TPC Regimen) in the

Treatment of Anemia, Splenomegaly, and Constitutional Symptoms Associated with Myelofibrosis with Myeloid Metaplasia (MMM). ASH Annual Meeting Abstracts 2006;108:2689–2689.

40. Tefferi A, Cortes J, Verstovsek S, et al. Lenalidomide therapy in myelofibrosis with myeloid metaplasia. Blood 2006;108:1158–1164.
41. Abgrall JF, Guibaud I, Bastie JN, et al. Thalidomide versus placebo in myeloid metaplasia with myelofibrosis: a prospective, randomized, double-blind, multicenter study. Haematologica 2006;91:1027–1032.
42. Steensma DP, Mesa RA, Li CY, et al. Etanercept, a soluble tumor necrosis factor receptor, palliates constitutional symptoms in patients with myelofibrosis with myeloid metaplasia: results of a pilot study. Blood 2002;99:2252–2254.
43. Muller GW, Chen R, Huang SY, et al. Amino-substituted thalidomide analogs: potent inhibitors of TNF-alpha production. Bioorg Med Chem Lett 1999;9:1625–1630.
44. Schey SA, Fields P, Bartlett JB, et al. Phase I study of an immunomodulatory thalidomide analog, CC-4047, in relapsed or refractory multiple myeloma. J Clin Oncol 2004;22:3269–3276.
45. Giles F, List A, Carrol M, et al. PTK787/ZK 222584, a small molecule tyrosine kinase receptor inhibitor of vascular endothelial growth factor (VEGF), has modest activity in myelofibrosis with myeloid metaplasia. Leuk Res, in press.
46. Tefferi A, Barosi G, Mesa RA, et al. International Working Group (IWG) consensus criteria for treatment response in myelofibrosis with myeloid metaplasia, for the IWG for Myelofibrosis Research and Treatment (IWG-MRT). Blood 2006;108:1497–1503.
47. Giles FJ, Cooper MA, Silverman L, et al. Phase II study of SU5416—a small-molecule, vascular endothelial growth factor tyrosine-kinase receptor inhibitor—in patients with refractory myeloproliferative diseases. Cancer 2003;97:1920–1928.
48. O'Farrell AM, Abrams TJ, Yuen HA, et al. SU11248 is a novel FLT3 tyrosine kinase inhibitor with potent activity in vitro and in vivo. Blood 2003;101:3597–3605.
49. Fiedler W, Serve H, Dohner H, et al. A phase II study of SU11248 in the treatment of patients with refractory or resistant acute myeloid leukemia (AML) or not amenable to conventional therapy for the disease. Blood 2005;105:986–993.
50. Yingling JM, Blanchard KL, Sawyer JS. Development of TGF-beta signalling inhibitors for cancer therapy. Nat Rev Drug Discov 2004;3:1011–1022.
51. Schlingensiepen K, Bischof A, Egger T, et al. The TGF-beta1 antisense oligonucleotide AP 11014 for the treatment of non-small-cell lung, colorectal, and prostate cancer: preclinical studies. Proc Am Soc Clin Oncol 2004;23:(abstr 3132).
52. Sawyer JS, Beight DW, Britt KS, et al. Synthesis and activity of new aryl- and heteroaryl-substituted 5,6-dihydro-4 H-pyrrolo[1,2-b]pyrazole inhibitors of the transforming growth factor-beta type I receptor kinase domain. Bioorg Med Chem Lett 2004;14:3581–3584.
53. Gellibert F, Woolven J, Fouchet MH, et al. Identification of 1,5-naphthyridine derivatives as a novel series of potent and selective TGF-beta type I receptor inhibitors. J Med Chem 2004;47:4494–4506.
54. Callahan JF, Burgess JL, Fornwald JA, et al. Identification of novel inhibitors of the transforming growth factor beta1 (TGF-beta1) type 1 receptor (ALK5). J Med Chem 2002;45:999–1001.

55. Uhl M, Aulwurm S, Wischhusen J, et al. SD-208, a novel transforming growth factor beta receptor I kinase inhibitor, inhibits growth and invasiveness and enhances immunogenicity of murine and human glioma cells in vitro and in vivo. Cancer Res 2004;64:7954–7961.

56. Mesa RA, Tefferi A, Elliott MA, et al. A phase II trial of pirfenidone (5-methyl-1-phenyl-2-[1 H]-pyridone), a novel anti-fibrosing agent, in myelofibrosis with myeloid metaplasia. Br J Haematol 2001;114:111–113.

57. Komura E, Tonetti C, Penard-Lacronique V, et al. Role for the nuclear factor kappaB pathway in transforming growth factor-beta1 production in idiopathic myelofibrosis: possible relationship with FK506 binding protein 51 overexpression. Cancer Res 2005;65:3281–3289.

58. Rameshwar P, Narayanan R, Qian J, et al. NF-kappa B as a central mediator in the induction of TGF-beta in monocytes from patients with idiopathic myelofibrosis: an inflammatory response beyond the realm of homeostasis. J Immunol 2000;165: 2271–2277.

59. Wagner-Ballon O, Gastinne T, Tulliez M, et al. Proteasome inhibitor bortezomib can inhibit bone marrow fibrosis development in a murine model of myelofibrosis. Blood 2005;106:(abstr 2582).

60. Raza A, Lisak L, Tahir S, et al. Myelodysplastic syndrome patients show a variety of hematologic responses to the proteosome inhibitor bortezomib (PS-341). Blood 2002;100:a4906.

61. Kantarjian H, Sawyers C, Hochhaus A, et al. Hematologic and cytogenetic responses to imatinib mesylate in chronic myelogenous leukemia. N Engl J Med 2002;346: 645–652.

62. Kvasnicka HM, Thiele J. Bone marrow angiogenesis: methods of quantification and changes evolving in chronic myeloproliferative disorders. Histol Histopathol 2004;19:1245–1260.

63. Tefferi A, Mesa RA, Gray LA, et al. Phase 2 trial of imatinib mesylate in myelofibrosis with myeloid metaplasia. Blood 2002;99:3854–3856.

64. Cortes J, Ault P, Koller C, et al. Efficacy of imatinib mesylate in the treatment of idiopathic hypereosinophilic syndrome. Blood 2003;101:4714–4716.

65. Cortes J, Giles F, O'Brien S, et al. Results of imatinib mesylate therapy in patients with refractory or recurrent acute myeloid leukemia, high-risk myelodysplastic syndrome, and myeloproliferative disorders. Cancer 2003;97: 2760–2766.

66. le Bousse-Kerdiles M, Desteke C, Guerton B, et al. Glivec/STI571 treatment stimulates megakaryopoiesis and normalizes PDGF receptor beta kinase expression in thrombocytopenic patients with myeloid metaplasia with myelofibrosis. Blood 2005;106:(abstr 2599).

67. Lombardo LJ, Lee FY, Chen P, et al. Discovery of *N*-(2-chloro-6-methyl-phenyl)-2-(6-(4-(2-hydroxyethyl)-piperazin-1-yl)-2-methylpyrimidin-4-ylamino)thiazole-5-carboxamide (BMS-354825), a dual Src/Abl kinase inhibitor with potent antitumor activity in preclinical assays. J Med Chem 2004;47:6658–6661.

68. Reilly JT. Pathogenesis of idiopathic myelofibrosis: present status and future directions [review] [114 refs]. Br J Haematol 1994;88:1–8.

69. Beaupre DM, Kurzrock R. RAS and leukemia: from basic mechanisms to gene-directed therapy. J Clin Oncol 1999;17:1071–1079.

70. Du W, Lebowitz PF, Prendergast GC. Cell growth inhibition by farnesyltransferase inhibitors is mediated by gain of geranylgeranylated RhoB. Mol Cell Biol 1999;19:1831–1840.
71. Cortes J, Albitar M, Thomas D, et al. Efficacy of the farnesyl transferase inhibitor R115777 in chronic myeloid leukemia and other hematologic malignancies. Blood 2003;101:1692–1697.
72. Mesa RA, Camoriano JK, Geyer SM, et al. A phase 2 consortium (p2c) trial of R115777 (Tipifarnib) in myelofibrosis with myeloid metaplasia. Blood 2004; 104:a1509.
73. Kurzrock R, Fenaux P, Raza A, et al. High-risk myelodysplastic syndrome (MDS): First results of international phase II study with oral farnesyltransferase inhibitor R115777 (ZARNESTRATM). ASH Annual Meeting Abstracts 2004;104:68–68.
74. Gotlib J, Loh M, Lancet JE, et al. Phase I/II study of tipifarnib (Zarnestra, farnesyltransferase inhibitor (FTI) R115777) in patients with myeloproliferative disorders (MPDs): interim results. Blood 2003;102:a3425.
75. O'Brien S, Kipps TJ, Faderl S, et al. A phase I trial of the small molecule pan-Bcl-2 family inhibitor GX15–070 administered intravenously (iv) every 3 weeks to patients with previously treated chronic lymphocytic leukemia (CLL). Blood 2005;106:(abstr 446).
76. Baylin SB, Herman JG, Graff JR, et al. Alterations in DNA methylation: a fundamental aspect of neoplasia. Adv Cancer Res 1998;72:141–196.
77. Martyre MC, Steunou V, LeBousse-Kerdiles MC, et al. Lack of alteration in GATA-1 expression in CD34$^+$ hematopoietic progenitors from patients with idiopathic myelofibrosis [comment]. Blood 2003;101:5087–5088; Author reply, 5088–5089.
78. Issa JP, Gharibyan V, Cortes J, et al. Phase II study of low-dose decitabine in patients with chronic myelogenous leukemia resistant to imatinib mesylate. J Clin Oncol 2005;23:3948–3956.
79. James C, Ugo V, Le Couedic JP, et al. A unique clonal JAK2 mutation leading to constitutive signalling causes polycythaemia vera. Nature 2005;434:1144–1148.
80. Baxter EJ, Scott LM, Campbell PJ, et al. Acquired mutation of the tyrosine kinase JAK2 in human myeloproliferative disorders. Lancet 2005;365:1054–1061.
81. Levine RL, Wadleigh M, Cools J. Activating mutation in the tyrosine kinase JAK2 in polycythemia vera, essential thrombocythemia, and myelofibrosis with myeloid metaplasia. Cancer Cell 2005;7:387–397.
82. Kralovics R, Passamonti F, Buser AS, et al. A gain-of-function mutation of JAK2 in myeloproliferative disorders. N Engl J Med 2005;352:1779–1790.
83. Tefferi A, Lasho TL, Schwager SM, et al. The JAK2(V617F) tyrosine kinase mutation in myelofibrosis with myeloid metaplasia: lineage specificity and clinical correlates. Br J Haematol 2005;131:320–328.
84. Pardanani AD, Levine RL, Lasho T, et al. MPL515 mutations in myeloproliferative and other myeloid disorders: a study of 1182 patients. Blood 2006;108:3472–3476.
85. Pikman Y, Lee BH, Mercher T, et al. MPLW515 L is a novel somatic activating mutation in myelofibrosis with myeloid metaplasia. PLoS Med 2006;3:e270.
86. Scott LM, Tong W, Levine RL, et al. JAK2 exon 12 mutations in polycythemia vera and idiopathic erythrocytosis. N Engl J Med 2007;356:459–468.
87. Pardanani A, Hood J, Lasho T, et al. TG101209, a Selective JAK2 Kinase Inhibitor, Suppresses Endogenous and Cytokine-Supported Colony Formation from

Hematopoietic Progenitors Carrying JAK2V617F or MPLW515 K/L Mutations. ASH Annual Meeting Abstracts 2006;108:2680–2680.

88. Grandage VL, Everington T, Linch DC, et al. Go6976 is a potent inhibitor of the JAK 2 and FLT3 tyrosine kinases with significant activity in primary acute myeloid leukaemia cells. Br J Haematol 2006;135:303–316.

89. Li Z, Xu M, Xing S, et al. Erlotinib effectively inhibits JAK2V617F activity and polycythemia vera cell growth. J Biol Chem 2006;282:3428–3432.

90. Giles F, Freedman SJ, Xiao A, et al. MK-0457, a Novel Multikinase Inhibitor, Has Activity in Refractory AML, Including Transformed JAK2 Positive Myeloproliferative Disease (MPD), and in Philadelphia-Positive ALL. ASH Annual Meeting Abstracts 2006;108:1967–1967.

91. Dobrzanski P, Hexner E, Serdikoff C, et al. CEP-701 Is a JAK2 Inhibitor Which Attenuates JAK2/STAT5 Signaling Pathway and the Proliferation of Primary Cells from Patients with Myeloproliferative Disorders. ASH Annual Meeting Abstracts 2006;108:3594–3594.

92. Sayyah J, Ostrov D, Sayeski P. Identification and Characterization of a Novel Jak2 Tyrosine Kinase Inhibitor. ASH Annual Meeting Abstracts 2006;108:3604–3604.

93. Mesa RA, Powell H, Lasho T, et al. JAK2(V617F) and leukemic transformation in myelofibrosis with myeloid metaplasia. Leuk Res 2006;30:1457–1460.

94. Theocharides A, Boissinot M, Garand R, et al. Myeloid Blasts in Transformed JAK2-V617F Positive Myeloproliferative Disorders Are Frequently Negative for the JAK2-V617F Mutation. ASH Annual Meeting Abstracts 2006;108:375–375.

95. Druker BJ, Talpaz M, Resta DJ, et al. Efficacy and safety of a specific inhibitor of the BCR-ABL tyrosine kinase in chronic myeloid leukemia. N Engl J Med 2001;344:1031–1037.

9

Contemporary Diagnosis and Management of Systemic Mastocytosis

Peter Valent

*Division of Hematology & Hemostaseology, Medical University of Vienna,
Vienna, Austria*

Cem Akin

*Division of Allergy and Clinical Immunology, University of Michigan, Ann Arbor,
Michigan, U.S.A.*

Hans-Peter Horny

Institute of Pathology, Klinikum Ansbach, Ansbach, Germany

Dean D. Metcalfe

Laboratory of Allergic Diseases, NIAID/NIH, Bethesda, Maryland, U.S.A.

SUMMARY

Systemic mastocytosis (SM) is a clonal disease of mast cells (MCs) and their
progenitors. Clinical symptoms arise from MC-derived mediators and/or from
local MC infiltration, which in rare cases can be aggressive or even devastating. The clinical presentation, course, and prognosis in SM are variable. The
WHO discriminates the following disease variants: indolent SM (ISM), aggressive
SM (ASM), SM with associated clonal hematological non–MC-lineage disease
(AHNMD), and mast cell leukemia (MCL). The *KIT* mutation D816V is found
in all SM categories, including SM-AHNMD, where the mutation is sometimes

detectable in the AHNMD component of the disease. Other molecular defects are usually found in patients with SM-AHNMD, and reflect the nature of the associated malignancy. Therapeutic options in ISM include the use of antihistamines and other "mediator-targeting" drugs as well as bisphosphonates for those who develop osteoporosis. Patients with ASM are candidates for cytoreductive drugs (e.g., interferon-alpha or cladribine, 2CdA) or targeted drugs. Among the latter, imatinib works in the unusual patient, where no *KIT* mutations at codon 816 are found. For "codon 816 patients," investigational therapies with new tyrosine kinase inhibitors, such as midostaurin (PKC412) or dasatinib, may yield better results. For patients with rapidly progressing ASM or MCL, intensive chemotherapy and stem cell transplantation should be considered. In patients with SM-AHNMD, separate treatment plans for the SM- and AHNMD components of the disease need to be established. Examples are chemotherapy for AML in SM-AML, or imatinib in SM with concomitant FIP1L1/PDGFRA[+] eosinophilic leukemia.

ORIGIN, DISTRIBUTION, AND PHYSIOLOGY OF MAST CELLS

MCs are hematopoietic cells that display unique functional properties and express a distinct composition of mediators and antigens. In contrast to basophil granulocytes, MCs are long-lived cells with an estimated life span of at least 6 months. Mature MCs reside in diverse organs in connective tissues, often in the vicinity of smaller or larger blood vessels or nerve fibers. In tissue sections stained with basic dyes, MCs are easily identified by the presence of metachromatic granules. Notably, MCs store and generate an array of vasoactive and immunomodulating mediators, including histamine, heparin, and cytokines, including tumor necrosis factor alpha (Table 1) (1–3). These mediators are released when MCs are stimulated through the high-affinity IgE receptor (FcɛRI), stem cell factor (SCF) receptor (KIT), certain IgG receptors, or complement receptors. Other mediators, such as tryptase, are not only released upon cell activation, but are also secreted constitutively from MC (1–3). Therefore, a baseline tryptase level can be measured in the serum as a MC-related marker, and the level is believed to correlate with the total body burden of MC in normal subjects (normal serum tryptase level ranges between 0 and 15 ng/mL) and patients with mastocytosis (1–3).

MCs are derived from hematopoietic progenitor cells, which reside in the bone marrow, but also circulate in the peripheral blood (4–10). From here, MC progenitors can transmigrate into tissues and undergo differentiation and maturation. Several cytokines and the microenvironment are considered to contribute to the development of MC in various organs. Although MC heterogeneity has been described and has been related to the different microenvironments and local cytokine networks in mice, less is known about factors and cytokines controlling terminal maturation of MC in the human system. The most important cytokine supporting differentiation of early MC progenitors is mast cell growth factor, also known as SCF and KIT-ligand (4–10). This stromal cell–derived cytokine

Table 1 Mast Cell Mediators and Related Findings in Patients with SM

Mediator(s)	Site of action	Clinical features and symptoms frequently detected in SM
Histamine	H_1-receptors on vascular cells and other cells	Vascular instability, headache, edema, flushing, (acute) urticaria
	H_2-receptors on epithelial and other cells in the Gl tract	Gastric acid, hypersecretion, peptic ulcer disease, diarrhea, abdominal pain, cramping
	H_3-receptors in brain and Gl tract	Neurologic abnormalities, abdominal pain, diarrhea
Heparin	ATIII-cofactor, anticoagulant, cofactor for tPA, bFGF, and other growth factors	Coagulation abnormalities, bleeding diathesis, fibrosis, angiogenesis, osteopenia/osteoporosis
PGD_2, LTC_4, and other leukotrienes	PG and LT receptors on vascular and perivascular cells and other cell types	Edema, (acute) urticaria, flushing, bronchoconstriction, abdominal discomfort, cramping
VEGF	VEGF receptors on endothelial cells in diverse organs	Edema, increased angiogenesis in the bone marrow and other organs (in SM infiltrates)
bFGF	bFGF receptors on fibroblasts, endothelial cells, and other cell types	Bone marrow fibrosis, tissue fibrosis, increased angiogenesis, osteosclerosis
Tryptases	Diverse effects on fibroblasts, endothelial cells, leukocytes, and other mesenchymal cells	Fibrosis, angiogenesis, tissue remodeling, degradation of matrix molecules, abnormal coagulation, bone resorption
tPA	Plasmin activation	Hyperfibrinolysis
TNF-α	TNF receptors on endothelial cells and other cell types, cachexia, and vascular instability	Endothelial cell activation and CAM expression with resulting leukocyte-accumulation, fever
TGF-ß	TGF-ß receptors on various cells in tissues	Tissue fibrosis, abnormal bone remodeling, osteopenia

(cont.)

Table 1   (Cont.)

Mediator(s)	Site of action	Clinical features and symptoms frequently detected in SM
Interleukins (IL-1/-2/-3/-5/-6/-9/-10/-13)	IL-receptors on leukocytes and other cell types	Leukocyte differentiation and activation, eosinophilia, accumulation of eosinophils, growth and accumulation of lymphocytes in bone marrow, tissue fibrosis and activation of various stromal cells, myeloid hyperplasia
Chemokines (IL-8, MCP-1, Mip-1α, and others)	Chemokine receptors on leukocytes and stromal cells	Activation and chemotaxis of leukocytes, accumulation of lymphocytes, monocytes, eosinophils

Abbreviations: GI, gastrointestinal; PG, prostaglandin; LT, leukotriene; VEGF, vascular endothelial growth factor; bFGF, basic fibroblast growth factor; tPA, tissue-type plasminogen activator; TNF, tumor necrosis factor; TGF, transforming growth factor; IL, interleukin; GM-CSF, granulocyte-macrophage colony-stimulating factor; MCP-1, monocyte chemoattractant protein-1; Mip-1α, macrophage inflammatory protein-1α.

promotes the development of MC from their uncommitted and MC-committed progenitors (4–10). Correspondingly, MC progenitors as well as mature MC express KIT (8). This tyrosine kinase receptor is encoded by the *KIT* proto-oncogene. Several lines of evidence suggest that both KIT and SCF are critically involved in the regulation of the growth and differentiation of MC. Most significantly, defects in the *kit* gene or *scf* gene in mice are associated with MC deficiency (11,12). By contrast, "gain-of-function mutations" in *KIT* lead to autonomous (SCF-independent) growth and survival of MC (13). Such mutations, particularly *KIT* D816V, are frequently detected in SM (14–19).

PATHOGENESIS OF MASTOCYTOSIS

A pathogenetic hallmark of SM, shared by all subvariants, is the focal accumulation (clustering) of MC in internal organs (20–22). In high-grade MC neoplasms, MC and their progenitors may also show increased proliferative capacity. However, to date, little is known concerning pathogenetic factors that contribute to the development of SM variants and to disease progression. In cutaneous mastocytosis, a disease which is confined to the skin (and which often resolves spontaneously), the *KIT* mutation D816V is only found in a subgroup of patients and it is unclear in these mutation-positive patients, whether the disease is programmed to persist and to become systemic (23).

In SM, the vast majority of all patients display *KIT* D816V, supporting the clonal nature of the disease (14–19,24–26). A number of recent observations suggest that *KIT* D816V is an important "hit" contributing to MC differentiation and abnormal clustering of neoplastic cells, whereas *KIT* D816V per se is not able to act as a (mast cell) proliferation-enhancing oncogene (24,27). Thus, *KIT* D816V may play an important (possibly causative) role in indolent SM, where the pathologic hallmark is MC differentiation and clustering (but not MC proliferation), whereas in advanced MC neoplasms (ASM, MCL), in which *KIT* D816V is detectable, other (probably KIT-independent) factors may contribute to increased MC proliferation. These additional factors may relate to distinct signaling pathways and the individual genetic background of these patients.

It has also been suggested that, apart from D816V, other *KIT* mutations play a role in rare cases of SM (Table 2) (28–30). In addition, chromosome defects, single gene mutations, and gene polymorphisms have been discussed as contributing to the pathogenesis of SM (31–34). Many of these defects are detected in patients who have an additional myeloid neoplasm apart from SM, that is, an AHNMD (Table 2). Most of these defects have recently been linked to distinct myeloid neoplasms and have been, or will shortly be, defined as disease criteria by the WHO. Examples are the FIP1L1/PDGFRA fusion gene, JAK2 V617F, and AML1/ETO (Table 2) (24,31). Based on the specific clinical situation, these markers have to be applied in cases with suspected AHNMD. Likewise, in patients with SM and constant marked eosinophilia (SM-eo), it is appropriate to examine neoplastic cells for the presence of FIP1L1/PDGFRA (apart from other relevant molecular markers) (24,31), and in patients where FIP1L1/PDGFRA is demonstrable, the diagnosis SM-CEL, a subvariant of AHNMD, should be established. Table 2 provides a summary of chromosomal and gene defects that have been identified in patients with SM.

Another intriguing aspect in SM is the abnormal expression of adhesion antigens on neoplastic MC (35–38). In fact, several antigens specifically expressed on neoplastic MC in SM, such as CD2 (LFA-2), represent cell adhesion molecules. Since MC also express CD58 (LFA-3), the ligand of CD2, it has been hypothesized that CD2–CD58-dependent aggregation of MC contributes to abnormal MC clustering in SM (36). Moreover, MC in SM also express other cell-adhesion molecules, such as ß1 integrins or ICAM-1 (CD54), which may also contribute to cluster formation (37).

DIAGNOSTIC CRITERIA AND WHO CLASSIFICATION

Traditionally, mastocytosis is divided into cutaneous mastocytosis (CM) and SM. Localized MC tumors in tissues (mastocytoma and MC sarcoma) are very rare

Table 2 Gene Defects, Polymorphisms, and Chromosome Abnormalities Detected in Patients with Systemic Mastocytosis

Defect	Reported in patients with (frequency)
(a) *KIT* somatic mutations	
D816V	All variants of SM, 70–90% of all cases with ISM, most with BMM, SSM, and SM-AHNMD, also in a majority of cases with ASM and about 50% of cases with MCL and MCS
D816Y	SM (rare)
D816H	SM (rare)
I817V	SM (very rare)
D820G	SM (very rare)
V560G	SM (very rare)
D816F	SM (very rare)
(b) *KIT* germline mutations	
F522C	SM (very rare)
del419	SM (very rare, familial variant)
K509I	SM (very rare, familial variant)
(c) Gene polymorphisms	
IL-4Rα Q576R	SM (ISM)
(d) AHNMD-related gene defects	
FIP1L1/PDGFRA	SM-CEL (rare)
JAK2 V617F	SM-CIMF (rare), SM-PV, SM-ET (very rare)
BCR/ABL	SM-CML (very rare)
AML1/ETO	SM-AML M2 (rare)
PML/RARα	SM-AML M3 (very rare)
CBFβ/NYH11	SM-AML M4eo (very rare)
Ig-rearrangements	SM-NHL (rare)
paraproteinemia	SM-NHL (rare), SM-myeloma (rare)
(e) Karyotype abnormalities	
del 20(q12)	SM, SM-AHNMD (very rare)
+9	SM, SM-AHNMD (very rare)
Ph+	SM-CML (very rare)
t(8;21)	SM-AML M2 (rare)
t(15;17)	SM-AML M3 (very rare)
inv 16	SM-AML M4eo (very rare)
+8, −7, and others	SM-MDS (very rare)

(20–22). CM has its usual onset before puberty (39). By contrast, most adult patients are diagnosed with SM. In these individuals, the diagnosis should be established by a bone marrow examination (20–22,40,41), although other organs, such as the liver or the gastrointestinal tract, may also be affected (42–44). In contrast to SM, CM often shows spontaneous regression (45).

SM is a persistent disease in which the *KIT* mutation D816V is usually detected (14–19,25,26,46). In some SM patients, this mutation is not only found in MC, but also in non–MC-lineage hematopoietic cells (18,19,46). Based on such data, SM is now accepted to be a myeloproliferative disorder. This concept is consistent with the observation that MC derive from myelopoietic progenitors (4–7) and with the relatively high incidence of associated hematologic clonal non-MC-lineage diseases (AHNMD), including secondary acute myeloid leukemia (AML), which can occur in these patients (47–51).

During the last few years, substantial progress has been made in the morphological, phenotypic, and genetic characterization of neoplastic MC. Based on these advances, an update in the classification for mastocytosis has been proposed (50,51). This classification is based on specific criteria that help in the differentiation between SM and CM, between SM and myelomastocytic disorders, and between SM and a reactive increase in MC (50,51). Respective criteria have been termed SM criteria and are divided into major SM criteria and minor SM criteria (50,51). If at least one major and one minor criterion or at least three minor criteria are fulfilled, the final diagnosis is SM (Table 3).

Histology of the Bone Marrow (Major Criterion)

The crucial step in the diagnostic evaluation of adult patients is a thorough histologic examination of the bone marrow (40,41,50–54). Indeed, the major SM criterion is the presence of compact dense multifocal MC infiltrates in the bone marrow biopsy section (Table 3). The most suitable markers for MC detection in such biopsies are tryptase and KIT (Table 3) (52–54). Thus, antibodies against tryptase or KIT detect even small-sized compact or diffuse MC infiltrates (52–54). Compact MC infiltrates are diagnostic and are sometimes also detected in extramedullary visceral organs. However, the bone marrow should always be regarded as the primary site of investigation in suspected SM.

Apart from compact sharply demarcated MC infiltrates, other types of MC infiltrates have also been reported, with correlation between MC patterns and the subtype of SM (41,52–54). Notably, in advanced MC disorders (ASM, MCL), MC infiltrates often are diffuse or are compact with a significant diffuse component (mixed pattern). In patients with ASM or MCL, the remaining bone marrow architecture is typically altered by the MC infiltrate, whereas this is not the case in ISM (41). Here, MC infiltration does not lead to an alteration in the architecture of the remaining (surrounding) normal bone marrow, even if some MC are diffusely spread in these areas (41,52–54).

Table 3   Criteria for Systemic Mastocytosis (SM[a]) and Recommended Techniques

Criterion	Definition	Technique recommended
Major[a]	Multifocal dense infiltrates of MC in bone marrow histology sections or histologies of another extracutaneous organ(s) (> 15 MC in aggregates)	Tryptase staining (IHC), KIT staining (IHC), Giemsa, CAE
Minor[a]	Abnormal morphology of MC in compact MC infiltrates in tissues sections in the bone marrow or another extracutaneous organ(s) or: abnormal morphology of MC (type I) in bone marrow smears (> 25%: histology or smear)	Tryptase staining (IHC), KIT staining (IHC), Giemsa (IHC), Giemsa (bone marrow smear), CAE
	KIT mutation at codon 816 in extracutaneous organ(s)	Use bone marrow cells! RFLP, PNA clamping
	Expression of CD2 and/or CD25 on KIT[+] mast cells in an extracutaneous organ	Multicolor flow cytometry and IHC: KIT, CD25, tryptase (CD2 often negative)
	Serum total tryptase > 20 ng/mL (does not count in patients who have AHNMD-type disease)	Fluoroimmune enzyme assay (FIA)

[a]If at least one major and one minor or at least three minor criteria are fulfilled, the diagnosis of SM can be established (50,51).
Abbreviations: SM, systemic mastocytosis; IHC, immunohistochemistry; MC, mast cell(s); AHNMD, associated clonal non–mast cell–lineage disease.

MINOR DIAGNOSTIC CRITERIA

Minor criteria of SM include the morphology of MC (spindle shaped, atypical MC type I), the phenotype of MC (expression of CD2 and/or CD25), elevated serum tryptase (> 20 ng/mL), and a *KIT* codon 816 mutation, usually *KIT* D816V (Table 3) (50,51). If at least one major and one minor or at least three minor SM criteria are fulfilled, the diagnosis SM is established (Table 3). The application of minor SM criteria is crucial to the diagnosis SM, as MC may also increase and even form focal infiltrates in reactive states, at local tumor sites, or in myelo-mastocytic leukemia (55,56). In the latter condition, which is often confused with basophilic leukemia (even by experienced hematopathologists), an increase in diffusely spread MC in the bone marrow is found, but cytological or biochemical evidence of SM, that is, SM criteria (1 major + 1 minor or 3 minor) are not demonstrable (56).

Major and minor SM criteria are listed in Table 3. Table 4 shows the differential diagnoses to be considered in suspected SM.

Table 4 Systemic Mastocytosis—Differential Diagnoses[a]

(a) Disorders mimicking effects of mast cell–derived mediators
     Vascular instability (plus hypotension and shock)
     Endocrinologic disorders (diabetes, adrenal tumors, VIPoma, carcinoid, . . .)
     Neurological and psychiatric diseases (encephalopathy, neuritis, . . .)
     Gastrointestinal disorders (Crohn's disease, ulcerative colitis, celiac disease, . . .)
     Infectious diseases (parasitic infections, hepatitis, others)

(b) Mast cell activation in various diseases
     Monoclonal mast cell activation syndrome (MMAS)[b]
     Allergies, atopic disorders
     Benign cutaneous flushing
     Idiopathic anaphylaxis
     Chronic urticaria
     Drug effects on mast cells

(c) Local mast cell hyperplasia
     NHL (immunocytomas) with reactive focal increase in mast cells
     Cutaneous tumors (melanomas, basal cell carcinoma, others)
     Chronic inflammation (autoimmune disorders, intestinal ulcer, . . .)
     Treatment with recombinant stem cell factor (SCF)
     Thromboembolic disorders (perivascular accumulation of MC)

(d) Myelomastocytic overlap syndromes
     Myelomastocytic leukemia
     (myeloid neoplasm with increase in MCs but criteria to diagnose SM not fulfilled)
     Tryptase-positive acute myeloid leukemia (AML)
     KIT+ AML with blast cells expressing CD2 (FAB AML-M4eo, some M3)
     AML with aberrant expression of *KIT* point mutations at codon 816[c]
     Chronic myeloid leukemia with accumulation of tryptase[+] cells
     Idiopathic myelofibrosis with focal accumulation of mast cells
     Acute or chronic basophilic leukemia

---

[a]SM criteria are sufficient to discriminate SM from these differential diagnoses.
[b]MMAS is a condition defined by the presence of one or two minor SM criteria and typical (SM-like) symptoms, such as anaphylaxis (e.g., after insect stings).
[c]Often occult SM (i.e., after eradication of AML, frank SM is diagnosed).

Cytological Properties of Mast Cells in Bone Marrow Smears and Morphologic Grading

The bone marrow smear in suspected SM may show an increased MC number, an abnormal morphology of MC, or additional cytomorphological abnormalities, such as myelodysplasia, eosinophilia, or an increase in blasts, which in turn, raises the suspicion of an AHNMD (50,51). In normal bone marrow, the percentage of MC is < 0.1%. In SM, the percentage usually is higher. A percentage of MC of > 10% in the bone marrow smear is associated with a poor prognosis and often is indicative of aggressive disease (50,51,57). If the percentage of MC exceeds

20%, the diagnosis is MCL, provided that SM criteria are met (50,57). Based on consensus criteria, four distinct types of mast cells and their progenitors are defined: the metachromatically granulated blast (metachromatic blast), the promastocyte (atypical MC type II = MC with bi- or multilobed nuclei), the atypical MC type I, and mature MC (mononuclear MC) (Fig. 1) (50,57). Immature MC are frequently recorded in bone marrow smears in patients with ASM or MCL (50,57). In ISM, bone marrow MC are more mature, albeit they do show characteristic morphological abnormalities, including cytoplasmic extensions, oval nuclei, and a hypogranulated cytoplasm (= "atypical MC type I") (57).

Aberrant Expression of Leukocyte Antigens in/on Mast Cells in SM

MC exhibit a characteristic phenotype in normal tissues, as well as in SM (35–38,58,59). In most patients with SM, several CD antigens are overexpressed on bone marrow MC compared to normal MC (35,37). Most significantly, MC in patients with SM frequently coexpress CD2 and CD25, two surface antigens that are not found on normal MC (35,37,38). Because of this, aberrant expression of at least one of these two antigens on MC is employed as a minor criterion of SM (50,51). Expression of CD2 and CD25 in bone marrow MC is investigated by flow cytometry (35,37) or by immunohistochemistry (58,59). In both instances, CD25 is the more sensitive parameter and is expressed in MC in almost all cases of SM.

Serum Tryptase Levels in SM

Tryptase is a well-established and important disease-related marker, which should be determined in all patients with suspected SM (1–3). In healthy individuals, the total tryptase level ranges between < 1 and 15 ng/mL (median: approximately 5 ng/mL) (1–3). In most patients with CM (no systemic involvement), tryptase levels are normal (1–3). The same holds true for most cases with "isolated" bone marrow mastocytosis = BMM. By contrast, in most patients with (typical) SM, tryptase levels exceed 20 ng/mL (50,51). Note, however, that elevated tryptase levels are not only detected in SM, but also in other myeloid neoplasms, especially in myeloid leukemias (60–62). Moreover, serum tryptase levels may transiently increase during a severe anaphylactic reaction (62,63). Thus, tryptase per se cannot be regarded as a specific diagnostic test for SM. Based on this limitation, a persistently elevated serum tryptase level of > 20 ng/mL is employed as a minor criterion of SM, provided that an AHNMD was excluded (50,51).

Recommended Molecular and Cytogenetic Tests

In all patients with SM, molecular studies of bone marrow cells should include an analysis of *KIT* for codon-816 mutations, using appropriate assays such as PNA clamping or restriction fragment length polymorphism analysis (RFLP) (14–16,23,25,26). It has to be emphasized that such analysis should always be performed on bone marrow cells. If the test is negative, sequencing of *KIT*

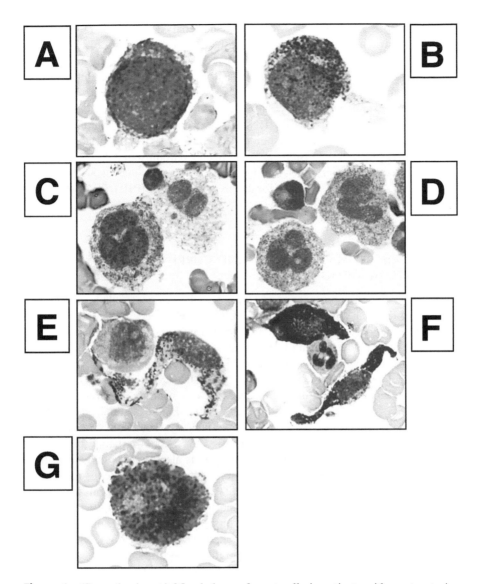

Figure 1 (See color insert.) Morphology of mast cells in patients with mastocytosis. Metachromatic blasts and mast cells were detected in Wright–Giemsa-stained bone marrow smears in patients with mastocytosis. (**A, B**) metachromatically granulated blast cells (metachromatic blasts) found in the bone marrow smear in a patient with mast cell leukemia; (**C, D**) immature mast cells with bi- or polylobed nuclei (promastocytes = atypical mast cell type II) detected in patients with mast cell leukemia; (**E, F**) atypical mast cells type I (spindle-shaped, hypogranulated cytoplasm, oval nuclei) in patients with indolent systemic mastocytosis; and (**G**) typical mature tissue mast cell (round, well granulated with a round central nucleus) in a patient with indolent systemic mastocytosis.

may reveal other mutations. However, sequence analysis may yield false-negative results because of low sensitivity. By contrast, a false-negative RFLP is unusual unless MC infiltrates in the bone marrow are very small or MC are outnumbered by leukemic (D816V-negative) cells. In such patients, the mutation may only be detected when enriched (sorted or microdissected) MC are analyzed, or the bone marrow is reexamined after successful chemotherapy (as with occult SM).

In patients with suspected AHNMD, bone marrow cells should not only be examined for *KIT* mutations, but should also be subjected to appropriate molecular analyses seeking specific fusion genes or specific chromosomal defects related to hematopoietic neoplasm. Likewise, in patients with coexisting eosinophilia, bone marrow cells should be examined for the presence of the FIP1L1/PDGFRA fusion gene (31). In SM-AML, the t(8;21) is often detected (Table 2).

CATEGORIES OF MASTOCYTOSIS AND CURRENT THERAPEUTIC OPTIONS

The delineation of subcategories of CM is based on macroscopic inspection and biopsy of lesional skin (39,64,65). Based on these aspects, three major variants have been defined: maculopapular CM (urticaria pigmentosa), diffuse CM, and solitary mastocytoma of skin (39,50,51,64,65).

In patients with SM, a number of specific questions must be addressed in order to define the subtype of disease. Aggressive SM is characterized by progressive infiltration of internal organs by MC, with resulting impairment of organ function. Respective clinical findings are termed C-Findings (Table 5) (50,51,66). Mast cell infiltration with associated organomegaly should not be regarded as organopathy (C-Finding) unless accompanied by signs of impaired organ function (Table 5) (50,51). Note that organomegaly is also found in patients with an indolent or an uncertain (smouldering) course (46,50,51), and then is regarded as a B-Finding (50). B- and C-Findings are listed in Table 5. In patients with a suspected AHNMD, WHO criteria for SM and for AHNMD are employed to define the subvariant (50,51). It may on occasion be difficult to discriminate between SM-AML, MCL, and myelomastocytic leukemia (50,51). MCL is a rare subentity of SM, where SM criteria are fulfilled and there is a diffuse leukemic infiltration of hematopoietic tissues by immature neoplastic MC (50,51,66–68). In contrast to ISM, patients with MCL, and most with ASM, do not exhibit typical skin lesions (66–68). Table 6 shows the current consensus classification of SM, which is essentially based on the WHO consensus classification of mastocytosis (50,51).

An important aspect of mastocytosis is the frequent occurrence of mediator-related symptoms. These symptoms may be mild, but may also be severe or even life-threatening (69–73). It is important to be aware that such severe symptoms (SM_{SY}) can occur in any subvariant of mastocytosis, and that the symptoms per se are not regarded as indication/signs of aggressive disease (not regarded as C-Findings). The following sections provide a brief overview of distinct variants of

Table 5 B- and C-Findings

B-Findings = Indication of high burden of MCs, and expansion of the genetic defect into various myeloid lineages

1. Infiltration grade (MCs) in bone marrow > 30% in histology and: serum total tryptase levels > 200 ng/mL
2. Hypercellular marrow with loss of fat cells, discrete signs of dysmyelopoiesis without substantial cytopenias or WHO criteria for an MDS or MPD
3. Organomegaly: palpable hepatomegaly, splenomegaly, or lymphadenopathy (on CT or US: > 2 cm) without impaired organ function

C-Findings = Indication of impaired organ function due to MC infiltration (has to be confirmed by biopsy in most cases)

1. Cytopenia(s): ANC < 1000/μL or Hb < 10 g/dL or Plt < 100,000/μL
2. Hepatomegaly with ascites and impaired liver function
3. Palpable splenomegaly with hypersplenism
4. Malabsorption with hypalbuminemia and weight loss
5. Skeletal lesions: large-sized osteolyses and/or severe osteoporosis causing pathologic fractures
6. Life-threatening organopathy in other organ systems that is definitively caused by an infiltration of the tissue by neoplastic MCs

Abbreviation: MCs, mast cells.

Table 6 Classification of Systemic Mastocytosis

Variant term	Abbreviation	Subvariants
Indolent systemic mastocytosis	ISM	
Isolated bone marrow mastocytosis[a]	BMM[a]	
Smouldering systemic mastocytosis[a]	SSM[a]	
Systemic mastocytosis with an associated clonal hematologic non–mast cell–lineage disease	SM-AHNMD	- SM-AML
		- SM-MDS
		- SM-MPD
		- SM-CEL
		- SM-CMML
		- SM-NHL
		- SM-myeloma
Aggressive systemic mastocytosis	ASM	
Mast cell leukemia	MCL	- Typical MCL
		- Aleukemic MCL

The current classification of SM is essentially based on the WHO consensus classification of masto-cytosis (50,51) with a recent update (69).
[a]In the original WHO classification, these variants have been described as provisional subvariants of ISM.

mastocytosis recognized by the WHO, with special reference to diagnostic criteria and available treatment options.

Cutaneous Mastocytosis (CM)

In CM, MC infiltration is confined to the skin (39,64). Most patients are children. By contrast, in most adults with skin lesions, a systemic variant of mastocytosis is diagnosed. Thus, the skin lesions of CM cannot be distinguished from that found in SM, either by macroscopic examination or by histology or molecular tests. Most patients with CM and most with SM have a characteristic maculopapular rash (39,64). In a smaller group of patients, usually those with CM, skin lesions are diffuse or nodular (39,64,65). A positive Darier's sign (urtication on stroking of lesional skin) is a typical finding. Blistering of the skin may also be observed, but is unusual. The diagnosis of CM is thus based on typical skin lesions, a skin biopsy, and lack of SM criteria (50,51,69). The serum tryptase usually is below < 20 ng/mL. For further information about subtypes, prognosis, and the management of CM, we refer the reader to the available literature (39,64,69).

Indolent Systemic Mastocytosis (ISM)

The most frequently diagnosed variant of SM is ISM. This condition is defined by SM criteria and the absence of all of the following: (a) signs of smouldering disease (B-Findings), (b) aggressive disease (C-Findings), (c) mast cell leukemia (less than 20% MC in bone marrow smears), and (d) an AHNMD. Most, but not all, patients with ISM display UP-like skin lesions. The clinical course in ISM is indolent, and the prognosis is good with a normal life expectancy, unless transformation into a high-grade MC disorder occurs (50,51). Fortunately, this is rarely seen. Mediator-related symptoms and osteopathy (i.e., osteopenia, osteoporosis) are often recorded, and may be the predominant medical problem (69). The bone marrow is almost always affected (40,41,50,51). The infiltration grade usually is low, and infiltrates are sharply demarcated from normal marrow (40,41). Typically, MC in bone marrow smears are atypical MC type I (57). Apart from the marrow, MC infiltrates may also be detected in other organs, including the liver, spleen, and the gastrointestinal tract. MC usually exhibit CD2 and CD25, and contain the *KIT* mutation D816V (50,51). The serum tryptase usually is > 20 ng/mL (1–3,50,51). Patients with ISM are treated with "mediator-targeting" drugs, including antihistamines, but not with cytoreductive agents (Table 7) (50,51,69,72,73). In those with osteoporosis or severe osteopenia, the administration of an oral (or i.v.) bisphosphonate should be recommended (69). Skin lesions in ISM may also require treatment (74). In most cases, transient responses are seen after PUVA (74).

Isolated Bone Marrow Mastocytosis (BMM)

This is a rare subentity of SM characterized by the absence of skin lesions and lack of multiorgan involvement (50,51,69). It is often overlooked, or misdiagnosed

Table 7 Cytoreductive Treatment Options for Patients with Systemic Mastocytosis (SM)

Disease variant	Treatment options
Typical indolent systemic mastocytosis (ISM)	No cytoreductive treatment required (exception: consider IFN-α2b for severe osteoporosis even if no histology documenting ASM is available, these cases are considered as "probably ASM")
Smouldering systemic mastocytosis (SSM)	Watch and wait in most cases. However, in select cases (rapidly progressive B-findings), IFN-α2b ± glucocorticoids can be considered.
SM-AHNMD	Treat AHNMD as if no SM is present and also treat SM as if no AHNMD is found. If splenomegaly and hypersplenism prohibit therapy, consider splenectomy.
Examples:	
SM-CEL+FIP1L1/PDGFRA	STI571 (Imatinib)
SM-AML	Chemotherapy or palliative drugs
SM-MDS	Palliative in most cases
Aggressive systemic mastocytosis (ASM) with slow progression	IFN-α2b ± glucocorticoids. If splenomegaly and hypersplenism prohibit therapy, consider splenectomy. In patients without detectable c-kit mutation D816V, STI571 (Imatinib) can be considered
ASM-rapid progression and patients who do not respond to IFN-α2b	Polychemotherapy (± IFN-α2b); consider bone marrow transplantation in select cases. If splenomegaly and hypersplenism prohibit therapy, consider splenectomy. For select cases, cladribine (2CdA) or other cytoreductive drugs can be considered. Consider hydroxyurea as a palliative drug.
Mast cell leukemia (MCL)	Polychemotherapy (± 2CDA; ± IFN-α2b). Consider bone marrow transplantation. If splenomegaly and hypersplenism prohibit therapy, consider splenectomy. Consider hydroxyurea as a palliative drug.

Abbreviation: IFN, interferon; SM-AHNMD, systemic mastocytosis with an associated hematologic clonal non–mast cell–lineage disease.

as unexplained anaphylaxis, unexplained osteoporosis, an unexplained endocrine syndrome, etc. Whereas BMM has so far been considered as a provisional entity, most recent data and outcomes of recent conferences support the conclusion that this condition should be regarded as a separate variant of SM (69). It is also important to differentiate bone marrow mastocytosis from ASM or MCL, where skin lesions are also absent (50,51,66,69). In contrast to ASM and MCL, the serum tryptase level in BMM is often < 20 ng/mL. In most patients, no therapy is required. In a subgroup, however, antimediator-type drugs and bisphosphonates need to be considered.

Smouldering Systemic Mastocytosis (SSM)

SSM is another subentity of SM (24,46,50,51,69). As with BMM, SSM should now also be regarded as a separate variant of SM (69), where previously, SSM was considered a subentity of ISM (50). In contrast to ISM, B-Findings ($\geq$ 2) are noted in SSM (Table 5). B-Findings reflect a high burden of MC and extension of the clonal disease to several myeloid lineages (24,46). Clinically, the smouldering state has an uncertain prognosis and a variable clinical course. In a group of patients, the course is long lasting and silent. In others, an AHNMD or ASM is diagnosed after a variable latency period. Typically, patients with SSM exhibit a bone marrow infiltration grade of more than 30% MC (dense infiltrates) and a serum tryptase level > 200 ng/mL (46). Discrete signs of myelodysplasia or myeloproliferation in the bone marrow are also present in most cases. In addition, palpable organomegaly (liver or spleen) or lymphadenopathy due to MC infiltration may be present (46). However, impairment of organ function (C-Findings) is not observed in SSM. The bone marrow in SSM typically contains mixed infiltrates composed of areas with dense focal accumulations of MC and an additional diffuse component (46). The *KIT* mutation D816V is usually detectable not only in MC, but also in other myeloid lineages and sometimes even in B lymphocytes (18,19,46). Treatment of SSM is identical to that in patients with ISM. However, SSM patients should be observed closely for signs of progression or occurrence of an AHNMD.

SM with Associated Clonal Hematologic Non–Mast Cell–Lineage Disease (SM-AHNMD)

In a group of patients with SM, an AHNMD is identified, thus leading to the diagnosis of SM–AHNMD (47–51,75–77). In these cases, WHO criteria for AHNMD and WHO criteria for SM are fulfilled. In the majority of patients, a myeloid neoplasm, such as a myeloproliferative disorder or a myeloid leukemia, develops (47–51). Myelodysplastic syndromes may also be diagnosed. One of the most frequently identified AHNMD is CMML. The occurrence of a lymphoid neoplasm, such as multiple myeloma or a lymphoma (usually B lineage), is less frequently diagnosed. In all cases, the SM component must be defined and subclassified in the same way as if no AHNMD was recorded.

In all patients with SM-AHNMD, separate treatment plans for SM and the AHNMD component of the disease should be established. Notably, SM is treated as if no AHNMD is present, and AHNMD is treated as if no SM had been diagnosed (Table 7). Likewise, in patients with SM and associated chronic eosinophilia (SM-CEL) expressing FIP1L1/PDGFRA, imatinib is an appropriate therapy and responses may be the same compared to patients with CEL without coexisting SM (31,75,76). In patients with SM-AML, polychemotherapy (that would be given in patients with AML without SM) may induce complete hematologic remission of AML (24,48,77).

An important aspect in SM-AHNMD is that the SM component may present as ISM or ASM, which in turn, has implications for defining the treatment plan. In some patients, cytoreductive drugs may show beneficial effects for both ASM and the AHNMD.

Aggressive Systemic Mastocytosis (ASM)

ASM is characterized by organopathy resulting from the pathologic and sometimes rapidly devastating infiltration of various organs by neoplastic MC, and the subsequent impairment of organ function (24,50,51,66). In contrast to MCL, the bone marrow smear shows less than 20% MC (50,51). In contrast to ISM and SSM, C-Findings, reflecting compromised organ function, due to histologically proven aggressive MC infiltration, are detectable in ASM (Table 5). In particular, patients show one of the following: (a) significant cytopenia(s); (b) impairment of liver function due to MC infiltration, often with ascites; (c) osteolyses with pathologic fractures; (d) malabsorption with weight loss; (e) splenomegaly with hypersplenism; or (f) life-threatening impairment of organ function in other organ systems (50,51,66). The most frequently affected organ systems are the liver, bone marrow, and the skeletal system. UP-like skin lesions are usually absent in ASM (50,51,66). The histology of the bone marrow shows a variable degree of infiltration, with MC infiltrates often exhibiting a mixed (dense focal + diffuse) pattern. The bone marrow cytology often shows major MC atypia with occurrence of promastocytes and metachromatic blasts (50,51,57). Serum tryptase levels may become quite high. Patients with ASM are candidates for treatment with cytoreductive drugs (Table 7). Patients with a relatively slow progression are usually treated with glucocorticoids (prednisone) and interferon alpha (IFN-α) (24,50,66,69,78–81). Prednisone (50–75 mg p. o. daily) may be initiated a few days before IFN-α is administered (3 million I.U. s.c. three times a week). During the first days of treatment, the patient should be carefully monitored. After a few weeks, the interferon dosage can usually be escalated to 3–5 million units per day, and prednisone tapered to a low maintenance dose (12.5 mg/day or less) or even discontinued. In patients with severe osteopathy, IFN-α can be administered together with bisphosphonates but without corticosteroids. Patients with ASM with rapid disease progression, signs of progression to MCL, or failure to respond to IFN-α, are candidates for 2CdA or polychemotherapy (Table 7) (24,69,82,83). The use of targeted drugs in ASM has also been considered. Imatinib (STI571) has been described to be effective in some of these patients. In fact, several SM patients with wild-type *KIT* or *KIT* mutations other than D816V appear to respond to imatinib. However, most patients with ASM have *KIT* D816V, which appears to be resistant against imatinib (84–86). Therefore, imatinib cannot be recommended for routine use in patients with ASM or MCL. However, a number of novel tyrosine kinase inhibitors are available, and some, such as midostaurin (PKC412) and dasastinib (BMS354825), appear to inhibit the growth of neoplastic MC harboring *KIT* D816V (85–91). These drugs are currently being tested in clinical trials in order to define their activity in patients with ASM and MCL.

Mast Cell Leukemia (MCL) and Mast Cell Sarcoma (MCS)

MCL is a rare aggressive MC neoplasm defined by increased numbers of MC in bone marrow smears ($\geq$ 20%) and by circulating MC (20–22,24,50,51,66–68). Patients typically suffer from rapidly progressive organopathy involving the liver, bone marrow, and other organs. The bone marrow typically shows a diffuse plus dense infiltration with MC (41,50,66–68). MCs are often immature, show a blast-like morphology, and/or have polylobed nuclei (promastocytes) (50,57). In typical MCL, MCs account for more than 10% of blood leukocytes (50,57). In a smaller group of patients, pancytopenia occurs and MCs account for less than 10% (aleukemic variant of MCL) (50,51). In many patients, MC express CD2 and CD25. The *c-kit* mutation D816V may be detected. The prognosis in MCL is poor. Most patients survive less than 1 year and respond poorly to chemotherapy (24,50,51,66–68). A curative therapy for MCL is currently not available. Chemotherapeutic regimens employing substances otherwise used for treatment of AML (with or without 2CdA) may be considered (Table 7) (50,69). Another experimental option is bone marrow transplantation, although no experience exists concerning responses and mortality.

Mast cell sarcoma (MCS) is an extremely rare form of mastocytosis. To date, the authors are aware of only three well-documented cases (92–94). The disease is defined by a local destructive sarcoma-like growth of a tumor consisting of highly atypical MC. At initial diagnosis, no systemic involvement is found. However, secondary generalization with involvement of visceral organs and hematopoietic tissues has been described. The terminal phase may be indistinguishable from ASM or MCL (92–94). The prognosis in MCS is grave.

CONCLUDING REMARKS

During the last few years, major advances in mastocytosis research have been made including the identification of molecular markers and drug targets in neoplastic mast cells and the formulation of diagnostic criteria. In addition, standard diagnostic techniques and response criteria are available, and several potentially effective drugs are currently in cinical trials, with the goal to improve the outcome in ASM and MCL.

ACKNOWLEDGMENT

This work was supported by the Fonds zur Förderung der Wissenschaftlichen Forschung, FWF, Austria, and by the Division of Intramural Research, NIAID/NIH.

REFERENCES

1. Schwartz LB, Sakai K, Bradford TR, et al. The alpha form of human tryptase is the predominant type present in blood at baseline in normal subjects and is elevated in those with systemic mastocytosis. J Clin Invest 1995;96: 2702–2710.
2. Akin C, Metcalfe DD. Surrogate markers of disease in mastocytosis. Int Arch Allergy Immunol 2002;127:133–136.
3. Sperr WR, Jordan JH, Fiegl M, et al. Serum tryptase levels in patients with mastocytosis: correlation with mast cell burden and implication for defining the category of disease. Int Arch Allergy Immunol 2002;128:136–141.
4. Kirshenbaum AS, Goff JP, Kessler SW, et al. Effects of IL-3 and stem cell factor on the appearance of human basophils and mast cells from CD34$^+$ pluripotent progenitor cells. J Immunol 1992;148:772–777.
5. Kirshenbaum AS, Goff JP, Semere T, et al. Demonstration that human mast cells arise from a progenitor cell population that is CD34$^+$, c-kit$^+$, and expresses aminopeptidase N (CD13). Blood 1999;94:2333–2342.
6. Agis H, Willheim M, Sperr WR, et al. Monocytes do not make mast cells when cultured in the presence of SCF. Characterization of the circulating mast cell progenitor as a c-kit$^+$, CD34$^+$, Ly$^-$, CD14$^-$, CD17$^-$, colony-forming cell. J Immunol 1993;151:4221–4227.
7. Rottem M, Okada T, Goff JP, et al. Mast cells cultured from peripheral blood of normal donors and patients with mastocytosis originate from a CD34$^+$/FcεRI$^-$ cell population. Blood 1994;84:2489–2496.
8. Valent P. The riddle of the mast cell: c-kit ligand as missing link? Immunol Today 1994;15:111–114.
9. Irani AM, Nilsson G, Miettinen U, et al. Recombinant human stem cell factor stimulates differentiation of human mast cells from dispersed fetal liver cells. Blood 1992;80:3009–3016.
10. Valent P, Spanblöchl E, Sperr WR, et al. Induction of differentiation of human mast cells from bone marrow and peripheral blood mononuclear cells by recombinant human stem cell factor (SCF)/kit ligand (KL) in long-term culture. Blood 1992;80:2237–2245.
11. Kitamura Y, Go S, Hatanaka S. Decrease of mast cells in W/W^v mice and their increase by bone marrow transplantation. Blood 1978;52:447–452.
12. Kitamura Y, Go S. Decreased production of mast cells in Sl/Sl^d mice. Blood 1979;53:492–497.
13. Furitsu T, Tsujimura T, Tono T, et al. Identification of mutations in the coding sequence of the proto-oncogene c-kit in a human mast cell leukemia cell line causing ligand-independent activation of the c-kit product. J Clin Invest 1993;92: 1736–1744.
14. Nagata H, Worobec AS, Oh CK, et al. Identification of a point mutation in the catalytic domain of the protooncogene *c-kit* in peripheral blood mononuclear cells of patients who have mastocytosis with an associated hematologic disorder. Proc Natl Acad Sci U S A 1995;92:10560–10564.
15. Longley BJ, Tyrrell L, Lu SZ, et al. Somatic *c-kit* activating mutation in urticaria pigmentosa and aggressive mastocytosis: establishment of clonality in a human mast cell neoplasm. Nat Genet 1996;12:312–314.

16. Longley BJ, Metcalfe DD, Tharp M, et al. Activating and dominant inactivating *c-kit* catalytic domain mutations in distinct forms of human mastocytosis. Proc Natl Acad Sci U S A 1999;96:1609–1614.

17. Büttner C, Henz BM, Welker P, et al. Identification of activating *c-kit* mutations in adult-, but not childhood-onset indolent mastocytosis: a possible explanation for divergent clinical behaviour. J Invest Dermatol 1998;111:1227–1231.

18. Akin C, Kirschenbaum AS, Semere T, et al. Analysis of the surface expression of c-kit and occurrence of the c-kit Asp816Val activating mutation in T cells, B cells, and myelomonocytic cells in patients with mastocytosis. Exp Hematol 2000;28:140–147.

19. Yavuz AS, Lipsky PE, Yavuz S, et al. Evidence for the involvement of a hematopoietic progenitor cell in systemic mastocytosis from single cell analysis of mutations in the *c-kit* gene. Blood 2002;100:661–665.

20. Parwaresch MR, Horny H-P, Lennert K. Tissue mast cells in health and disease. Pathol Res Pract 1985;179:439–461.

21. Metcalfe DD. Classification and diagnosis of mastocytosis: current status. J Invest Dermatol 1991;96:2S–4S.

22. Valent P. Biology, classification, and treatment of human mastocytosis. Wien Klin Wochenschr 1996;108:385–397.

23. Sotlar K, Escribano L, Landt O, et al. One-step detection of *c-kit* point mutations using peptide nucleic acid-mediated polymerase chain reaction clamping and hybridization probes. Am J Pathol 2003;162:737–746.

24. Valent P, Akin C, Sperr WR, et al. Diagnosis and treatment of systemic mastocytosis: state of the art. Br J Haematol 2003;122:695–717.

25. Fritsche-Polanz R, Jordan JH, Feix A, et al. Mutation analysis of *C-KIT* in patients with myelodysplastic syndromes without mastocytosis and cases of systemic mastocytosis. Br J Haematol 2001;113:357–364.

26. Akin C. Molecular diagnosis of mast cell disorders: a paper from the 2005 William Beaumont Hospital Symposium on Molecular Pathology. J Mol Diagn 2006;8: 412–419.

27. Ferrao PT, Gonda TJ, Ashman LK. Constitutively active mutant D816VKit induces megakayocyte and mast cell differentiation of early haemopoietic cells from murine foetal liver. Leuk Res 2003;27:547–555.

28. Pignon JM, Giraudier S, Duquesnoy P, et al. A new c-kit mutation in a case of aggressive mast cell disease. Br J Haematol 1997;96:374–376.

29. Akin C, Fumo G, Yavuz AS, et al. A novel form of mastocytosis associated with a transmembrane *c-Kit* mutation and response to imatinib. Blood 2003;103:3222–3225.

30. Pullarkat VA, Pullarkat ST, Calverley DC, Brynes RK. Mast cell disease associated with acute myeloid leukemia: detection of a new *c-kit* mutation Asp816His. Am J Hematol 2000;65:307–309.

31. Pardanani A, Ketterling RP, Brockman SR, et al. CHIC2 deletion, a surrogate for FIP1L1-PDGFRA fusion, occurs in systemic mastocytosis associated with eosinophilia and predicts response to imatinib mesylate therapy. Blood 2003;102:3093–3096.

32. Swolin B, Rodjer S, Roupe G. Cytogenetic studies and in vitro colony growth in patients with mastocytosis. Blood 1987;70:1928–1932.

33. Lishner M, Confino-Cohen R, Mekori YA, et al. Trisomies 9 and 8 detected by fluorescence in situ hybridization in patients with systemic mastocytosis. J Allergy Clin Immunol 1996;98:199–204.

34. Daley T, Metcalfe DD, Akin C. Association of the Q576R polymorphism in the interleukin-4 receptor alpha chain with indolent mastocytosis limited to the skin. Blood 2001;98:880–882.
35. Escribano L, Orfao A, Diaz-Agustin B, et al. Indolent systemic mast cell disease in adults: immunophenotypic characterization of bone marrow mast cells and its diagnostic implication. Blood 1998;91:2731–2736.
36. Schernthaner GH, Jordan JH, Ghannadan M, et al. Expression, epitope analysis, and functional role of the LFA-2 antigen detectable on neoplastic mast cells. Blood 2001;98:3784–3792.
37. Escribano L, Díaz-Agustín B, Bellas C, et al. Utility of flow cytometric analysis of mast cells in the diagnosis and classification of adult mastocytosis. Leuk Res 2001;25:563–570.
38. Valent P, Schernthaner GH, Sperr WR, et al. Variable expression of activation-linked surface antigens on human mast cells in health and disease. Immunol Rev 2001;179:74–81.
39. Wolff K, Komar M, Petzelbauer P. Clinical and histopathological aspects of cutaneous mastocytosis. Leuk Res 2001;25:519–528.
40. Horny H-P, Parwaresch MR, Lennert K. Bone marrow findings in systemic mastocytosis. Hum Pathol 1985;16:808–814.
41. Horny H-P, Valent P. Diagnosis of mastocytosis: general histopathological aspects, morphological criteria, and immunohistochemical findings. Leuk Res 2001;25: 543–551.
42. Horny H-P, Ruck M, Kaiserling E. Spleen findings in generalized mastocytosis. A clinicopathologic study. Cancer 1992;70:459–468.
43. Horny H-P, Kaiserling E, Campbell M, Parwaresch MR, Lennert K. Liver findings in generalized mastocytosis. A clinicopathologic study. Cancer 1989;63:532–538.
44. Metcalfe DD. The liver, spleen, and lymph nodes in mastocytosis. J Invest Dermatol 1991;96:45S–46S.
45. Caplan RM. The natural course of urticaria pigmentosa. Arch Dermatol 1963;87: 146–157.
46. Valent P, Akin C, Sperr WR, et al. Smouldering mastocytosis: a new type of systemic mastocytosis with slow progression. Int Arch Allergy Immunol 2002;127: 137–139.
47. Horny H-P, Ruck M, Wehrmann M, et al. Blood findings in generalized mastocytosis: evidence of frequent simultaneous occurrence of myeloproliferative disorders. Br J Haematol 1990;76:186–193.
48. Sperr WR, Horny H-P, Lechner K, et al. Clinical and biologic diversity of leukemias occuring in patients with mastocytosis. Leuk Lymphoma 2000;37: 473–486.
49. Travis WD, Li CY, Yam LT, et al. Significance of systemic mast cell disease with associated hematologic disorders. Cancer 1988;62:965–972.
50. Valent P, Horny H-P, Escribano L, et al. Diagnostic criteria and classification of mastocytosis: a consensus proposal. Conference Report of "Year 2000 Working Conference on Mastocytosis." Leuk Res 2001;25:603–625.
51. Valent P, Horny H-P, Li CY, et al. Mastocytosis (mast cell disease). In: Jaffe ES, Harris NL, Stein H, Vardiman JW, eds. World Health Organization (WHO) Classification of Tumours. Pathology & Genetics. Tumours of Haematopoietic and Lymphoid Tissues. Lyon, France: IARC Press, Vol 1. 2001, pp. 291–302.

52. Horny H-P, Sillaber C, Menke D, et al. Diagnostic utility of staining for tryptase in patients with mastocytosis. Am J Surg Pathol 1998;22:1132–1140.
53. Fukuda T, Kamashima T, Tsuura Y, et al. Expression of the c-kit gene product in normal and neoplastic mast cells but not in neoplastic basophil/mast cell precursors from chronic myelogenous leukaemia. J Pathol 1995;177:139–146.
54. Li WV, Kapadia SB, Sonmez-Alpan E, et al. Immunohistochemical characterization of mast cell disease in paraffin sections using tryptase, CD68, myeloperoxidase, lysozym, and CD20 antibodies. Mod Pathol 1996;9:982–988.
55. Prokocimer M, Polliack A. Increased bone marrow mast cells in preleukemic syndromes, acute leukemia, and lymphoproliferative disorders. Am J Clin Pathol 1981;75:34–38.
56. Valent P, Sperr WR, Samorapoompichit P, et al. Myelomastocytic overlap syndromes: biology, criteria, and relationship to mastocytosis. Leuk Res 2001;25:595–602.
57. Sperr WR, Escribano L, Jordan JH, et al. Morphologic properties of neoplastic mast cells: delineation of stages of maturation and implication for cytological grading of mastocytosis. Leuk Res 2001;25:529–536.
58. Jordan JH, Walchshofer S, Jurecka W, et al. Immunohistochemical properties of bone marrow mast cells in systemic mastocytosis: evidence for expression of CD2, CD117/Kit, and bcl-x$_L$. Hum Pathol 2001;32:545–552.
59. Sotlar K, Horny HP, Simonitsch I, et al. CD25 indicates the neoplastic phenotype of mast cells: a novel immunohistochemical marker for the diagnosis of systemic mastocytosis (SM) on routinely processed bone marrow biopsy specimens. Am J Surg Pathol 2004;28:1319–1325.
60. Sperr WR, Stehberger B, Wimazal F, et al. Serum tryptase measurements in patients with myelodysplastic syndromes. Leuk Lymphoma 2002;43:1097–1105.
61. Sperr WR, Jordan JH, Baghestanian M, et al. Expression of mast cell tryptase by myeloblasts in a group of patients with acute myeloid leukemia. Blood 2001;98:2200–2209.
62. Schwartz LB. Clinical utility of tryptase levels in systemic mastocytosis and associated hematologic disorders. Leuk Res 2001;25:553–562.
63. Schwartz LB, Metcalfe DD, Miller JS, et al. Tryptase levels as an indicator of mast-cell activation in systemic anaphylaxis and mastocytosis. N Engl J Med 1987;316:1622–1626.
64. Hartmann K, Henz BM. Cutaneous mastocytosis—clinical heterogeneity. Int Arch Allergy Immunol 2002;127:143–146.
65. Willemze R, Ruiter DJ, Scheffer E, et al. Diffuse cutaneous mastocytosis with multiple cutaneous mastocytomas. Report of a case with clinical, histopathological, and ultrastructural aspects. Br J Dermatol 1980;102:601–607.
66. Valent P, Akin C, Sperr WR, et al. Aggressive systemic mastocytosis and related mast cell disorders: current treatment options and proposed response criteria. Leuk Res 2003;27:635–641.
67. Dalton R, Chan L, Batten E, et al. Mast cell leukemia: evidence for bone marrow origin of the pathological clone. Br J Haematol 1986;64:397–406.
68. Travis WD, Li CY, Hogaland HC, et al. Mast cell leukemia: report of a case and review of the literature. Mayo Clin Proc 1986;61:957–966.
69. Valent P, Akin C, Escribano L, et al. Standards and standardization in mastocytosis: consensus statements on diagnostics, treatment recommendations, and response criteria. Eur J Clin Invest 2007;37:435–453.

70. Austen KF. Systemic mastocytosis. N Engl J Med 1992;326:639–640.
71. Castells M, Austen KF. Mastocytosis: mediator-related signs and symptoms. Int Arch Allergy Immunol 2002;127:147–152.
72. Escribano L, Akin C, Castells M, et al. Mastocytosis: current concepts in diagnosis and treatment. Ann Hematol. 2002;81:677–690.
73. Worobec AS. Treatment of systemic mast cell disorders. Hematol Oncol North Am 2000;14:659–687.
74. Godt O, Proksch E, Streit V, Christophers E. Short- and long-term effectiveness of oral and bath PUVA therapy in urticaria pigmentosa and systemic mastocytosis. Dermatology 1997;195:35–39.
75. Pardanani A, Elliott M, Reeder T, et al. Imatinib for systemic mast-cell disease. Lancet 2003;362:535–536.
76. Tefferi A, Pardanani A. Imatinib therapy in clonal eosinophilic disorders, including systemic mastocytosis. Int J Hematol 2004;79:441–447.
77. Sperr WR, Walchshofer S, Horny HP, et al. Systemic mastocytosis associated with acute myeloid leukaemia: report of two cases and detection of the *c-kit* mutation Asp-816 to Val. Br J Haematol 1998;103:740–749.
78. Kluin-Nelemans HC, Jansen JH, Breukelman H, et al. Response to interferon alfa-2b in a patient with systemic mastocytosis. N Engl J Med 1992;326:619–623.
79. Worobec AS, Kirshenbaum AS, Schwartz LB, et al. Treatment of three patients with systemic mastocytosis with interferon alpha-2b. Leuk Lymphoma 1996;22:501–508.
80. Weide R, Ehlenz K, Lorenz W, et al. Successful treatment of osteoporosis in systemic mastocytosis with interferon alpha-2b. Ann Hematol 1996;72:41–43.
81. Hauswirth AW, Simonitsch-Klupp I, Uffmann M, et al. Response to therapy with interferon alpha-2b and prednisolone in aggressive systemic mastocytosis: report of five cases and review of the literature. Leuk Res 2004;28:249–257.
82. Tefferi A, Li CY, Butterfield JH, et al. Treatment of systemic mast-cell disease with cladribine. N Engl J Med 2001;344:307–309.
83. Kluin-Nelemans HC, Oldhoff JM, Van Doormaal JJ, et al. Cladribine therapy for systemic mastocytosis. Blood 2003;102:4270–4276.
84. Akin C, Brockow K, D'Ambrosio C, et al. Effects of tyrosine kinase inhibitor STI571 on human mast cells bearing wild-type or mutated forms of c-kit. Exp Hematol 2003;31:686–692.
85. Ma Y, Zeng S, Metcalfe DD, et al. The *c-KIT* mutation causing human mastocytosis is resistant to STI571 and other KIT kinase inhibitors; kinases with enzymatic site mutations show different inhibitor sensitivity profiles than wild-type kinases and those with regulatory type mutations. Blood 2002;99:1741–1744.
86. Frost MJ, Ferrao PT, Hughes TP, et al. Juxtamembrane mutant V560GKit is more sensitive to Imatinib (STI571) compared with wild-type c-kit whereas the kinase domain mutant D816VKit is resistant. Mol Cancer Ther 2002;1:1115–1124.
87. Growney JD, Clark JJ, Adelsperger J, et al. Activation mutations of human c-KIT resistant to imatinib are sensitive to the tyrosine kinase inhibitor PKC412. Blood 2005;106:721–724.
88. Gotlib J, Berube C, Growney JD, et al. Activity of the tyrosine kinase inhibitor PKC412 in a patient with mast cell leukemia with the D816V KIT mutation. Blood 2005;106:2865–2870.
89. Gleixner KV, Mayerhofer M, Aichberger KJ, et al. The tyrosine kinase-targeting drug PKC412 inhibits in vitro growth of neoplastic human mast cells expressing the

D816V-mutated variant of kit: comparison with AMN107, imatinib, and cladribine (2CdA), and evaluation of cooperative drug effects. Blood 2006;107:752–759.

90. von Bubnoff N, Gorantla SH, Kancha RK, et al. The systemic mastocytosis-specific activating c-Kit mutation D816V can be inhibited by the tyrosine kinase inhibitor AMN107. Leukemia 2005;19:1670–1671.
91. Shah NP, Lee FY, Luo R, et al. Dasatinib (BMS-354825) inhibits KITD816V, an imatinib-resistant activating mutation that triggers neoplastic growth in the majority of patients with systemic mastocytosis. Blood 2006;108:286–291.
92. Horny H-P, Parwaresch MR, Kaiserling E, et al. Mast cell sarcoma of the larynx. J Clin Pathol 1986;39:596–602.
93. Kojima M, Nakamura S, Itoh H, et al. Mast cell sarcoma with tissue eosinophilia arising in the ascending colon. Mod Pathol 1999;12:739–743.
94. Günther PP, Huebner A, Sobottka SB, et al. Temporary response of localized intracranial mast cell sarcoma to combination chemotherapy. J Pediatr Hematol Oncol 2001;23:134–138.

10

Primary Eosinophilic Disorders

Animesh Pardanani and Ayalew Tefferi
Division of Hematology, Mayo Clinic College of Medicine, Rochester, Minnesota, U.S.A.

INTRODUCTION

Eosinophils normally comprise less than 5% of the circulating nucleated cells in the peripheral blood. During normal hematopoiesis, eosinophils, like other hematopoietic cells, are derived from hematopoietic stem cells, but the identity of the precursor cell from which eosinophils are derived remains incompletely defined. While there are data supporting the presence of a hybrid precursor with combined characteristics of basophils and eosinophils (1,2), recent evidence suggests that eosinophil development diverges from that of other granulocytes at the granulocyte/monocyte progenitor stage, to yield a phenotypically distinct eosinophil progenitor cell population (3). Recent evidence also reveals cooperation between the transcription factors GATA-1, c/EBPα, and PU.1 (particularly GATA-1) to provide important instructive signals for eosinophil formation in vivo (4). For instance, GATA-1–deficient mice fail to develop eosinophil progenitors in fetal liver (5), and targeted disruption of a high-affinity GATA binding site in the GATA-1 promoter leads to selective loss of eosinophil development in vivo (6).

The cytokines interleukin (IL)-3, IL-5, and granulocyte monocyte-colony stimulating factor (GM-CSF) share a common β chain (but possess distinct α chains) and are encoded by closely linked genes on chromosome 5q31– these three cytokines play an important role in supporting eosinophil development in vivo (7,8) Of these cytokines, IL-5 is most specific for eosinophil formation as well as eosinophil mobilization from bone marrow and appears to be a late-acting factor in the network of cytokines that includes IL-3 and GM-CSF (3,8,9). Interestingly, IL-5 overexpression from a transgene is sufficient to cause

185

Table 1   Causes of Eosinophilia

1) **Congenital**
2) **Secondary**
   a) Infections
   b) Drugs and exposure to other toxins
   c) A nonmyeloid neoplasm, including lymphoma and metastatic cancer
   d) Endocrinopathies
   e) Connective tissue disease
   f) Vasculitides
   g) Miscellaneous group of pulmonary and inflammatory diseases
3) **Primary**
   a) Idiopathic eosinophilia (IE)
      i) Hypereosinophilic syndrome (HES)
   b) Lymphoproliferative variant IE
   Clonal
   i) Molecularly characterized
      (a) Chronic myeloid leukemia (*BCR-ABL*)
      (b) PDGFRA-rearranged eosinophilic leukemia/systemic mastocytosis
      (c) PDGFRB-rearranged eosinophilic leukemia/chronic myelomonocytic leukemia
      (d) Kit-mutated systemic mastocytosis
      (e) Stem cell leukemia and lymphoma syndrome (8p11 translocations)
   ii) Molecularly not characterized
      (a) Acute leukemia associated with eosinophilia
      (b) Myelodysplastic syndrome associated with eosinophilia
      (c) Classic myeloproliferative disorder associated with eosinophilia
      (d) Nonclassic myeloproliferative disorder associated with eosinophilia

massive, life-long eosinophilia, but without apparent deleterious health effects, in transgenic mice (10).

Blood eosinophilia is considered when the absolute eosinophil count (AEC) exceeds 0.5×10^9/L to 0.7×10^9/L (11). Rarely, eosinophilia might represent an autosomal dominant congenital disorder that is relatively indolent in its clinical course (12). Acquired eosinophilia is much more prevalent and is generally classified into "secondary" and "primary" acquired eosinophilia (Table 1) (11). Secondary eosinophilia is usually associated with infection (e.g., tissue-invasive helminths or human immunodeficiency virus) eosinophilogenic drugs, allergic/atopic conditions, connective tissue disorders, vasculitis, malignancy (solid tumors or hematopoietic malignancies), or endocrinopathies (13). A working diagnosis of "primary" eosinophilia is made if the clinical scenario does not suggest secondary eosinophilia.

From a pathogenetic standpoint, the term 'primary eosinophilia' indicates a cell-intrinsic mechanism, such as clonal expansion of eosinophils through acquisition of a somatic mutation (e.g., FIP1L1-PDGFRA), whereas 'secondary eosinophilia' represents a response to exogenous type 2 cytokines (cell-extrinsic mechanism). The latter might involve dysregulated production of IL-3, IL-5, and/or GM-CSF by various cell populations (i.e., mast cells, T-lymphocytes, and eosinophils) (14–16). Early studies have revealed the requirement for functionally competent lymphocytes, particularly T-lymphocytes, for the development of an eosinophilic response in secondary eosinophilia (17–19). In particular, CD4[+] T-helper lymphocytes that are functionally polarized to produce the "type 2" cytokine profile (especially IL-4, IL-5, and IL-13), and which also promote immunoglobulin (Ig)E isotype switching and enhanced mucosal immunity, play a key role in the host response to metazoan parasites, as well as in allergic and atopic disorders (20).

PRIMARY EOSINOPHILIA

Primary eosinophilia is generally considered as being either clonal or idiopathic. The distinction between "clonal" and "idiopathic" eosinophilia is operational and not necessarily biological. In clonal eosinophilia, overt evidence of neoplastic myeloproliferation is present and includes molecular (e.g., FIP1L1-PDGFRA) or cytogenetic abnormalities (Table 2) or bone marrow histological features that are reminiscent of otherwise defined myeloid neoplasms such as myeloproliferative disorders (MPD), including systemic mastocytosis (SM) (Table 1). However, this does not necessarily imply that idiopathic eosinophilia is nonclonal in nature. In fact, X-linked clonality studies have suggested otherwise (84,85). Similarly, disease transformation into either acute myeloid leukemia (AML) or another well-defined myeloid neoplasm in some patients with otherwise typical idiopathic eosinophilia supports the notion that some patients with "idiopathic" eosinophilia do harbor an underlying clonal myeloid malignancy (37,76,86,87).

Hypereosinophilic syndrome (HES) and "lymphoproliferative variant" idiopathic eosinophilia are subcategories of idiopathic eosinophilia (Table 1). HES is characterized by the presence of a sustained (> 6 months duration) AEC of more than 1.5×10^9/L and evidence for target organ damage. The WHO definition of HES requires, in addition, the absence of aberrant phenotype or clonal T cell population (88). Therefore, an HES-like phenotype with evidence of clonal, or phenotypically aberrant, T cells, should be referred to as "lymphoproliferative variant" idiopathic eosinophilia and some of the patients with the particular presentation progress into overt lymphoma (84,89,90). The term "HES" is erroneously used by some to describe patients with chronic eosinophilic leukemia (CEL), which is an HES phenotype associated with either a molecular/cytogenetic clonal marker or excess myeloblasts in blood (> 2%) or bone marrow (> 5%) (91).

CLONAL EOSINOPHILIA

For practical purposes, clonal eosinophilia can be classified into imatinib mesylate (IM)-sensitive and IM-resistant variants. The former are characterized by

Table 2 Cytogenetic Anomalies Reported in Association with Clonal Eosinophilic Disorders

Chromosome affected	Karyotype	Molecular phenotype	Clinico-pathological presentation	References
1	t (1; 4) (q44:q12)	PDGFRA-FIPILI	HES	(21)
	+1,dic (1; 7)(p10:q10)	rearrangement	aCML	(22)
	1,der (1; 7)(q10; p10)	Abnormality of PDGFRB	CMPD	(23)
	t (1; 5) (q21; q33)	c-kit mutations	CMPD	(24)
	t (1; 5) (q21; q31)		CMML	(24)
	t (1; 5) (q21; q33)		AML Eo	(24)
	t (1; 3; 5) (p36; p21; q33)		MDS	(24)
	t (1; 5) (q23; p14)			(25)
	Trisomy 1			(26)
2	t (2; 4) (p24; q12)	N-MYC-PDGFRA	HES	(27)
	t (2; 12; 5) (q37; q22; q33)	PDGFRB mutation	MDS	(27)
3	t (3; 4) (p13; q12)		HES	(28)
	t (3; 5) (p21; q31)		aCML	(24)
	t (3; 5) (p13; q13)		HES/CEL	(29)
4	t (4; 7) (q11; q32)		aCML	(30)
	t (4; 7) (q11; p13)	FIPILI-PDGFRA	MPD	(31)
	t (4; 16) (q11/12;p13)	BCR-PDGFRA	aCML	(32)
	del 4q12		HES	(33,34)
	t(4; 22) (q12; q11)		aCML	(35)
5	t (5; 9) (q11; q34)	ABL-TK	MPD	(36)
	t (5; 11) (p15; q13)	NIN-PDGFRB	CEL	(37)
	t(5; 14) (q33; q24)	HCMOGT-1B PDGFRB	aCML	(38)
	t (5; 17) (q33; p11)	TP53BP1-PDGFRB.	JMML	(39)
	t (5; 15) (q33; q22)	TEL (ETV6)-PDGFRB	aCML	(40)
		CEV14-PDGFRB	CMML	(41
	t (5; 12) (q33; p13)	HIP1-PDGFB	AML after clonal	(42)
	t (5; 14) (q33; q32)	H4-PDGFRB	evolution	(43)
	t(5; 7) (q33; q11.2)	RAB5-PDGFRB	CML	(44)
	t (5; 10) (q33; q11.2)		aCML	(45)
	t (5; 17) (q33; p13)		CMML	(46)
	t (5; 14) (q33;q32)		CMPD	(47)
	t(5;16) (q33;q22)		AML Eo	

Table 2 (Cont.)

Chromosome affected	Karyotype	Molecular phenotype	Clinico-pathological presentation	References
6	t (6; 11) (q27; q23)		HES/ CEL	(48)
	del (6) (q24)	FOP-FGFRI	EMS	(34)
	t (6;8) (p12; q12)			(49)
7	t (7; 12) (p11; q11)		HES	(50)
	−7 Monosomy 7		MPD	(51)
			AML Eo	(52)
8	t (8; 9) (p22; p23)	FIPILI-PDGFRA	CEL	(53)
	t (8; 9) (p21; p24)	ZNF198-FGFR1	HES	(54)
	Trisomy 8	CEP110-FGFR1	CEL	(55)
	+ 8 p23	BCR-FGFR1	CEL	(56)
	+I (8p)	FGFR1	HES	(57)
	+8; +9	HERVK-FGFR1	CEL	(58)
	+8; + 21		CEL	(59)
	t (8; 13) (p12; q12)		EMS	(60)
	t (8; 9) (p12; q33)		EMS	(61)
	t (8; 22) (p11; q11)		EMS	(62)
	t (8; 17) (p11; q25)		SM	(63)
	t (8; 19) (p12; q13.3)		EMS	
9	Ins (9; 4)		HES	(64)
	(934;q12q31)			
10	Trisomy 10		HES	(34)
	t(10;11) (p14;q21)		AML Eo	(65)
11	NA	NA	NA	
12	Ins (12;8) (p11; p11p22)	FGFR1 OP2-FGFR1	EMS	(66)
13	NA	NA	NA	
14	NA	NA	NA	
15	t (15; 21) (q13; q22)		MDS	(67)
	+ 15		CEL	(68)
	+ 15;−Y		CEL	(69)
16	t(16;21) (p11;q22)	NA	AML Eo	(70)
	Inv (16) (p13q22)	CBFb-MYH11	AML M4Eo	(71)
	t(16,16) (p13;q22)		AML M4 Eo	(71)
17	Isochromosome 17		HES	(72)
	Add (17) (q25)		HES	(73)
18	NA	NA	NA	
19	NA	NA	NA	
20	Del 20 (q11; q12)		HES	(74)
21	Trisomy 21		HES	(75)
22	NA	NA	NA	
X	NA	NA	NA	

(cont.)

Table 2   (Cont.)

Chromosome affected	Karyotype	Molecular phenotype	Clinico-pathological presentation	References
Y	−Y	c-N-ras activation	HES	(76)
	Short Y		CEL	(77)
	Y, del (15q22)		HES	(78)
Complex cytogenetics	XYY, t (3;5), +8,+mar	NA	HES	(79)
	4q+,-5,+mar	NA	CMPD	(80)
	der(7);-3,-11,-13,-15	NA	CEL	(81)
	-21,+14,+11;del (5)q31	NA	CEL	(82)
	+8,+19,+2q,-6q	NA	CEL with AT	(83)

Reproduced by permission from Tefferi, Patnaik, and Pardanani (13).
Abbreviations: HES, hypereosinophilic syndrome; CMPD, chronic myeloproliferative disorder; CEL, chronic eosinophilic leukemia; MDS myelodysplastic syndrome; EMS, eosinophilic mastocytosis; MS, mastocytosis; CML, chronic myelogenous leukemia; AML Eo, acute eosinophilic leukemia; CMML, chronic myelomonocytic leukemia; JMML, juvenile myelomonocytic leukemia; NA, data not available; AT, acute transformation.

mutations involving platelet-derived growth factor receptors (PDGFR) α (*PDGFRA* located on chromosome 4q12) and β (*PDGFRB* located on chromosome 5q31–q32) (Table 3). IM-resistant clonal eosinophilia includes both stem cell leukemia lymphoma (SCLL), which is invariably associated with various chromosomal translocations involving fibroblast growth factor receptor 1 (*FGFR1*) gene, and many other myeloid neoplasms that are molecularly not characterized (Table 1). Treatment in the latter group of disorders is dictated by the underlying myeloid neoplasm. In this section, we will discuss the three molecularly characterized clonal eosinophilias: PDGFRA-, PDGFRB-, and FGFR1-rearranged eosinophilic disorders.

PDGFRA-Rearranged Clonal Eosinophilia

Instigated by the serendipitous observation of IM-induced complete hematological remission seen in some patients with both an "HES" phenotype as well as an "SM" phenotype associated with eosinophilia (92,93), in 2003 Cools et al. cloned the FIP1L1-PDGFRA oncogene in such IM-sensitive patients with clonal eosinophilia (21). FIP1L1-PDGFRA is cytogenetically occult and results from an approximately 800 kb interstitial deletion within 4q12 that fuses the 5′ portion of *FIP1L1* to the 3′ portion of *PDGFRA* (21). Molecular studies showed that the breakpoint in *FIP1L1* is relatively promiscuous, while the *PDGFRA* breakpoint is restricted to exon 12, which encodes part of the protein-protein interaction module

Table 3 Mutations of Putative Pathogenetic Relevance in Clonal Eosinophilia

PDGFRA mutation	Phenotype	PDGFRB mutation	Phenotype	FGFR1 mutation	Phenotype
FIP1L1-PDGFRA del(14q12)	CEL-SM	**ETV6-PDGFRB** t(5;12)(q33;p13)	CMML-eos	**ZNF 198-FGFR1** t(8;13)(p11;q12)	SCLL
BCR-PDGFRA t(4;22)(q12;q11)	CEL, UMPD	**RABAPTIN-5-PDGFRB** t(5;17)(q33;p13)	CMML	**FOP-FGFR1** t(6;8)(p27;p11)	SCLL
		HCMOGT-1-PDGFRB t(5;17)(q33;p11.2)	JMML-eos		
KIF5B-PDGFRA t(4;10)(q12;p11)	CEL	**CEV14-PDGFRB** t(5;14)(q33;q32)	AML-eos	**FGFR1 OP2-PDGFRA** ins(12;8)(p11;p11p22)	SCLL
		NIN-PDGFRB t(5;14)(q33;q24)	UMPD-eos		
		KIAA1509-PDGFRB t(5;14)(q31;q32)	CMML-eos		
CDK5RAP2-PDGFRA ins(9;4)(q33;q12q25)	CEL	**TP53BP1-PDGFRB** t(5;15)(q33;q22)	UMPD-eos	**TIF1-FGFR1** t(7;8)(q34;p11)	SCLL
		PDE4DIP-PDGFRB t(1;5)(q23;q33)	UMPD-eos	**MYO18 A-FGFR1** t(8;17)(p11;q23)	SCLL
		HIP1-PDGFRB t(5;7)(q33;q11.2)	CMML-eos	**HERV-K-FGFR1** t(8;19)(p12;q13.3)	SCLL
		H4-PDGFRB t(5;10)(q33;q22)	UMPD	**BCR-FGFR1** t(8;22)(p11;q11)	aCML
				CEP110-FGFR1 t(8;9)(p12;q33)	SCLL

Abbreviations: PV, polycythemia vera; ET, essential thrombocythemia; PMF, primary myelofibrosis; AML, acute myeloid leukemia; UMPD, unclassified MPD; CEL-SM, chronic eosinophilic leukemia associated with systemic mastocytosis; CMML, chronic myelomonocytic leukemia; JMML, juvenile myelomonocytic leukemia; SCLL, stem cell leukemia-lymphoma syndrome.

with two fully conserved tryptophan (WW domain)-containing juxta-membrane (JM) region (21,33). The mutation results in constitutive activation of PDGFRA, thus providing a molecular explanation for the remarkable efficacy of IM in this disorder (21,92,94,95). Subsequent studies have demonstrated the stem cell origin of the FIP1L1-PDGFRA (96,97), and functional studies have demonstrated transforming properties of the mutation in cell lines and its ability to induce MPD-like phenotype in mice (98,99). Unlike most tyrosine kinase fusion oncogenes, the *FIP1L1*-encoded sequences are dispensable for cell transformation and there is no requirement for a dimerization motif in FIP1L1-PDGFRA. Instead, disruption of the autoinhibitory JM motif appears to be the basis for constitutive activation of PDGFRA kinase activity (100).

PDGFRA can also be activated by chromosomal translocations (Table 3); examples include KIF5B-PDGFRA, t(4:10)(q12;p11) (101), BCR-PDGFRA, t(4;22)(q12;q11) (35), and CDK5RAP2-PDGFRA, ins(9;4)(q33;q12q25) (102). Molecular studies on 2 patients, presenting with atypical chronic myelogenous leukemia (aCML) with eosinophilia, revealed an in-frame breakpoint cluster region (BCR*)* (breakpoints in intron 7 and exon 12)-to-PDGFRA (breakpoints in exon 12) fusion mRNA. Subsequently, another case with aCML evolving into pre-B acute lymphoblastic leukemia, with the BCR (exon 1)-to-PDGFRA (exon 13) fusion, was described and the patient achieved a complete hematological remission with IM treatment (103). More recently, Safley et al. reported another IM-sensitive aCML associated with eosinophilia, with the BCR (exon 17)-to-PDGFRA (exon 12) fusion (104). The PDGFRA breakpoints in most of these cases are tightly clustered in the JM region, pointing again to a key regulatory role for this domain.

The prevalence of FIP1L1-PDGFRA is variable and largely reflects the characteristics of the particular patient population screened. Reported mutational frequency in relatively large studies is approximately 10–15% in cohorts with unexplained eosinophilia of greater than 1.5×10^9/L (105–107) in general, and mutational frequency is higher in patients with myeloproliferative features (i.e., splenomegaly, bone marrow fibrosis, etc.) (108). In routine clinical practice, prevalence of the mutation might be as low as approximately 4% (106). FIP1L1-PDGFRA–positive patients with clonal eosinophilia have been labeled as myelo-proliferative variant of hypereosinophilic syndrome by some (109,110), and SM with associated eosinophilia (SM-CEL) by others (108,111). In our experience, 14 of 15 FIP1L1-PDGFRA–positive patients (93%) were identified as SM-CEL (one patient had CEL by WHO criteria) (106). SM-CEL indicates the presence of phenotypically and morphologically aberrant mast cells in almost all affected patients and a clinical presentation consistent with WHO-defined SM in some, including elevated serum tryptase in all affected patients (108). Consistent with this observation, subsequent studies were able to localize the mutation in mast cells as well as in other myeloid and lymphoid lineage cells (96). However, recent studies suggest that the mutation might be detected even in cases of AML, T cell lymphoma, or lymphomatoid papulosis, when associated with eosinophilia (107,

112). Similar to what has been seen with FIP1L1-PDGFRA–positive SM-CEL, the patients in the latter study responded well to IM. Therefore, the histologic distinction among FIP1L1-PDGFRA–positive cases with eosinophilia might be moot because of the uniform and predicted response to IM, whereas the particular observations underscore the importance of screening for FIP1L1-PDGFRA in all cases of primary eosinophilia.

IM at 100 mg/day is the treatment of choice for FIP1L1-PDGFRA–positive SM-CEL or other clonal eosinophilia and induces a complete hematologic and molecular remission in almost all affected patients (107,108). Therefore, it is of utmost therapeutic relevance to perform peripheral blood screening for FIP1L1-PDGFRA, using either FISH or RT-PCR, in all patients with primary eosinophilia (107). In mutation-positive patients, one can assess minimal residual disease by using quantitative molecular analysis (107). FIP1L1-PDGFRA mutation (T674I) that is homologous to the resistance-inducing, "gatekeeper" T315I mutation in *BCR-ABL* has been described (21,113,114) and in vitro salvage with other kinase inhibitors, including PKC412 (98) and sorafenib (115), has been demonstrated, whereas such activity has not been conclusively shown for nilotinib (116,117). Sorafenib has also been shown to overcome resistance from *ETV6-PDGFRB* mutant (118).

PDGFRB-Rearranged Eosinophilia

PDGFRB rearrangement was first characterized and published in 1994, where fusion of the tyrosine kinase encoding region of *PDGFRB* to the *ets*-like gene, *ETV6* (previously known as *TEL*) [ETV6-PDGFRB, t(5;12)(q33;p13)] was demonstrated in a patient with chronic myelomonocytic leukemia (CMML) (41). The fusion protein was transforming to cell lines and resulted in constitutive activation of PDGFRB signaling (119). Since then, several other PDGFRB fusion transcripts with similar and other (e.g., unclassified MPD associated with eosinophilia, CEL, aCML) disease phenotypes have been described (Table 3) (38–40,42,43,45,46,120,121). In general, PDGFRB is fused to the N-terminal segment of a partner protein that encodes for one or more oligomerization domains (34,122). PDGFRB mutations have been shown to induce cell line transformation (43,45,121) and MPD-like disease in mice (45). Similar to PDGFRA-rearranged cases, IM therapy, although usually employed at 400 mg/day, produces complete hematological remission in PDGFRB-rearranged clonal eosinophilia (38,40,46,120,123,124). In a recent study of 12 patients with PDGFRB-rearranged clonal eosinophilia, IM therapy was administered for a median of 47 months; 11 patients achieved hematological remission with 10 achieving complete cytogenetic remission as well (125). All 12 patients displayed prominent eosinophilia (i.e., AEC $> 1.5 \times 10^9$/L) at diagnosis. Molecular remission was demonstrated in the majority of responding patients. Initial IM doses in the particular study ranged from 200 to 800 mg/day with no difference in response patterns. The authors of the particular study obtained follow-up information from eight additional cases in the literature, treated with daily IM 200–400 mg/day, and documented durable remissions in 6 patients (125).

It is important to recognize that PDGFRB translocations are extremely rare. For example, a Mayo Clinic review of 56709 cytogenetic studies identified only 25 cases of t(5;12) (0.04%). In addition, in another cohort of 213 CMML patients, of which 205 had karyotype analysis, none were found to carry t(5;12), even though 34% had other cytogenetic abnormalities (126). Of equal importance is the fact that the mere finding of a 5q33-involving chromosomal translocation in patients with a myeloid disorder does not necessarily indicate that PDGFRB is involved (24). Conversely, involvement of 5q31 does not exclude PDGFRB involvement given that translocations may be complex at the molecular level. Hence, molecular studies are essential in patients with 5q31–33 translocations to confirm or exclude PDGFRB rearrangement, given the therapeutic relevance of such a finding.

FGFR1-Rearranged Eosinophilic Disorder

FGFR1 gene is located on chromosome 8p11 and is involved in various chromosomal translocations (Table 3) (49,59,61–63,66,127–135) that are usually associated with a clinical phenotype with features of both an aggressive, eosinophilia-associated myeloproliferative disorder and T-cell lymphoblastic lymphoma (136). The composite syndrome is known as either the 8p11 myeloproliferative syndrome (EMS) or SCLL syndrome and is molecularly characterized by fusion of various 5′ partner genes to the 3′ part of *FGFR1* making it constitutively active. The mutation is present in both myeloid and lymphoid lineage cells (59,127–130). Some of the FGFR1 fusion mutants have been shown to transform cell lines (61,137–139) and induce SCLL-(140) or CML-like (139) disease in mice, depending on the specific *FGFR1* partner gene; *ZNF198* or *BCR*, respectively (139). Consistent with this laboratory observation, some patients with BCR-FGFR1 mutation manifest a more indolent CML-like disease (61). These data implicate different signaling pathways originating from both the FGFR1 kinase as well as the fusion partner.

Clinically, EMS/SCLL runs a biphasic course—a relatively short chronic phase, followed by transformation into acute leukemia with a poor overall prognosis. At present, drug therapy is ineffective and allogeneic stem cell transplantation should be considered as soon as the particular diagnosis is established. There is an ongoing interest in the use of FGFR1-targeting small-molecule kinase inhibitors based on preliminary data regarding in vitro activity (141).

IDIOPATHIC EOSINOPHILIA

Hypereosinophilic Syndrome

HES is a subset of idiopathic eosinophilia that fulfills the conventional, although scientifically questionable, criteria of a persistent (> 6 months) and moderate to severe increase in AEC (> 1.5×10^9/L) associated with target organ damage (142). We believe both the assignment of the specific AEC threshold level and definition of "organ damage" are arbitrary and we prefer the general term of "idiopathic" eosinophilia using the threshold of 600×10^9/L and further stratify patients with or without "overt" organ manifestation. For now, we have arbitrarily assigned the term "pre-HES" for idiopathic eosinophilia that does not fulfill the conventional criteria for HES.

Over 90% of patients with HES are males, a scenario that is similar to the *PDGFR*-rearranged clonal eosinophilias (142,143). Clinical manifestations in HES include pruritus, urticaria, angioedema, erythematous papules, valvular disease, mural thrombi, cardiomyopathy, sensorimotor polyneuropathies, mononeuritis multiplex, isolated central nervous system vasculitis, optic neuritis, acute transverse myelitis, pulmonary infiltrates, pleural effusion, hepatosplenomegaly, gastroenteritis, sclerosing cholangitis, cytopenias, bone marrow fibrosis, and thrombotic microangiopathy (144–151). However, the major and most frequent tissue targets are the heart, the nervous system, the skin, the upper and lower respiratory tract, and the gastrointestinal system. It should also be noted that thromboembolic disease involving the cardiac chambers (152) as well as both venous (153) and arterial (154) vessels are not infrequent. HES is a potentially fatal disease, with less than 50% of the patients reporting a 10-year survival (150).

Initial evaluation of an "HES" case should include bone marrow examination with both cytogenetic and molecular (i.e., FISH or RT-PCR for FIP1L1-PDGFRA) studies. A diagnosis of either HES or idiopathic eosinophilia is made only after all causes of clonal eosinophilia are excluded. Also, in all cases, T-cell immunophenotyping and T-cell receptor antigen gene rearrangement analysis should be performed and if either clonal or immunophenotypically aberrant T-cells are discovered, a diagnosis of lymphoproliferative variant idiopathic eosinophilia is preferred. Initial evaluation should also include echocardiogram, chest x-ray, pulmonary function tests, and measurement of serum troponin levels. Increased level of serum cardiac troponin has been shown to correlate with the presence of cardiomyopathy in HES and recent studies have suggested a predictive role for drug-induced cardiogenic shock during treatment with IM (155,156).

Management of idiopathic eosinophilia, including HES, starts with deciding whether or not a particular patient requires specific therapy. In general, treatment is not indicated in the asymptomatic patient with normal troponin and no evidence of organ damage. Some of these patients might display severe eosinophilia (AEC $> 5 \times 10^9$/L), but there is no evidence that treatment based simply on AEC is beneficial to the patient. We currently prefer to closely monitor rather than to treat asymptomatic patients, regardless of the degree of eosinophilia. Accordingly, we recommend measurement of serum troponin level every 3–6 months and an echocardiogram every 6–12 months. The first-line drug of choice for symptomatic patients is prednisone (starting dose of 1 mg/kg/day). An overall response rate of more than 70% to prednisone is expected, but relapse is frequent with steroid taper (157). The second-line drug of choice at the moment is interferon alpha (IFN-α) (starting dose 3 million units three-times-a-week) (158–161). Patients intolerant to IFN-α can be treated with hydroxyurea instead (starting dose

500 mg twice-a-day) (157). Such therapy is however not associated with impressive results but benefits a substantial minority of corticosteroid-dependent patients. In true HES (i.e., FIP1L1/PDGFRA–negative), IM therapy is unlikely to produce durable complete remissions and is not recommended as either first- or second-line therapy (108). However, partial and occasionally complete remissions are sometimes seen and empiric treatment trial with IM 400 mg/day is reasonable in cases that are refractory to both corticosteroids and IFN-α (21,108). During IM therapy of HES, it is important to recognize the possibility of drug-induced acute cardiac shock (156,162). The specific complication is managed by the concomitant use of systemic corticosteroid therapy, for 1–2 weeks, which is recommended in the presence of either elevated serum troponin level or an abnormal echocardiogram (156).

We currently prefer monoclonal antibody therapy for HES that is both refractory to usual therapy and life-threatening. There are currently two drugs in this regard; mepolizumab, which targets IL-5 and alemtuzumab, which targets the CD52 antigen that is expressed by eosinophils but not neutrophils. Both are effective in controlling blood eosinophilia as well as disease symptoms, at least in the short term. Recommended starting doses are 30 mg s.c. every week for alemtuzumab (163,164) and monthly 1 mg/kg i.v. infusion for mepolizumab (165–168). Other therapies used for refractory HES include myeloablative and nonmyeloablative ASCT (169–171), chlorambucil (148), etoposide (172), cyclosporine (173), vincristine alone (57) or in combination with mercaptopurine (174), cladribine alone (175) or in combination with cytarabine (175,176), and combination of cytarabine and 6-thioguanine (177).

Lymphoproliferative Variant Idiopathic Eosinophilia

T cells were first implicated as being pathogenetically contributory in "HES" when CD4$^+$ T-cell clones secreting "eosinophil colony-stimulating factor(s)" were identified in a patient with unexplained eosinophilia (178). Subsequently, another study demonstrated the presence, in a patient with "HES," of a T-cell clone with aberrant phenotype (CD4$^+$CD3$^-$) that spontaneously produced IL-5 and IL-4, but not IL-2 and interferon-gamma (IFN-γ) (179). More recently, Simon et al. reported that 16 of 60 (~27%) patients with idiopathic eosinophilia had circulating T-cells with a variably abnormal immunophenotype (11 were CD4$^+$8$^-$, 3 CD4$^-$8$^+$, and 2 CD4$^-$8$^-$, most with aberrancies of other T-cell markers) (89). Of these, 8 (50%) patients exhibited clonal rearrangements of the T-cell receptor (TCR), and the aberrant T-cells were shown to produce significant amounts of IL-5 in vitro. The prevalence of a circulating T-cell clone in patients with idiopathic eosinophilia is unknown, but may be as high as approximately 30% (33).

In a study of 99 patients with "idiopathic" eosinophilia, from my institution, 8 patients (~8%) were found to carry an occult T-cell clone, based on abnormal T-cell immunophenotype and/or clonal TCR gene rearrangements, in peripheral blood, bone marrow, skin, and/or lymph node (180). Most patients had cutaneous involvement manifest as a dermal and epidermal T-cell infiltrate with intense eosinophilia (7 of 8 patients), often with elevated serum IgE level (5 of 7 patients), and three patients had organopathy from visceral disease (interstitial nephritis, pneumonia, and sinusitis). In 2 patients, a prolonged eosinophilic prodrome (3 and > 8 years) evolved to a cutaneous peripheral T-cell lymphoma.

In essence, this entity (described as "lymphoproliferative variant" of HES (L-HES) by some (181) is poorly understood, and is thought to represent a premalignant T-cell clonal disorder of variable severity with predominantly cutaneous involvement, and with the potential for progression to a full-blown T-cell malignancy in a proportion of cases. Reaching a diagnosis is frequently challenging and requires a high-index of suspicion supported by appropriate and comprehensive molecular testing of multiple tissue specimens, as well as close collaboration between the specialties (i.e., dermatology, dermatopathology, hematology, and hematopathology). Screening for clonal T-cells is based on immunophenotyping of circulating lymphocytes as well as analysis for clonal TCR rearrangements with southern blot and/or PCR. Detection of increased levels of IgE and/or IL-5 in the serum is helpful in these cases, but neither test is sensitive or specific for the diagnosis of L-HES (181). Other specialized studies, including FACS-sorting of aberrant lymphocytes with TCR gene rearrangement and cytogenetic analyses on sorted lymphocytes, or analysis of secreted cytokine profile, either within single cells (by flow cytometry) or in supernatants of cultured lymphocytes, may only be available in reference laboratories.

Treatment for lymphoproliferative variant idiopathic eosinophilia is based on anecdotal experience. In the aforementioned study from our institution, 2 patients with significant disease morbidity, including adenopathy, renal insufficiency, lung infiltrates, and dermatitis, received treatment with single-agent, low-dose oral cyclophosphamide or methotrexate and achieved complete clinical remission within 3 months. Although both patients continued to enjoy a durable remission off therapy at last follow-up (after 1 and 5 years of active treatment), eradication of the T-cell clone has not been documented by molecular studies. Two patients required only symptom control as therapy, whereas 2 other patients were managed primarily with variable doses of prednisone. Of importance, 2 patients were treated with IM and neither responded to the drug. It should be noted that lymphoproliferative variant idiopathic eosinophilia does not display FIP1L1-PDGFRA. Other therapeutic approaches of unproven benefit include cyclosporine that might interfere with synthesis and/or activity of eosinophilopoietic cytokines (e.g., IL-5). Although use of humanized monoclonal anti–IL-5 antibodies (e.g., mepolizumab) is an option, the response to such therapy is generally transient (167). Other steroid-sparing options include the use of IFN-α, although this is often poorly tolerated.

CONCLUDING REMARKS

It is no longer acceptable to misuse the term "HES," which should be reserved for cases that do not display any evidence of either clonal myelopoiesis (i.e., based on molecular, cytogenetic, or histological markers) or clonal or phenotypically aberrant T-cells. The appropriate terms for the latter two entities are "clonal eosinophilia" and "lymphoproliferative variant idiopathic eosinophilia." This contention is consistent with the current WHO criteria for the diagnosis of HES. Along these lines, IM therapy is usually ineffective in the treatment of true HES, as defined by the WHO criteria, and should not be offered as first-line treatment in such cases. However, one should screen for the presence of FIP1L1-PDGFRA during the initial evaluation of all cases of primary eosinophilia; its presence mandates treatment with IM. It is of practical relevance to recognize that FIP1L1-PDGFRA does not occur in the absence of prominent blood eosinophilia. In other words, one should not perform FIP1L1-PDGFRA mutation screening in the evaluation of either mild eosinophilia or SM that is not associated with blood eosinophilia. The pathogenesis of true HES remains elusive at the present time. In this regard, known mechanisms of disease in clonal eosinophilia should provide guidance for focused research. In the meantime, preliminary information from the therapeutic use of both alemtuzumab and mepolizumab are encouraging and offer a much-needed option for salvage therapy in refractory HES, as well as some cases of clonal eosinophilia. However, the long-term effects of such a therapy are not known and patients receiving such therapy should be followed closely.

REFERENCES

1. Denburg JA, Telizyn S, Messner H, et al. Heterogeneity of human peripheral blood eosinophil-type colonies: evidence for a common basophil-eosinophil progenitor. Blood 1985;66:312–318.
2. Boyce JA, Friend D, Matsumoto R, et al. Differentiation in vitro of hybrid eosinophil/basophil granulocytes: autocrine function of an eosinophil developmental intermediate. J Exp Med 1995;182:49–57.
3. Iwasaki H, Mizuno S, Mayfield R, et al. Identification of eosinophil lineage-committed progenitors in the murine bone marrow. J Exp Med 2005;201:1891–1897.
4. McNagny K, Graf T. Making eosinophils through subtle shifts in transcription factor expression. J Exp Med 2002;195:F43–F47.
5. Hirasawa R, Shimizu R, Takahashi S, et al. Essential and instructive roles of GATA factors in eosinophil development. J Exp Med 2002;195:1379–1386.
6. Yu C, Cantor AB, Yang H, et al. Targeted deletion of a high-affinity GATA-binding site in the GATA-1 promoter leads to selective loss of the eosinophil lineage in vivo. J Exp Med 2002;195:1387–1395.
7. Sanderson CJ. Interleukin-5, eosinophils, and disease. Blood 1992;79:3101–3109.
8. Clutterbuck EJ, Hirst EM, Sanderson CJ. Human interleukin-5 (IL-5) regulates the production of eosinophils in human bone marrow cultures: comparison and interaction with IL-1, IL-3, IL-6, and GMCSF. Blood 1989;73:1504–1512.
9. Collins PD, Marleau S, Griffiths-Johnson DA, et al. Cooperation between interleukin-5 and the chemokine eotaxin to induce eosinophil accumulation in vivo. J Exp Med 1995;182:1169–1174.

10. Dent LA, Strath M, Mellor AL, et al. Eosinophilia in transgenic mice expressing interleukin 5. J Exp Med 1990;172:1425–1431.
11. Brigden M, Graydon C. Eosinophilia detected by automated blood cell counting in ambulatory North American outpatients. Incidence and clinical significance. Arch Pathol Lab Med 1997;121:963–967.
12. Klion AD, Law MA, Riemenschneider W, et al. Familial eosinophilia: a benign disorder? Blood 2004;103:4050–4055.
13. Tefferi A, Patnaik MM, Pardanani A. Eosinophilia: secondary, clonal, and idiopathic. Br J Haematol 2006;133:468–492.
14. Strath M, Sanderson CJ. Detection of eosinophil differentiation factor and its relationship to eosinophilia in Mesocestoides corti-infected mice. Exp Hematol 1986;14:16–20.
15. Yamaguchi Y, Matsui T, Kasahara T, et al. In vivo changes of hemopoietic progenitors and the expression of the interleukin 5 gene in eosinophilic mice infected with Toxocara canis. Exp Hematol 1990;18:1152–1157.
16. Hamid Q, Azzawi M, Ying S, et al. Expression of mRNA for interleukin-5 in mucosal bronchial biopsies from asthma. J Clin Invest 1991;87:1541–1546.
17. Basten A, Beeson PB. Mechanism of eosinophilia. II. Role of the lymphocyte. J Exp Med 1970;131:1288–1305.
18. Nielsen K, Fogh L, Andersen S. Eosinophil response to migrating Ascaris suum larvae in normal and congenitally thymus-less mice. Acta Pathol Microbiol Scand [B] Microbiol Immunol 1974;82:919–920.
19. Hsu CK, Hsu SH, Whitney RA, Jr., et al. Immunopathology of schistosomiasis in athymic mice. Nature 1976;262:397–399.
20. Romagnani S. Th1 and Th2 in human diseases. Clin Immunol Immunopathol 1996;80:225–235.
21. Cools J, DeAngelo DJ, Gotlib J, et al. A tyrosine kinase created by fusion of the PDGFRA and FIP1L1 genes as a therapeutic target of imatinib in idiopathic hypercosinophilic syndrome. N Engl J Med 2003;348:1201–1214.
22. Forrest DL, Horsman DE, Jensen CL, et al. Myelodysplastic syndrome with hyper-eosinophilia and a nonrandom chromosomal abnormality dic(1;7): confirmation of eosinophil clonal involvement by fluorescence in situ hybridization. Cancer Genet Cytogenet 1998;107:65–68.
23. Park CY, Chung CH, Park YJ. Chronic eosinophilic leukemia with 46,XY,1,der(1;7)(q10;p10) translocation. Ann Hematol 2004;83:547–548.
24. Baxter EJ, Kulkarni S, Vizmanos JL, et al. Novel translocations that disrupt the platelet-derived growth factor receptor beta (PDGFRB) gene in BCR-ABL–negative chronic myeloproliferative disorders. Br J Haematol 2003;120:251–256.
25. Zermati Y, De Sepulveda P, Feger F, et al. Effect of tyrosine kinase inhibitor STI571 on the kinase activity of wild-type and various mutated c-kit receptors found in mast cell neoplasms. Oncogene 2003;22:660–664.
26. Harrington DS, Peterson C, Ness M, et al. Acute myelogenous leukemia with eosinophilic differentiation and trisomy-1. Am J Clin Pathol 1988;90:464–469.
27. Musto P, Falcone A, Sanpaolo G, et al. Heterogeneity of response to imatinib-mesylate (Glivec) in patients with hypereosinophilic syndrome: implications for dosing and pathogenesis. Leuk Lymphoma 2004;45:1219–1222.

28. Myint H, Chacko J, Mould S, et al. Karyotypic evolution in a granulocytic sarcoma developing in a myeloproliferative disorder with a novel (3;4) translocation. Br J Haematol 1995;90:462–464.

29. Shanske AL, Kalman A, Grunwald H. A myeloproliferative disorder with eosinophilia associated with a unique translocation (3;5). Br J Haematol 1996;95: 524–526.

30. Duell T, Mittermuller J, Schmetzer HM, et al. Chronic myeloid leukemia associated hypereosinophilic syndrome with a clonal t(4;7)(q11;q32). Cancer Genet Cytogenet 1997;94:91–94.

31. Schoffski P, Ganser A, Pascheberg U, et al. Complete haematological and cytogenetic response to interferon alpha-2a of a myeloproliferative disorder with eosinophilia associated with a unique t(4;7) aberration. Ann Hematol 2000;79:95–98.

32. Hild F, Fonatsch C. Cytogenetic peculiarities in chronic myelogenous leukemia. Cancer Genet Cytogenet 1990;47:197–217.

33. Roche-Lestienne C, Lepers S, Soenen-Cornu V, et al. Molecular characterization of the idiopathic hypereosinophilic syndrome (HES) in 35 French patients with normal conventional cytogenetics. Leukemia 2005;19:792–798.

34. Gotlib J. Molecular classification and pathogenesis of eosinophilic disorders: 2005 update. Acta Haematol 2005;114:7–25.

35. Baxter EJ, Hochhaus A, Bolufer P, et al. The t(4;22)(q12;q11) in atypical chronic myeloid leukaemia fuses BCR to PDGFRA. Hum Mol Genet 2002;11:1391–1397.

36. Bakhshi S, Hamre M, Mohamed AN, et al. t(5;9)(q11;q34): A novel familial transloca-tion involving Abelson oncogene and association with hypereosinophilia. J Pediatr Hematol Oncol 2003;25:82–84.

37. Yoo TJ, Orman SV, Patil SR, et al. Evolution to eosinophilic leukemia with a t(5:11) translocation in a patient with idiopathic hypereosinophilic syndrome. Cancer Genet Cytogenet 1984;11:389–384.

38. Vizmanos JL, Novo FJ, Roman JP, et al. NIN, a gene encoding a CEP110-like centrosomal protein, is fused to PDGFRB in a patient with a t(5;14)(q33;q24) and an imatinib-responsive myeloproliferative disorder. Cancer Res 2004;64: 2673–2676.

39. Morerio C, Acquila M, Rosanda C, et al. HCMOGT-1 is a novel fusion partner to PDGFRB in juvenile myelomonocytic leukemia with t(5;17)(q33;p11.2). Cancer Res 2004;64:2649–2651.

40. Grand FH, Burgstaller S, Kuhr T, et al. p53-binding protein 1 is fused to the platelet-derived growth factor receptor beta in a patient with a t(5;15)(q33;q22) and an imatinib-responsive eosinophilic myeloproliferative disorder. Cancer Res 2004;64:7216–7219.

41. Golub TR, Barker GF, Lovett M, et al. Fusion of PDGF receptor beta to a novel ets-like gene, tel, in chronic myelomonocytic leukemia with t(5;12) chromosomal translocation. Cell 1994;77:307–316.

42. Abe A, Emi N, Tanimoto M, et al. Fusion of the platelet-derived growth factor receptor beta to a novel gene CEV14 in acute myelogenous leukemia after clonal evolution. Blood 1997;90:4271–4277.

43. Ross TS, Bernard OA, Berger R, et al. Fusion of Huntingtin interacting protein 1 to platelet-derived growth factor beta receptor (PDGFbetaR) in chronic myelomono-cytic leukemia with t(5;7)(q33;q11.2). Blood 1998;91:4419–4426.

44. Kulkarni S, Heath C, Parker S, et al. Fusion of H4/D10S170 to the platelet-derived growth factor receptor beta in BCR-ABL–negative myeloproliferative disorders with a t(5;10)(q33;q21). Cancer Res 2000;60:3592–3598.
45. Magnusson MK, Meade KE, Brown KE, et al. Rabaptin-5 is a novel fusion partner to platelet-derived growth factor beta receptor in chronic myelomonocytic leukemia. Blood 2001;98:2518–2525.
46. Levine RL, Wadleigh M, Sternberg DW, et al. KIAA1509 is a novel PDGFRB fusion partner in imatinib-responsive myeloproliferative disease associated with a t(5;14)(q33;q32). Leukemia 2005;19:27–30.
47. Bhambhani K, Inoue S, Tyrkus M, et al. Acute myelomonocytic leukemia type M4 with bone marrow eosinophilia and t(5;16)(q33;q22). Cancer Genet Cytogenet 1986;20:187–188.
48. Suzuki S, Chiba K, Toyoshima N, et al. Chronic eosinophilic leukemia with t(6;11)(q27;q23) translocation. Ann Hematol 2001;80:553–556.
49. Popovici C, Zhang B, Gregoire MJ, et al. The t(6;8)(q27;p11) translocation in a stem cell myeloproliferative disorder fuses a novel gene, FOP, to fibroblast growth factor receptor 1. Blood 1999;93:1381–1389.
50. da Silva MA, Heerema N, Schwenk GR, Jr., et al. Evidence for the clonal nature of hypereosinophilic syndrome. Cancer Genet Cytogenet 1988;32:109–115.
51. Humphrey MJ, Hutter, Tom WW. Hypereosinophilia in a monosomy 7 myeloproliferative disorder in childhood. Am J Hematol 1981;11:107–110.
52. Song HS PS. A case of monosomy-7 eosinophilic leukemia and neurofibromatosis terminated with disseminated crytpococcosis. Korean J Intern Med 1987;2:131–134.
53. Vandenberghe P, Wlodarska I, Michaux L, et al. Clinical and molecular features of FIP1L1-PDFGRA (+) chronic eosinophilic leukemias. Leukemia 2004;18:734–742.
54. Weinfeld A, Westin J, Swolin B. Ph1-negative eosinophilic leukaemia with trisomy 8. Case report and review of cytogenetic studies. Scand J Haematol 1977;18:413–420.
55. Kook H CD, Noh H-Y. Chronic eosinophilic leukemia with unique chromosomal abnormality, add 8p23, in a 14-month girl: Treatment with imatinib mesylate (abstract). Blood 2002;100:344b.
56. Egesten A, Hagerstrand I, Kristoffersson U, et al. Hypereosinophilic syndrome in a child mosaic for a congenital triplication of the short arm of chromosome 8. Br J Haematol 1997;96:369–373.
57. Spry CJ. The hypereosinophilic syndrome: clinical features, laboratory findings, and treatment. Allergy 1982;37:539–551.
58. Kueck BD, Smith RE, Parkin J, et al. Eosinophilic leukemia: a myeloproliferative disorder distinct from the hypereosinophilic syndrome. Hematol Pathol 1991;5:195–205.
59. Popovici C, Adelaide J, Ollendorff V, et al. Fibroblast growth factor receptor 1 is fused to FIM in stem-cell myeloproliferative disorder with t(8;13). Proc Natl Acad Sci U S A 1998;95:5712–5717.
60. Guasch G, Mack GJ, Popovici C, et al. FGFR1 is fused to the centrosome-associated protein CEP110 in the 8p12 stem cell myeloproliferative disorder with t(8;9)(p12;q33). Blood 2000;95:1788–1796.

61. Demiroglu A, Steer EJ, Heath C, et al. The t(8;22) in chronic myeloid leukemia fuses BCR to FGFR1: transforming activity and specific inhibition of FGFR1 fusion proteins. Blood 2001;98:3778–3783.

62. Sohal J, Chase A, Mould S, et al. Identification of four new translocations involving FGFR1 in myeloid disorders. Genes Chrom Cancer 2001;32:155–163.

63. Guasch G, Popovici C, Mugneret F, et al. Endogenous retroviral sequence is fused to FGFR1 kinase in the 8p12 stem-cell myeloproliferative disorder with t(8;19)(p12;q13.3). Blood 2003;101:286–288.

64. Schoch C, Schnittger S, Bursch S, et al. Comparison of chromosome banding analysis, interphase- and hypermetaphase-FISH, qualitative and quantitative PCR for diagnosis, and for follow-up in chronic myeloid leukemia: a study on 350 cases. Leukemia 2002;16:53–59.

65. Broustet A, Bernard P, Dachary D, et al. Acute eosinophilic leukemia with a translocation (10p+;11q-). Cancer Genet Cytogenet 1986;21:327–333.

66. Grand EK, Grand FH, Chase AJ, et al. Identification of a novel gene, FGFR1 OP2, fused to FGFR1 in 8p11 myeloproliferative syndrome. Genes Chromosomes Cancer 2004;40:78–83.

67. Brito-Babapulle F. Clonal eosinophilic disorders and the hypereosinophilic syndrome. Blood Rev 1997;11:129–145.

68. Oliver JW, Deol I, Morgan DL, et al. Chronic eosinophilic leukemia and hypereosinophilic syndromes. Proposal for classification, literature review, and report of a case with a unique chromosomal abnormality. Cancer Genet Cytogenet 1998;107:111–117.

69. Weide R, Rieder H, Mehraein Y, et al. Chronic eosinophilic leukaemia (CEL): a distinct myeloproliferative disease. Br J Haematol 1997;96:117–123.

70. Mecucci C, Bosly A, Michaux JL, et al. Acute nonlymphoblastic leukemia with bone marrow eosinophilia and structural anomaly of chromosome 16. Cancer Genet Cytogenet 1985;17:359–363.

71. Le Beau MM, Larson RA, Bitter MA, et al. Association of an inversion of chromosome 16 with abnormal marrow eosinophils in acute myelomonocytic leukemia. A unique cytogenetic-clinicopathological association. N Engl J Med 1983;309: 630–636.

72. Mitelman F, Panani A, Brandt L. Isochromosome 17 in a case of eosinophilic leukaemia. An abnormality common to eosinophilic and neutrophilic cells. Scand J Haematol 1975;14:308–312.

73. Rotoli B, Catalano L, Galderisi M, et al. Rapid reversion of Loeffler's endocarditis by imatinib in early-stage clonal hypereosinophilic syndrome. Leuk Lymph 2004;45:2503–2507.

74. Brigaudeau C, Liozon E, Bernard P, et al. Deletion of chromosome 20q associated with hypereosinophilic syndrome. A report of two cases. Cancer Genet Cytogenet 1996;87:82–84.

75. Kusanagi Y, Ochi H, Matsubara K, et al. Hypereosinophilic syndrome in a trisomy 21 fetus. Obstet Gynecol 1998;92:701–702.

76. Needleman SW, Mane SM, Gutheil JC, et al. Hypereosinophilic syndrome with evolution to myeloproliferative disorder: temporal relationship to loss of Y chromosome and c-N-ras activation. Hematol Pathol 1990;4: 149–155.

77. Flannery EP, Dillon DE, Freeman MV, et al. Eosinophilic leukemia with fibrosing endocarditis and short Y chromosome. Ann Intern Med 1972;77: 223–228.

78. Goffman TE, Mulvihill JJ, Carney DN, et al. Fatal hypereosinophilia with chromosome 15q- in a patient with multiple primary and familial neoplasms. Cancer Genet Cytogenet 1983;8:197–202.

79. Bitran JD, Rowley JD, Plapp F, et al. Chromosomal aneuploidy in a patient with hypereosinophilic syndrome. Evidence for a malignant disease. Am J Med 1977;63:1010–1014.

80. Ellman L, Hammond D, Atkins L. Eosinophilia, chloromas, and a chromosome abnormality in a patient with a myeloproliferative syndrome. Cancer 1979;43: 2410–2413.

81. Wolz DE, Granato JE, Giles HR, et al. A unique chromosomal abnormality in idiopathic hypereosinophilic syndrome presenting with cardiac involvement. Am Heart J 1993;126:246–248.

82. Bigoni R, Cuneo A, Roberti MG, et al. Cytogenetic and molecular cytogenetic characterization of 6 new cases of idiopathic hypereosinophilic syndrome. Haematologica 2000;85:486–491.

83. Cools J, Quentmeier H, Huntly BJ, et al. The EOL-1 cell line as an in vitro model for the study of FIP1L1-PDGFRA–positive chronic eosinophilic leukemia. Blood 2004;103:2802–2805.

84. Chang HW, Leong KH, Koh DR, et al. Clonality of isolated eosinophils in the hypereosinophilic syndrome. Blood 1999;93:1651–1657.

85. Malcovati L, La Starza R, Merante S, et al. Hypereosinophilic syndrome and cyclic oscillations in blood cell counts. A clonal disorder of hematopoiesis originating in a pluripotent stem cell. Haematologica 2004;89:497–499.

86. Brown NJ, Stein RS. Idiopathic hypereosinophilic syndrome progressing to acute myelomonocytic leukemia with chloromas. South Med J 1989;82:1303–1305.

87. Owen J, Scott JG. Transition of the hypereosinophilic syndrome to myelomonocytic leukemia. Can Med Assoc J 1979;121:1489–1491.

88. Bain B, Pierre R, Imbert M, et al. Chronic eosinophilic leukemia and the hypereosinophilic syndrome. In: Jaffe ES, Harris NL, Stein H, et al., eds. World Health Organization Classification of Tumors: Tumours of the Haematopoietic and Lymphoid Tissues. Lyon, France: International Agency for Research on Cancer (IARC) Press, 2001, pp. 29–31.

89. Simon HU, Plotz SG, Dummer R, et al. Abnormal clones of T-cells producing interleukin-5 in idiopathic eosinophilia. N Engl J Med 1999;341: 1112–1120.

90. Butterfield JH. Diverse clinical outcomes of eosinophilic patients with T-cell receptor gene rearrangements: the emerging diagnostic importance of molecular genetics testing. Am J Hematol 2001;68:81–86.

91. Bain BJ. Relationship between idiopathic hypereosinophilic syndrome, eosinophilic leukemia, and systemic mastocytosis. Am J Hematol 2004;77:82–85.

92. Gleich GJ, Leiferman KM, Pardanani A, et al. Treatment of hypereosinophilic syndrome with imatinib mesilate. Lancet 2002;359:1577–1578.

93. Pardanani A, Elliott M, Reeder T, et al. Imatinib for systemic mast-cell disease. Lancet 2003;362:535–536.

94. Schaller JL, Burkland GA. Case report: rapid and complete control of idiopathic hypereosinophilia with imatinib mesylate. MedGenMed 2001;3:9.
95. Ault P, Cortes J, Koller C, et al. Response of idiopathic hypereosinophilic syndrome to treatment with imatinib mesylate. Leuk Res 2002;26:881–884.
96. Robyn J, Lemery S, McCoy JP, et al. Multilineage involvement of the fusion gene in patients with FIP1L1/PDGFRA-positive hypereosinophilic syndrome. Br J Haematol 2006;132:286–292.
97. Tefferi A, Lasho TL, Brockman SR, et al. FIP1L1-PDGFRA and c-kit D816V mutation-based clonality studies in systemic mast cell disease associated with eosinophilia. Haematologica 2004;89:871–873.
98. Cools J, Stover EH, Boulton CL, et al. PKC412 overcomes resistance to imatinib in a murine model of FIP1L1-PDGFRalpha-induced myeloproliferative disease. Cancer Cell 2003;3:459–469.
99. Griffin JH, Leung J, Bruner RJ, et al. Discovery of a fusion kinase in EOL-1 cells and idiopathic hypereosinophilic syndrome. Proc Natl Acad Sci U S A 2003;100: 7830–7835.
100. Stover EH, Chen J, Folens C, et al. Activation of FIP1L1-PDGFRalpha requires disruption of the juxtamembrane domain of PDGFRalpha and is FIP1L1-independent. Proc Natl Acad Sci U S A 2006;103:8078–8083.
101. Score J, Curtis C, Waghorn K, et al. Identification of a novel imatinib responsive KIF5B-PDGFRA fusion gene following screening for PDGFRA overexpression in patients with hypereosinophilia. Leukemia 2006;20:827–832.
102. Walz C, Curtis C, Schnittger S, et al. Transient response to imatinib in a chronic eosinophilic leukemia associated with ins(9;4)(q33;q12q25) and a CDK5RAP2-PDGFRA fusion gene. Genes Chrom Cancer 2006;45(10):950–956.
103. Trempat P, Villalva C, Laurent G, et al. Chronic myeloproliferative disorders with rearrangement of the platelet-derived growth factor alpha receptor: a new clinical target for STI571/Glivec. Oncogene 2003;22:5702–5706.
104. Safley AM, Sebastian S, Collins TS, et al. Molecular and cytogenetic characterization of a novel translocation t(4;22) involving the breakpoint cluster region and platelet-derived growth factor receptor-alpha genes in a patient with atypical chronic myeloid leukemia. Genes Chrom Cancer 2004;40:44–50.
105. Bacher U, Reiter A, Haferlach T, et al. A combination of cytomorphology, cytogenetic analysis, fluorescence in situ hybridization, and reverse transcriptase polymerase chain reaction for establishing clonality in cases of persisting hypereosinophilia. Haematologica 2006;91:817–820.
106. Pardanani A, Ketterling RP, Li CY, et al. FIP1L1-PDGFRA in eosinophilic disorders: prevalence in routine clinical practice, long-term experience with imatinib therapy, and a critical review of the literature. Leuk Res 2006;30: 965–970.
107. Jovanovic JV, Score J, Waghorn K, et al. Low-dose imatinib mesylate leads to rapid induction of major molecular responses and achievement of complete molecular remission in FIP1L1-PDGFRA–positive chronic eosinophilic leukemia. Blood 2007;109(11):4635–4640.
108. Pardanani A, Brockman SR, Paternoster SF, et al. FIP1L1-PDGFRA fusion: prevalence and clinicopathologic correlates in 89 consecutive patients with moderate to severe eosinophilia. Blood 2004;104:3038–3045.

109. Klion AD, Noel P, Akin C, et al. Elevated serum tryptase levels identify a subset of patients with a myeloproliferative variant of idiopathic hypereosinophilic syndrome associated with tissue fibrosis, poor prognosis, and imatinib responsiveness. Blood 2003;101:4660–4666.

110. Klion AD, Robyn J, Akin C, et al. Molecular remission and reversal of myelofibrosis in response to imatinib mesylate treatment in patients with the myeloproliferative variant of hypereosinophilic syndrome. Blood 2004;103:473–478.

111. Pardanani A, Ketterling RP, Brockman SR, et al. CHIC2 deletion, a surrogate for FIP1L1-PDGFRA fusion, occurs in systemic mastocytosis associated with eosinophilia and predicts response to imatinib mesylate therapy. Blood 2003;102:3093–3096.

112. McPherson T, Cowen EW, McBurney E, et al. Platelet-derived growth factor receptor-alpha-associated hypereosinophilic syndrome and lymphomatoid papulosis. Br J Dermatol 2006;155:824–826.

113. von Bubnoff N, Sandherr M, Schlimok G, et al. Myeloid blast crisis evolving during imatinib treatment of an FIP1L1-PDGFR alpha-positive chronic myeloproliferative disease with prominent eosinophilia. Leukemia 2005;19:286–287.

114. Ohnishi H, Kandabashi K, Maeda Y, et al. Chronic eosinophilic leukaemia with FIP1L1-PDGFRA fusion and T674I mutation that evolved from Langerhans cell histiocytosis with eosinophilia after chemotherapy. Br J Haematol 2006;134(5):547–549.

115. Lierman E, Folens C, Stover EH, et al. Sorafenib (BAY43–9006) is a potent inhibitor of FIP1L1-PDGFR{alpha} and the imatinib resistant FIP1L1-PDGFR{alpha} T674I mutant. Blood 2006;108(4):1374–1376.

116. Stover EH, Chen J, Lee BH, et al. The small molecule tyrosine kinase inhibitor AMN107 inhibits TEL-PDGFRbeta and FIP1L1-PDGFRalpha in vitro and in vivo. Blood 2005;106:3206–3213.

117. von Bubnoff N, Gorantla SP, Thone S, et al. The FIP1L1-PDGFRA T674I mutation can be inhibited by the tyrosine kinase inhibitor AMN107 (nilotinib). Blood 2006;107:4970–4971; author reply, 4972.

118. Lierman E, Lahortiga I, Van Miegroet H, et al. The ability of sorafenib to inhibit oncogenic PDGFRbeta and FLT3 mutants and overcome resistance to other small molecule inhibitors. Haematologica 2007;92:27–34.

119. Carroll M, Tomasson MH, Barker GF, et al. The TEL/platelet-derived growth factor beta receptor (PDGF beta R) fusion in chronic myelomonocytic leukemia is a transforming protein that self-associates and activates PDGF beta R kinase-dependent signaling pathways. Proc Natl Acad Sci USA 1996;93:14845–14850.

120. Wilkinson K, Velloso ER, Lopes LF, et al. Cloning of the t(1;5)(q23;q33) in a myeloproliferative disorder associated with eosinophilia: involvement of PDGFRB and response to imatinib. Blood 2003;102:4187–4190.

121. Schwaller J, Anastasiadou E, Cain D, et al. H4(D10S170), a gene frequently rearranged in papillary thyroid carcinoma, is fused to the platelet-derived growth factor receptor beta gene in atypical chronic myeloid leukemia with t(5;10)(q33;q22). Blood 2001;97:3910–3918.

122. Pardanani A, Tefferi A. Imatinib targets other than BCR/ABL and their clinical relevance in myeloid disorders. Blood 2004;104:1931–1939.

123. Apperley JF, Gardembas M, Melo JV, et al. Response to imatinib mesylate in patients with chronic myeloproliferative diseases with rearrangements of the platelet-derived growth factor receptor beta. N Engl J Med 2002;347:481–487.
124. Walz C, Metzgeroth G, Haferlach C, et al. Characterization of three new imatinib-responsive fusion genes in chronic myeloproliferative disorders generated by disruption of the platelet-derived growth factor receptor beta gene. Haematologica 2007;92:163–169.
125. David M, Cross NC, Burgstaller S, et al. Durable responses to imatinib in patients with PDGFRB fusion gene-positive and BCR-ABL-negative chronic myeloproliferative disorders. Blood 2007;109:61–64.
126. Onida F, Kantarjian HM, Smith TL, et al. Prognostic factors and scoring systems in chronic myelomonocytic leukemia: a retrospective analysis of 213 patients. Blood 2002;99:840–849.
127. Xiao S, Nalabolu SR, Aster JC, et al. FGFR1 is fused with a novel zinc-finger gene, ZNF198, in the t(8;13) leukaemia/lymphoma syndrome. Nat Genet 1998;18:84–87.
128. Smedley D, Hamoudi R, Clark J, et al. The t(8;13)(p11;q11–12) rearrangement associated with an atypical myeloproliferative disorder fuses the fibroblast growth factor receptor 1 gene to a novel gene RAMP. Hum Mol Genet 1998;7:637–642.
129. Still IH, Chernova O, Hurd D, et al. Molecular characterization of the t(8;13)(p11;q12) translocation associated with an atypical myeloproliferative disorder: evidence for three discrete loci involved in myeloid leukemias on 8p11. Blood 1997;90:3136–3141.
130. Reiter A, Sohal J, Kulkarni S, et al. Consistent fusion of ZNF198 to the fibroblast growth factor receptor-1 in the t(8;13)(p11;q12) myeloproliferative syndrome. Blood 1998;92:1735–1742.
131. Chaffanet M, Popovici C, Leroux D, et al. t(6;8), t(8;9), and t(8;13) translocations associated with stem cell myeloproliferative disorders have close or identical breakpoints in chromosome region 8p11–12. Oncogene 1998;16:945–949.
132. Mugneret F, Chaffanet M, Maynadie M, et al. The 8p12 myeloproliferative disorder. t(8;19)(p12;q13.3): a novel translocation involving the FGFR1 gene. Br J Haematol 2000;111:647–649.
133. Fioretos T, Panagopoulos I, Lassen C, et al. Fusion of the BCR and the fibroblast growth factor receptor-1 (FGFR1) genes as a result of t(8;22)(p11;q11) in a myeloproliferative disorder: the first fusion gene involving BCR but not ABL. Genes Chrom Cancer 2001;32:302–310.
134. Pini M, Gottardi E, Scaravaglio P, et al. A fourth case of BCR-FGFR1 positive CML-like disease with t(8;22) translocation showing an extensive deletion on the derivative chromosome 8p. Hematol J 2002;3:315–316.
135. Belloni E, Trubia M, Gasparini P, et al. 8p11 myeloproliferative syndrome with a novel t(7;8) translocation leading to fusion of the FGFR1 and TIF1 genes. Genes Chrom Cancer 2005;42:320–325.
136. Macdonald D, Reiter A, Cross NC. The 8p11 myeloproliferative syndrome: a distinct clinical entity caused by constitutive activation of FGFR1. Acta Haematol 2002;107:101–107.
137. Ollendorff V, Guasch G, Isnardon D, et al. Characterization of FIM-FGFR1, the fusion product of the myeloproliferative disorder-associated t(8;13) translocation. J Biol Chem 1999;274:26922–26930.

138. Guasch G, Ollendorff V, Borg JP, et al. 8p12 stem cell myeloproliferative disorder: the FOP-fibroblast growth factor receptor 1 fusion protein of the t(6;8) translocation induces cell survival mediated by mitogen-activated protein kinase and phosphatidylinositol 3-kinase/Akt/mTOR pathways. Mol Cell Biol 2001;21: 8129–8142.

139. Roumiantsev S, Krause DS, Neumann CA, et al. Distinct stem cell myeloproliferative/T lymphoma syndromes induced by ZNF198-FGFR1 and BCR-FGFR1 fusion genes from 8p11 translocations. Cancer Cell 2004;5:287–298.

140. Guasch G, Delaval B, Arnoulet C, et al. FOP-FGFR1 tyrosine kinase, the product of a t(6;8) translocation, induces a fatal myeloproliferative disease in mice. Blood 2004;103:309–312.

141. Chen J, Deangelo DJ, Kutok JL, et al. PKC412 inhibits the zinc finger 198-fibroblast growth factor receptor 1 fusion tyrosine kinase and is active in treatment of stem cell myeloproliferative disorder. Proc Natl Acad Sci U S A 2004;101: 14479–14484.

142. Chusid MJ, Dale DC, West BC, et al. The hypereosinophilic syndrome: analysis of fourteen cases with review of the literature. Medicine (Baltimore) 1975;54:1–27.

143. Yildiran A, Ikinciogullari A. Pediatric hypereosinophilic syndrome (HES) clinically differs from adult HES, but there is a lack of confirmatory laboratory data. J Pediatr 2005;147:869.

144. Fauci AS, Harley JB, Roberts WC, et al. NIH conference. The idiopathic hypereosinophilic syndrome. Clinical, pathophysiologic, and therapeutic considerations. Ann Intern Med 1982;97:78–92.

145. Harley JB, Fauci AS, Gralnick HR. Noncardiovascular findings associated with heart disease in the idiopathic hypereosinophilic syndrome. Am J Cardiol 1983;52: 321–324.

146. Moore PM, Harley JB, Fauci AS. Neurologic dysfunction in the idiopathic hypereosinophilic syndrome. Ann Intern Med 1985;102:109–114.

147. Liapis H, Ho AK, Brown D, et al. Thrombotic microangiopathy associated with the hypereosinophilic syndrome. Kidney Int 2005;67:1806–1811.

148. Weller PF, Bubley GJ. The idiopathic hypereosinophilic syndrome. Blood 1994;83:2759–2779.

149. Ommen SR, Seward JB, Tajik AJ. Clinical and echocardiographic features of hypereosinophilic syndromes. Am J Cardiol 2000;86:110–113.

150. Lefebvre C, Bletry O, Degoulet P, et al. Prognostic factors of hypereosinophilic syndrome. Study of 40 cases. Ann Med Interne (Paris) 1989;140:253–257.

151. Leiferman KM, O'Duffy JD, Perry HO, et al. Recurrent incapacitating mucosal ulcerations. A prodrome of the hypereosinophilic syndrome. Jama 1982;247: 1018–1020.

152. Kocaturk H, Yilmaz M. Idiopathic hypereosinophilic syndrome associated with multiple intracardiac thrombi. Echocardiography 2005;22:675–676.

153. Liao YH, Su YW, Tsay W, et al. Association of cutaneous necrotizing eosinophilic vasculitis and deep vein thrombosis in hypereosinophilic syndrome. Arch Dermatol 2005;141:1051–1053.

154. Ponsky TA, Brody F, Giordano J, et al. Brachial artery occlusion secondary to hypereosinophilic syndrome. J Vasc Surg 2005;42:796–799.

155. Sato Y, Taniguchi R, Yamada T, et al. Measurement of serum concentrations of cardiac troponin T in patients with hypereosinophilic syndrome: a sensitive non-invasive marker of cardiac disorder. Intern Med 2000;39:350.
156. Pitini V, Arrigo C, Azzarello D, et al. Serum concentration of cardiac troponin T in patients with hypereosinophilic syndrome treated with imatinib is predictive of adverse outcomes. Blood 2003;102:3456–3457; author reply, 3457.
157. Parrillo JE, Fauci AS, Wolff SM. Therapy of the hypereosinophilic syndrome. Ann Intern Med 1978;89:167–172.
158. Butterfield JH, Gleich GJ. Interferon-alpha treatment of six patients with the idiopathic hypereosinophilic syndrome. Ann Intern Med 1994;121:648–653.
159. Baratta L, Afeltra A, Delfino M, et al. Favorable response to high-dose interferon-alpha in idiopathic hypereosinophilic syndrome with restrictive cardiomyopathy—case report and literature review. Angiology 2002;53:465–470.
160. Yoon TY, Ahn GB, Chang SH. Complete remission of hypereosinophilic syndrome after interferon-alpha therapy: report of a case and literature review. J Dermatol 2000;27:110–115.
161. Ceretelli S, Capochiani E, Petrini M. Interferon-alpha in the idiopathic hypereosinophilic syndrome: consideration of five cases. Ann Hematol 1998;77:161–164.
162. Pardanani A, Reeder T, Porrata LF, et al. Imatinib therapy for hypereosinophilic syndrome and other eosinophilic disorders. Blood 2003;101:3391–3397.
163. Sefcick A, Sowter D, DasGupta E, et al. Alemtuzumab therapy for refractory idiopathic hypereosinophilic syndrome. Br J Haematol 2004;124:558–559.
164. Pitini V, Teti D, Arrigo C, et al. Alemtuzumab therapy for refractory idiopathic hypereosinophilic syndrome with abnormal T cells: a case report. Br J Haematol 2004;127:477.
165. Koury MJ, Newman JH, Murray JJ. Reversal of hypereosinophilic syndrome and lymphomatoid papulosis with mepolizumab and imatinib. Am J Med 2003;115: 587–589.
166. Plotz SG, Simon HU, Darsow U, et al. Use of an anti-interleukin-5 antibody in the hypereosinophilic syndrome with eosinophilic dermatitis. N Engl J Med 2003;349:2334–2339.
167. Klion AD, Law MA, Noel P, et al. Safety and efficacy of the monoclonal anti-interleukin-5 antibody SCH55700 in the treatment of patients with hypereosinophilic syndrome. Blood 2004;103:2939–2941.
168. Kim YJ, Prussin C, Martin B, et al. Rebound eosinophilia after treatment of hypereosinophilic syndrome and eosinophilic gastroenteritis with monoclonal anti-IL-5 antibody SCH55700. J Allergy Clin Immunol 2004;114: 1449–1455.
169. Ueno NT, Anagnostopoulos A, Rondon G, et al. Successful non-myeloablative allogeneic transplantation for treatment of idiopathic hypereosinophilic syndrome. Br J Haematol 2002;119:131–134.
170. Cooper MA, Akard LP, Thompson JM, et al. Hypereosinophilic syndrome: long-term remission following allogeneic stem cell transplant in spite of transient eosinophilia post-transplant. Am J Hematol 2005;78:33–36.
171. Juvonen E, Volin L, Koponen A, et al. Allogeneic blood stem cell transplantation following non-myeloablative conditioning for hypereosinophilic syndrome. Bone Marrow Transplant 2002;29:457–458.

172. Smit AJ, van Essen LH, de Vries EG. Successful long-term control of idiopathic hypereosinophilic syndrome with etoposide. Cancer 1991;67:2826–2827.
173. Nadarajah S, Krafchik B, Roifman C, et al. Treatment of hypereosinophilic syndrome in a child using cyclosporine: implication for a primary T-cell abnormality. Pediatrics 1997;99:630–633.
174. Marshall GM, White L. Effective therapy for a severe case of the idiopathic hypereosinophilic syndrome. Am J Pediatr Hematol Oncol 1989;11:178–183.
175. Ueno NT, Zhao S, Robertson LE, et al. 2-chlorodeoxyadenosine therapy for idiopathic hypereosinophilic syndrome. Leukemia 1997;11:1386–1390.
176. Jabbour E, Verstovsek S, Giles F, et al. 2-chlorodeoxyadenosine and cytarabine combination therapy for idiopathic hypereosinophilic syndrome. Cancer 2005;104: 541–546.
177. Eakin DL, Gill DP, Weiss GB. Response of hypereosinophilic syndrome to 6-thioguanine and cytarabine. Cancer Treat Rep 1982;66:545–547.
178. Raghavachar A, Fleischer S, Frickhofen N, et al. T lymphocyte control of human eosinophilic granulopoiesis. Clonal analysis in an idiopathic hypereosinophilic syndrome. J Immunol 1987;139:3753–3758.
179. Cogan E, Schandene L, Crusiaux A, et al. Brief report: clonal proliferation of type 2 helper T cells in a man with the hypereosinophilic syndrome. N Engl J Med 1994;330:535–538.
180. Vaklavas C, Tefferi A, Butterfield J, et al. "Idiopathic" eosinophilia with an occult T-cell clone: prevalence and clinical course. Leuk Res 2006;31(5):691–694.
181. Roufosse F, Cogan E, Goldman M. Recent advances in pathogenesis and management of hypereosinophilic syndromes. Allergy 2004;59:673–689.

11

Myelodysplastic/Myeloproliferative Diseases (Overlap Syndromes)

John M. Bennett

Professor of Laboratory Medicine and Pathology, James P. Wilmot Cancer Center, University of Rochester Medical Center, Rochester, New York, U.S.A.

Curtis A. Hanson

Professor of Laboratory Medicine and Pathology, Mayo Clinic College of Medicine, Rochester, Minnesota, U.S.A.

INTRODUCTION

For at least four decades, hematologists and hematopathologists have distinguished two broad classes of chronic clonal hematopoietic neoplasms: those that are primarily dysplastic (increased rates of programmed cell death or apoptosis but often accompanied with a component of stem cell proliferation) referred to as the "myelodysplastic syndromes" (MDS) (1), and those that are primarily proliferative with a selective myeloid predominance that involves either the erythroid cell line [polycythemia vera (PV)]; granulocytic cell line [chronic myelogenous leukemia (CML), atypical chronic myeloid leukemia (aCML), chronic myelomonocytic leukemia (CMML), chronic eosinophilic leukemia, chronic neutrophilic leukemia, and juvenile myelomonocytic leukemia (JMML)]; and the megakaryocytic cell line [essential thrombocythemia (ET) and possibly primary myelofibrosis (PMF)] (2). As these diseases progress toward acute leukemia (often referred to as transformation), the morphologic common pathway includes dysplastic granulocytes and increased $CD34^+/117^+$ blasts. The identification, therefore, of a molecular abnormality such as *BCR-ABL* {t(9;22)} may be the only way to recognize the original chronic-phase diagnosis (3).

Until recently, no specific genetic aberration has been recognized that would allow a ready separation of MDS from the *BCR-ABL*–negative myeloproliferative disorders (MPDs); a leukocyte count threshold of 13 × 10^9/L has been used to arbitrarily distinguish "proliferative" from "myelodysplastic" variants in certain cases, including CMML. The frequency of N-RAS gene mutations, particularly in CMML, has been striking (4), but not either diagnostic or specific to the particular entity. The recent description of an activating somatic mutation of the Janus tyrosine kinase 2 (JAK2V617F) gene in over 90% of patients with PV and close to 50% in ET and PMF has helped to understand better the pathogenesis of the *BCR-ABL*–negative MPDs (5). In MDS, the vast majority of cases are negative for JAK2V617F but, as will be discussed below, in a few well-defined subgroups, the specific mutation has been described in a substantial number of cases that feature histological changes that are characteristic of both MDS and MPD (6). Such "overlap syndromes" [i.e., CMML, JMML, aCML, and refractory anemia with ringed sideroblasts and thrombocytosis (RARS-T)] are recognized by the World Health Organization (WHO) classification system for myeloid neoplasms and are discussed further in this chapter (7).

As background, in 1994, the French–American–British (FAB) Cooperative Leukemia Study Group (8) proposed guidelines for the separation of CML, aCML, and CMML. In a series of workshops, all 15 cases of CML were correctly predicted from the peripheral blood films, as were about 75% of those of either CMML or aCML. The particular study identified basophilia and immature granulocytes as the most important features for CML, immature granulocytes and dysplasia for aCML, and monocytosis for CMML. However, certain cases remained relatively difficult to distinguish among the three entities, and bone marrow histology was largely unhelpful in this regard. Therefore, it was recommended that cytogenetic studies be performed routinely to identify *BCR-ABL* and other translocations, such as t(5;12) or t (5;10) (9).

CHRONIC MYELOMONOCYTIC LEUKEMIA

Current diagnosis of CMML requires the presence of at least 1 × 10^9/L monocytes in the peripheral blood, less than 20% bone marrow blasts, and morphologic dysplasia in erythroid and/or granulocyte lineage. In the WHO system, CMML is included in the section of mixed myelodysplastic/myeloproliferative syndromes (10). The justification for this "movement" was that although the FAB group had placed this entity within MDS, approximately half of the cases present with leukocyte counts above 13 × 10^9/L and 25% of those with only slight degrees of monocytosis but significant dysplasia of erythroid, granulocyte, and megakaryocyte lineage cells will progress to a proliferative form in time. Of interest is that true "dysplasia" of monocytes has proved to be an elusive goal among morphologists and the percentage of monoblasts is usually low. In fact, in the bone marrow, monocytes may be difficult to recognize without performing nonspecific esterase stains. Another challenge in the evaluation of CMML is determining the degree of immaturity in a blood or bone marrow aspirate specimen as there is frequently a morphologic spectrum from mature monocytes to promonocytes to, eventually, monoblasts. Immunophenotyping has not proven to be useful in aiding in this separation and thus it remains a microscopic evaluation process. In the bone marrow biopsy, it should be noted that nodules of monocytes may some-times be observed that can be confused with lymphoid cells. These nodules stain selectively with CD123 and TCL-1, which are commonly thought of as markers of plasmacytoid dendritic cells (Fig. 1).

When CMML presents with a normal leukocyte count, the prognosis is dependent on the percentage of blasts in the bone marrow and the degree of cellular dysplasia, including the presence of ringed sideroblasts (11). In addition, the WHO elected to divide CMML into two prognostic categories, CMML-I and CMML-II, similar to the separation of refractory anemia with excess blasts (RAEB) into RAEB-I and RAEB-II. Within this framework, CMML-I was considered in the presence of less than 10% bone marrow blasts and less than 5% peripheral blood blasts; CMML-II is characterized by either 10–19% bone marrow blasts or 5–19% peripheral blood blasts (12). In order to validate this proposal, we have recently reviewed over 300 patients with primary CMML in the Dusseldorf MDS Registry (13); 78% were diagnosed as CMML-I and their median survival was 20 months compared to 15 months in patients with CMML-II ($p = 0.001$). Simi-larly, the cumulative risk of AML was significantly higher in CMML-II as opposed to CMML-I (63% vs. 18% at 5 years). Interestingly, and not surprisingly, sur-vival was longer in CMML-dysplastic ($< 13 \times 10^9$/L) as opposed to CMML-proliferative (leukocyte count of $> 13 \times 10^9$/L; 29 months vs. 15 months).

ATYPICAL CHRONIC MYELOID LEUKEMIA

aCML has been one of the more controversial clinicopathologic entities in terms of nomenclature; some refer to it as unclassified MPD and others as *BCR-ABL*–negative CML. In general, it is important to distinguish aCML from Ph(−) but *BCR-ABL*–positive CML; the latter behaves similar to Ph(+) and *BCR-ABL*–positive CML in terms of both clinical presentation and treatment response. The peripheral blood in aCML features left-shifted dysplastic granulocytosis without monocytosis. Bone marrow is markedly hypercellular, as is the case with CML, with prominent granulocytic dysplasia and minimal monocytosis or basophilia (Fig. 2). By definition, bone marrow blast percentage is less than 20% and *BCR-ABL* is absent. No specific immunophenotypic or cytogenetic aberrations have been noted. The number of series have been few, but survival and progression to AML are similar to CMML (8).

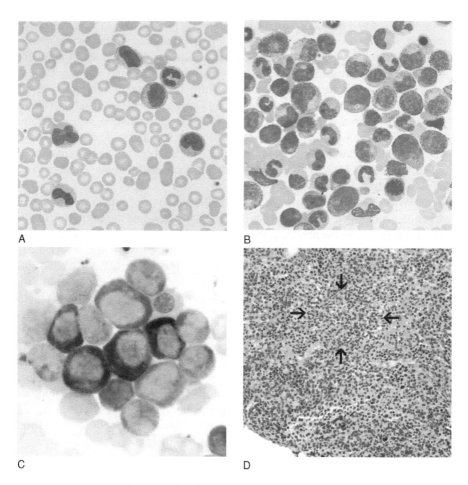

A   B

C   D

Figure 1   (See color insert.) Chronic myelomonocytic leukemia. (**A**) Peripheral blood smear showing a leukocytosis and a spectrum of monocyte maturation. (**B**) Hypercellular bone marrow aspirate with a marked granulocytic and monocytic expansion. (**C**) A combined chloroacetate esterase/butyrate esterase stain showing: chloroacetate esterase positive granulocytic precursors (blueish stain), butyrate esterase positive monocytes (reddish-brown stain), and combined chloroacetate/butyrate esterase positive hybrid myelomonocytic cells (both blueish and reddish brown stains). These latter cells are commonly identified in CMML, thus contributing to the difficulty in morphologic cell identification. (**D**) A packed bone marrow biopsy with a granulocytic and monocytic hyperplasia. There is monocytic nodule present (outlined by arrows).

JUVENILE MYELOMONOCYTIC LEUKEMIA

The diagnostic criteria for JMML proposed by the WHO were accepted with some modifications by a consensus group in 2003 (14). Diagnostic features required both clinical and molecular criteria. Major criteria included splenomegaly, monocytosis $> 1 \times 10^9$/L, a leukocyte count $> 10 \times 10^9$/L, presence of RAS, NF1, or PTPN11

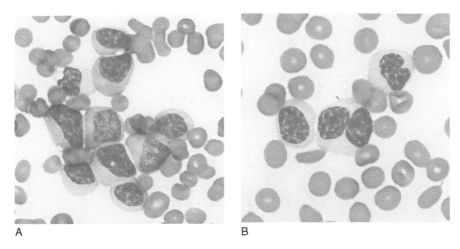

A   B

Figure 2 (See color insert.) Atypical chronic myeloid leukemia. Peripheral blood smear showing: (**A**) left-shifted granulocytosis and (**B**) dysplastic neutrophils with hypolobulation and hypogranulation.

gene mutations, bone marrow blasts < 20%, and absence of *BCR-ABL*. If any of these are absent, then demonstration of GM-CSF hypersensitivity of myeloid precursors is required. Hemoglobin F is usually increased for age, and the presence or absence of monosomy 7 is not relevant for diagnosis, although seen in many cases. Morphologically promonocytes are considered as blasts. More than 75% of JMML cases occur before the age of 3 years and survival is poor unless treatment includes allogenic stem cell transplantation. Altered RAS signaling is a characteristic feature of JMML and is mediated by one of the mutually exclusive mutations involving RAS, PTPN11, or NF1. Approximate incidences in this regard are 30%, 20%, and 15%.

Refractory Anemia with Ringed Sideroblasts and Thrombocytosis

It is now well-established that some patients with refractory anemia with ringed sideroblasts (RARS) or even refractory anemia (RA) with del(5q) could present with a striking elevation of the platelet count, usually above 600×10^9/L. Associated with this elevation is an increase in marrow megakaryocytes whose morphology might resemble those seen in ET (Fig. 3). The WHO classification committee for myeloid neoplasms recognizes such cases and has placed them under the provisional category of RARS-T. It is important to underscore that such designations should be restricted to cases with the presence of dyserythropoiesis as well as ET-like dysmegakaryopoiesis. In other words, the presence of ringed sideroblasts in otherwise typical ET or PMF does not change the diagnosis to RARS-T. Regardless, the platelet count is rarely high enough to warrant therapy exclusive of what would be proposed for the treatment of the underlying MDS. Of great interest has been the observation that the detection rate of JAK2V617F mutation in RARS-T

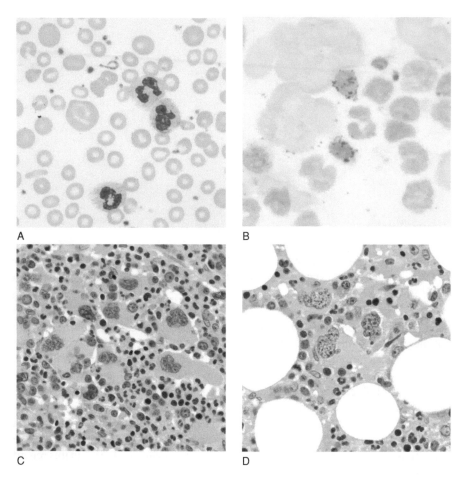

Figure 3   (See color insert.) Refractory anemia with ringed sideroblasts and thrombocytosis. (**A**) Peripheral blood smear showing a thrombocytosis with occasional atypical platelets and a neutrophilia. (**B**) Iron stain of bone marrow aspirate showing two ringed sideroblasts. (**C**) and (**D**) Hypercellular bone marrow biopsy showing a panhyperplasia and prominent atypical megakaryocytes. The megakaryocytes form loose clusters in the marrow biopsy.

is significantly higher than what is seen in typical MDS ($< 3\%$); mutational frequencies of greater than 50% have been described (15). Patients with del(5q) can also present with thrombocytosis and JAK2V617F has also been described in such cases, especially in the presence of a higher platelet count (6).

SUMMARY

Many of the features described above are more common to patients with MDS rather than MPD. However, the elevated leukocyte and/or platelet counts necessitate reconsidering the treatment approach. The International Prognostic Scoring System does not apply in these patients because they were generally excluded from the original series. Conservative approaches for management are recommended, until the bone marrow blast percentage begins to approach 10% or greater, and then, where appropriate allogeneic bone marrow transplantation can be considered. For patients with del(5q), however, lenalidomide therapy is the current treatment of choice.

REFERENCES

1. Bennett JM, Catovsky D, Daniel MT, et al. Proposals for the classification of the myelodysplastic syndromes. Br J Haematol 1982;51:189–199.
2. Vardiman J, Brunning RD, Harris NL. Chronic myeloproliferative diseases: introduction. In: Jaffe ES, Harris NL, Stein H, et al., eds. World Health Organization Classification of Tumors—Pathology and Genetics of Tumors of the Hematopoietic and lymphoid Tissues, 1st ed. Lyon: IARC press, 2001, pp. 29–31.
3. Shepherd PC, Ganesan TS, Galton DAG. Haematological classification of the chronic myeloid leukemias. Baillieres Clin Haematol 1987;1:887–906.
4. Cogswell PC, Morgan R, Dunn M, et al. Mutations of the RAS protooncogens in chronic myelogenous leukemia: a high frequency of RAS mutations in BCR/ABL rearrangement-negative chronic myelogenous leukemia. Blood 1989;74:2629–2633.
5. Tefferi A, Gilliland DG. The JAK2V617F tyrosine kinase mutation in myeloproliferative disorders: status report and immediate implications for disease classification and diagnosis. Mayo Clin Proc 2005;80:947–958.
6. Szpurka H, Tiu R, Murugesan G, et al. Refractory anemia with ringed sideroblasts associated with marked thrombocytosis (RARS-T), another myeloprolifcrative condition charactcrized by JAK2V627F mutation. Blood 2006;108:2173–2181.
7. Bain B, Vardiman J, Imbert M, et al. Myelodysplastic/myeloproliferative disease, unclassifiable. In: Jaffe ES, Harris NL, Stein H, et al., eds. WHO Classification of Tumors—Pathology and Genetics of Tumors of the Hemtopoietic and Lymphoid Tissues, 1st ed. Lyon: IARC Press, 2001, pp. 58–59.
8. Bennett JM, Catovsky D, Daniel MT, et al. The chronic myeloid leukemias; guidelines for distinguishing chronic granulocytic leukemia, atypical chronic myeloid leukemia, and chronic myelomoncytic leukemia; proposals by the French-American-British Cooperative Leukemia Group. Br J Haematol 1994;87:746–754.
9. Golub TR, Barker GF, Lovett M, et al. Fusion of PDGF receptor beta to a novel ets-like gene, tel, in chronic myelomonocytic leukemia with t(5;12) chromosomal translocation. Cell 1994;77:307–316.
10. Bennett JM. The myelodysplastic/myeloproliferative disorders; the interface. Hematol Oncol Clin North Am 2003;17:1095–1100.
11. Storniolo AM, Moloney WC, Rosenthal DS, et al. Chronic myelomonocytic leukemia. Leukemia 1990;4:766–770.
12. Bennett JM. WHO classification of the acute leukemias and myelodysplastic syndromes. Int J Hematol 2000;72:131–133.
13. Germing U, Strupp C, Knipp S, et al. Chronic myelomonocytic leukemia (CMML) in the light of the WHO proposals. Haematologica 2007;92(7):974–977.

14. Hasle H, Niemeyer CM, Chessells JM, et al. A pediatric approach to the WHO classification of the myelodysplastic syndromes and myeloproliferative disorders. Leukemia 2003;17:277–282.
15. Renneville A, Quesnel B, Charpentier A, et al. High occurrence of JAK2 V617F mutation in refractory anemia with ringed sideroblasts associated with marked thrombocytosis. Leukemia 2006;20:2067–2070.

Index

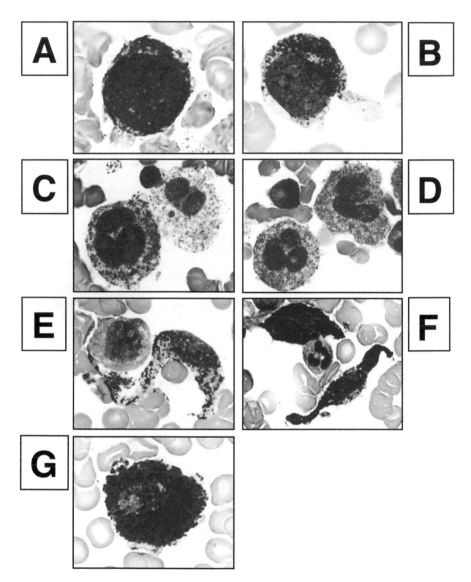

Figure 9.1 Morphology of mast cells in patients with mastocytosis. Metachromatic blasts and mast cells were detected in Wright–Giemsa-stained bone marrow smears in patients with mastocytosis: (**A, B**) metachromatically granulated blast cells (metachromatic blasts) found in the bone marrow smear in a patient with mast cell leukemia; (**C, D**) immature mast cells with bi- or polylobed nuclei (promastocytes = atypical mast cell type II) detected in patients with mast cell leukemia; (**E, F**) atypical mast cells type I (spindle-shaped, hypogranulated cytoplasm, oval nuclei) in patients with indolent systemic mastocytosis; and (**G**) typical mature tissue mast cell (round, well granulated with a round central nucleus) in a patient with indolent systemic mastocytosis. (See page 171.)

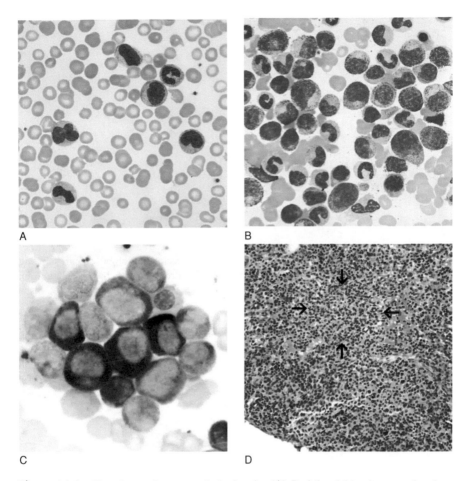

A

B

C

D

Figure 11.1 Chronic myelomonocytic leukemia. (**A**) Peripheral blood smear showing a leukocytosis and a spectrum of monocyte maturation. (**B**) Hypercellular bone marrow aspirate with a marked granulocytic and monocytic expansion. (**C**) A combined chloroacetate esterase/butyrate esterase stain showing: chloroacetate esterase positive granulocytic precursors (blueish stain), butyrate esterase positive monocytes (reddish-brown stain), and combined chloroacetate/butyrate esterase positive hybrid myelomonocytic cells (both blueish and reddish brown stains). These latter cells are commonly identified in CMML, thus contributing to the difficulty in morphologic cell identification. (**D**) A packed bone marrow biopsy with a granulocytic and monocytic hyperplasia. There is monocytic nodule present (outlined by arrows). (See page 214.)

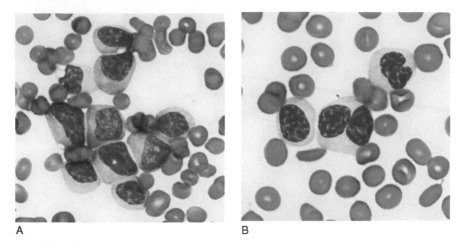

Figure 11.2 Atypical chronic myeloid leukemia. Peripheral blood smear showing: (**A**) left-shifted granulocytosis and (**B**) dysplastic neutrophils with hypolobulation and hypogranulation. (See page 215.)

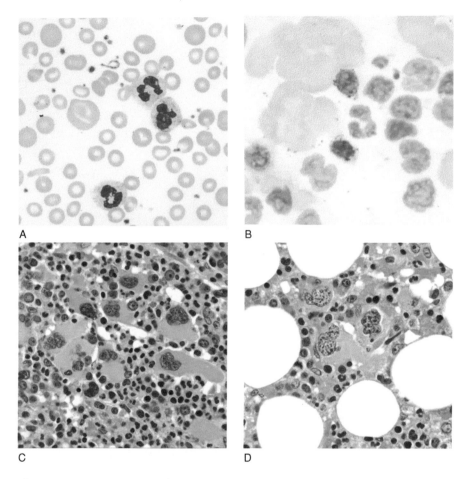

Figure 11.3 Refractory anemia with ringed sideroblasts and thrombocytosis. (**A**) Peripheral blood smear showing a thrombocytosis with occasional atypical platelets and a neutrophilia. (**B**) Iron stain of bone marrow aspirate showing two ringed sideroblasts. (**C, D**) Hypercellular bone marrow biopsy showing a panhyperplasia and prominent atypical megakaryocytes. The megakaryocytes form subtle clusters in the marrow biopsy. (See page 216.)

T - #0133 - 111024 - C238 - 229/152/11 - PB - 9780367452919 - Gloss Lamination